G000109809

Control of Hospital Infection

A PRACTICAL HANDBOOK

Control of Hospital Infection

A PRACTICAL HANDBOOK

Edited by
E. J. L. LOWBURY, G. A. J. AYLIFFE,
A. M. GEDDES *and* J. D. WILLIAMS

SECOND EDITION

LONDON

CHAPMAN AND HALL

First published 1975
by Chapman and Hall Ltd
11 New Fetter Lane, London EC4P 4EE
Second edition 1981
Reprinted 1982, 1988

© *1975, 1981 Chapman and Hall Ltd*

Printed by Antony Rowe Ltd, Chippenham, Wiltshire

ISBN 0 412 16300 4

British Library Cataloguing in Publication Data

Working Party on Control of Hospital Infection
Control of hospital infection. − 2nd ed.
1. Cross infection   2. Hospitals − Hygiene
I. Title   II. Lowbury, Edward Joseph Lister
614.4'4   RA969
ISBN 0−412−16300−4

Contents

v

Contents

Preface to the First Edition

This *Handbook* has been prepared as a guide for use by the staffs of hospitals. It is addressed to doctors, nurses, physiotherapists, radiographers and others who are involved in the treatment and care of patients, and in part also to administrators, architects, engineers, domestic superintendents and others whose work may influence the chances of infection among patients and staff.

Before the introduction of antiseptic and aseptic methods by Lister and others in the last century, major surgical infection ('hospital gangrene') was an overwhelming hazard and a common cause of death in hospitals. Although fulminating infection of this type was eliminated by the new measures, a residue of less dangerous infection persisted, and the development of new fields of surgery and therapy, including methods which interfere with the patients' immunity, has introduced new hazards of infection. Antibiotic treatment has brought relief against some of these infections, but it has often been frustrated by the emergence of antibiotic resistant bacteria. In addition to the hardship that it causes to patients (and sometimes to members of staff), hospital infection has, in the words of Sir Wilson Jameson, been 'a steady drain on the hospital purse and efficiency'. Abundant research in the past 25 years has shown that hospital infection can be greatly reduced by the correct application of a number of improved methods of asepsis and hygiene; but it is also a familiar experience that hospital infection is still common and that recommendations are often unknown or unobserved. The purpose of this *Handbook* is to offer the guidance and information needed for a more effective use of current knowledge on ways of controlling infection.

To be effective such a handbook must be understood clearly by all who wish to use it, and we have therefore tried to express, in as simple terms as we can, the elaborate and ever-developing strategy and tactics used in the control of hospital infection. This has involved calling many products by the proprietary names which are commonly used rather than (or as well as) by their official or chemical names; in many cases (e.g. the clear soluble phenolic compounds) no other names are available. When we refer to a disinfectant or antiseptic for a particular purpose, it must be regarded as an example, and one which we have examined; other products of which we have no information or personal experience may well be as effective — perhaps even more effective. Where our studies and those of others have shown one product or group of products to be more effective than others, we have naturally chosen that product or group of products; and occasionally where a commonly used product has been found, in careful studies, to fall short of expectation or to be ineffective, it has been necessary to mention this fact so that hospitals should choose a more effective product. The recommendations which we have made refer only to hospital practice and it must not be inferred that methods judged unsuitable for hospital use are not suitable for domestic and other purposes.

Cost as well as effectiveness must be considered, and we have therefore appended some information about retail prices at the time this *Handbook* was prepared, relating to a number of alternative products which we have found to be effective. Of course, prices will change frequently. Furthermore, it has not been possible to include the price structures which might apply to alternatives that we did not have the opportunity to assess, or to take account of special terms which might be available through contracting or bulk purchasing. Because such special terms may affect different materials to a different degree, we have presented some examples of the relative costs to hospitals of different compounds or mixtures which have been used for the same purpose. We feel that the information we have provided will be of some value to Health Authorities.

Hospital hygiene and aseptic practices have changed repeatedly with the arrival of new knowledge and the assessment of new materials. It is expected that many of the recommendations presented here will, in the course of time, be — and some may already have been — superseded by new and improved methods, which will call for a revision of the *Handbook*. Many alternative procedures are equally effective, and there should be no conflict in the choice between such alternatives. Sometimes the most effective method cannot be applied (e.g. because the equipment required is not available); under these circumstances a less desirable alternative must be recommended. It is important that the Bacteriologist, the Infection Control Officer and the Infection Control Nurse should be consulted on questions of uncertainty about procedures or principles; the Area Supplies Officer and the Area Pharmaceutical Officer should be consulted, and other officers as appropriate, in respect of costs. The handbook, supplemented by more recent information, will be used by the Infection Control Team in its handling of current infection problems.

Preface to the Second Edition

This book, originally conceived as a code of practice for one Region of the British National Health Service, has answered a much wider need and been found useful by hospital workers in many countries. In preparing a second edition the Editors have incorporated new knowledge, ideas and practices, and taken note of useful advice and comments made by readers of the first edition, to produce, we hope, an up-to-date and improved compilation. We have not changed the basic design of the book, which aims to provide hospital workers with practical guidance supported by a limited selection of relevant references — books, reviews and a few papers — for further reading; it is not, and does not aim to be, a fully documented textbook on hospital infection. As in the first edition, the Editors have called upon the expertise of a Working Party for advice and for some contributions to the text.

Since our first edition appeared there have been many improvements in procedure, and also some important changes in the pattern of infection; new (or rather, newly recognized) infections, such as Legionnaire's disease and Campylobacter enteritis, have been described, while others (notably smallpox) have receded. There has been, in many centres, a reduced incidence of cross-infection, especially of staphylococcal sepsis, and a decline in the presence of multiresistant 'hospital' staphylococci. In abdominal surgery endogenous infection, particularly with *Bacteroides* and other anaerobic bacteria normally present in human faeces, has been recognized as the major form of postoperative wound infection; its prevention by short-term chemoprophylaxis has been an important development in the control of hospital infection. There have been changes in availability and recommended choice of drugs and disinfectants, and considerable changes in their cost. Since our first edition, too, the responsibility of hospitals for the protection of staff against infective hazards has been strongly reinforced in Great Britain by the *Health and Safety at Work Act* of 1974 and the publication of the *Code of Practice for the Prevention of Infection in Clinical Laboratories and Postmortem Rooms* (Howie). There is still uncertainty about the application of some of the far-sighted improvements put forward in these publications, and it is important to recognize that a balance of hazard may exist — both for staff and for patients — between infection that might occur if some recommended procedures were not used and adverse effects (e.g. allergic or toxic reactions) that might occur as the result of using them. In situations involving such uncertainty, judgements based on clinical and microbiological expertise should be the deciding factor in the choice of procedures for the control of infection rather than adherence to rigid rules; the personal factor is of special importance in this field, and cannot be replaced by a code of practice. Nevertheless the Editors hope that this book will prove useful as a guide and reference to those who are called upon to make such decisions.

Acknowledgments

The Editors are grateful to all members of the Working Party for the material they have contributed and also to Sir Robert Williams, Dr J. C. Kelsey, and others who saw the first edition of the book before it was published and gave us valuable advice and information. Special thanks are due also to Mr George Dodwell for collating the various drafts from which the first edition was compiled; to Mr Peter Boileau, Miss Carole Jones and Miss Hilary Mellor for preparing the 'paste-up' of the second edition; to members of the Occupational Health Committee of the West Midlands Regional Health Authority under the chairmanship of Professor J. M. Bishop, for helpful suggestions; to Mr N. Cripps of the Regional Engineer's Department, W.M. Regional Health Authority; to Mrs M. Dyer, Mrs C. Fronczek and Mrs Linda Wortley for preparation of typescripts of the first edition, and to Mrs M. Dyer for typing additions and amendments to the text in the second edition.

West Midlands Regional Health Authority

Working Party on Control of Hospital Infection

Members and former† members

*E. J. L. Lowbury, OBE, MA, DM, DSc, LLD, FRCP, FRCS, FRCPath (Chairman)
L. W. Aldridge, FRCS
D. Ankrett, SRN
*G. A. J. Ayliffe, BSc, MD, FRCPath
F. A. J. Bridgwater, MB, Dip.Bact., FRCPath
P. P. Brown, MD, FRCPath, Dip.Bact.
G. Calder, BSc, MPS
Miss R. Challis, SRN
A. E. Chaplin, MD, FRCPath
P. Crees, FPS
T. H. Flewett, MD, FRCP, FRCPath
*A. M. Geddes, MB, ChB, FRCP(Ed.), MRCP(Lond.)
Miss M. E. Harris, SRN (Deceased)
F. C. Heath, MBE, FHA, FInstPS
C. H. L. Howells, BSc, MD, FRCPath
J. G. P. Hutchison, MD, FRCPath, FRCP(G)
B. Rhodes, BA, SRN, RNT
B. H. B. Robinson, MA, MB, FRCP
K. B. Rogers, MD, FRCPath
H. A. Thomas, SRN, RMN, RNT
J. L. Whitby, MB, FRCP, DTM&H, FRCPath
J. D. Williams, BSc, MD, MRCPath

Plus‡
A. D. Barnes, ChM, FRCS
B. J. Collins, AIMLS
R. H. George, MB, ChB, MRCPath

*Members of the editing sub-committee
†in italics
‡Members and co-opted members added to Working Party after publication of the first edition of the *Handbook*.

xii

C. A. Morris, BSc, MD, Dip.Bact.
T. J. Bradley, BSc, PhD, FPS, MIBiol
Ms L. J. Taylor, SRN, SCM

Co-opted for specific subjects:

Miss K. A. Barfield, SRN, RSCN, OHNC
D. R. Barry, MD, FRCP(Ed.), FRCPath, DO(RCS)
Miss C. Beavers, RSCN, SRN, SCM
P. Dawson-Edwards, FRCS
D. Hassell, SRN, RMN, QN, DNA(Aston), AMBIN
Miss E. A. Hunter, MADM
P. S. London, MBE, FRCS
W. H. Lowthorpe
M. W. N. Nicholls, MRCPath
M. J. Roper-Hall, ChM, FRCS, DOMS
J. S. Robinson, MD, FFA, RCS
T. H. Waterhouse, MA, LLB
G. Dodwell (Secretary to the Working Party)

Plus‡
D. W. Burdon, MB, MRCPath
P. Boileau (Administrator to the Working Party)
J. R. Babb, FIMLS
C. E. A. Deverill, AIMLS
J. E. Pearson, MB, BS, MRCS, DPH, MFCM
R. Wise, MB, MRCPath

Editors:

E. J. L. Lowbury, Hon. Visiting Professor of Medical Microbiology, University of Aston; formerly Hon. Director, Hospital Infection Research Laboratory, Dudley Road Hospital, Birmingham and Bacteriologist, MRC Burns Unit, Birmingham Accident Hospital; Consultant Adviser in Bacteriology to Birmingham Regional Hospital Board (1961-1974); Hon. Senior Clinical Lecturer and Research Fellow, Birmingham University; WHO Consultant in Hospital-acquired Infection, USA (1965).

G. A. J. Ayliffe, Director, Hospital Infection Research Laboratory, Dudley Road Hospital, Birmingham; Member of Scientific Staff, Medical Research Council Industrial Injuries and Burns Unit; Professor of Medical Microbiology, University of Birmingham.

A. M. Geddes, Consultant Physician in Communicable Diseases, East Birmingham Hospital; Hon. Senior Clinical Lecturer, Department of Medicine, University of Birmingham.

xiii

West Midlands Regional Health Authority

J. D. Williams, Professor of Medical Microbiology, London Hospital Medical College; Consultant Bacteriologist, The London Hospital.

CHAPTER ONE

Introduction

Definitions

The term *infection* is generally used to mean the deposition and multiplication of bacteria and other micro-organisms in tissues or on surfaces of the body where they can cause adverse effects; such adverse effects are often assumed in the definition. *Sepsis* means the presence of inflammation, pus formation and other signs of illness in wounds colonized by micro-organisms, and in tissues to which such infection has spread. Other types of infective illness are described by terms which refer to the site of infection (e.g. tonsillitis, peritonitis, pyelitis, gastro-enteritis, pneumonia) or to the specific disease, when this is distinctive (e.g. tuberculosis, measles, tetanus).

Hospital (or 'nosocomial'*) infection means infection acquired by patients while they are in hospital, or by members of hospital staff; the term *hospital-acquired* infection is sometimes used. This may be associated with sepsis or other forms of infective illness, either in hospital or after the patient returns home. *Cross-infection* means infection acquired in hospital from other people, either patients or staff. *Self- (or endogenous) infection* means infection caused by microbes which the patient carries on normal or septic areas of his own body, including organisms which these areas have acquired in hospital (i.e. self-infection supervening on cross-infection or on infection from the environment).

All infections of operation wounds are, for obvious reasons, hospital infections. In other sites, however, it is often impossible to say whether an infection was acquired by the patient in hospital or before he came into hospital. The term *hospital-associated infection* has been used to cover such infections, as well as those acquired in hospital.

A *source* of hospital infection may be defined as a place where *pathogenic* (i.e. potentially disease-producing) micro-organisms are growing or have grown, and from which they can be transmitted to patients (e.g. an infected wound, the nose or faeces of a carrier, contaminated food, contaminated solutions). A *reservoir* is a place where pathogens can survive outside the body and from which they could be transferred, directly or indirectly, to patients (e.g. static equipment, furniture, floors); the term is sometimes used interchangeably with the term *source*. A *vehicle* is a mobile object which can carry pathogenic organisms to a patient (e.g. dust particles, bedpans, blankets, toys etc.). The word *vector* is commonly used interchangeably with *vehicle*, but it is sometimes used in the specialized sense of an insect which carries pathogenic micro-organisms (i.e. an

*νοσοκομεῖον is the Greek (and nosocomium the Latin) word for hospital.

insect-vector) and should probably be restricted to this use. These categories overlap: e.g. a fluid in which bacteria multiply may be a 'vehicle' as well as a 'source' of infection, and will have acquired the organism from some antecedent 'source' (e.g. a patient with pseudomonas infection).

Incidence and importance of hospital infection

Many surveys have shown that an appreciable proportion (usually about 5-10%) of patients coming into hospital acquire some kind of clinical infection. The frequency and severity varies with the type of patient, the length of stay, the type of operation in surgical cases and various other factors. This continuous and apparently universal, though variable, incidence is described as *endemic infection*. But sometimes there is a large increase in the commonly occurring types of infection (e.g. postoperative wound sepsis) or the appearance of infection of a type not normally present in the hospital (e.g. salmonella infections in babies, or pseudomonas infections after eye surgery); this is called *epidemic infection*. Typing by serological, bacteriophage or bacteriocine methods shows endemic infections to be caused usually by a variety of types, while epidemic infection is usually due to a single type, which can often be traced to a source (e.g. a carrier of a virulent strain of *Staphylococcus aureus*, or a solution contaminated with *Pseudomonas aeruginosa*). If aseptic and hygienic measures in a hospital break down, the frequency of infection caused by multiple types of bacteria (i.e. 'endemic' infection as defined above) may increase to epidemic proportions.

The importance of hospital infection can be considered both in terms of the patient's illness, and of the prolonged occupancy of hospital beds. Illness due to hospital infection is today rarely a cause of death, though this may occur in patients with poor resistance (e.g. those with extensive burns) or from highly pathogenic organisms (e.g. some strains of serum hepatitis virus).

Factors involved in hospital infection

The occurrence and the effects of hospital infection depend basically on (1) the micro-organisms, (2) the host (patients or staff), (3) the environment, and (4) treatment.

The micro-organisms

Though virtually any infection may be acquired by patients or staff in hospital, there are certain pathogenic organisms which are particularly associated with hospital infection and some which rarely cause infection in other environments. Their role as a cause of hospital infection depends both on their pathogenicity or virulence (ability of the species or strain to cause disease) and on their numbers; it depends also on the patient's defences, and since many patients in hospital have diminished resistance because of their disease or treatment, organisms which are relatively harmless to healthy people may cause disease in hospital; such 'opportunistic' organisms, e.g. *Ps. aeruginosa (pyocyanea)*, are usually resistant to many antibiotics and able to flourish under conditions in which most disease-producing organisms cannot multiply.

In wound infection, antibiotic resistant *Staph. aureus* and various Gram-negative bacilli, including *Ps. aeruginosa*, have played a predominant role. Haemolytic streptococci of Group A (*Streptococcus pyogenes*), which were formerly a much feared cause of invasive and rapidly fatal wound infection, are today of relatively small importance as wound pathogens and have remained fully sensitive to penicillin; invasive streptococcal infection is today a rarity. In spite of its apparently diminished invasiveness, however, *Strep. pyogenes* is still more likely to cause the complete failure of skin grafts than other bacteria if it gains access to full skin thickness burns. Tetanus and gas gangrene are dangerous infections, which are very rare in spite of the fact that the bacteria that cause them are commonly found in dust and in human faeces. Their anaerobic growth requirements make it difficult or impossible for these organisms to colonize tissues with a good blood supply or exposed to the air. A group of anaerobes more commonly responsible for clinical infection in hospital is the family of non-sporing anaerobic bacilli, including *Bacteroides* spp. These organisms are normal inhabitants of the large intestine, where they greatly outnumber *Escherichia coli* and other aerobes. In lower intestinal operations *Bacteroides fragilis* has recently been recognized as a major pathogen, often causing peritonitis and wound infection together with aerobic organisms. In hypersusceptible patients receiving prolonged chemotherapy certain fungi and viruses have caused severe and sometimes fatal infections. Arthropod parasites (e.g. itch mites and lice) may be transmitted in hospital.

Outbreaks of infection (epidemic infection) may be caused by the agents of specific infectious diseases, usually due to the admission of an infected patient or the presence of a carrier in the ward. They may also occur through exceptional errors in asepsis or sterile supply (e.g. contamination of eye-drops or infusion fluids).

The host (patient or member of staff)

The susceptibility of the host and the virulence of the micro-organism are independent variables which have the same relevance to infection as the qualities of soil and seed have in agriculture.

A patient may have poor *general* resistance, e.g. in infancy, before antibodies have been formed and when the tissues that produce antibodies are imperfectly developed; or poor resistance associated with disease, such as uncontrolled diabetes, leukaemia or severe burns; or with poor nutrition; or with certain forms of treatment, such as the use of immunosuppressive drugs given to prevent the rejection of transplanted organs or in the chemotherapy of cancer.

The patient may also have poor *local* resistance because of imperfect blood supply to the tissues, or because of the presence of dead tissue or blood clot in which bacteria can grow without interference from the natural defences; foreign bodies including sutures and prostheses also increase the susceptibility of the tissues to local sepsis. Surgical operations and instrumentation (e.g. catheterization) allow access of bacteria to tissues which are normally protected against contamination; some of these — in particular the chambers of the eye, the meninges, the joints, the endocardium and the urinary tract — have very low

3

resistance to bacterial invasion and are, therefore, peculiarly susceptible to infection with 'opportunist' organisms.

Not only the patients, but the staff (including laboratory staff) are exposed to special hazards of infection with virulent organisms. The risk of infection among members of staff through contamination with blood and exudates of patients with serum hepatitis has received much attention in recent years.

The environment

The place where the patient is treated has an important influence on the likelihood of his acquiring infection and on the nature of such infection. A wide variety of micro-organisms, including virulent strains, is likely to be found in hospitals where many people, including some with infection, are aggregated; these organisms are likely to include a large proportion of antibiotic-resistant bacteria, which can flourish where antibiotic usage has led to the suppression of sensitive bacteria.

Different areas of the hospital have individual infection hazards. In the operating theatre there is a special hazard of wound infection because of the exposure, often for several hours, of susceptible tissues, and the presence of a number of potential human and inanimate sources. In wards the patients may be exposed for many weeks to contaminants from which surgical wounds will usually be protected by some form of cover, though this is imperfect in many patients — especially those with drains. Special hazards exist in neonatal wards through possible contamination of feeds, suction and resuscitation equipment etc., and because of the frequent handling of infants; and similar problems exist in intensive care units and burn wards. Cross-infection with antibiotic-resistant bacteria is a special hazard of wards. In Infectious Diseases Hospitals there is a special hazard of infection with the agents of acute communicable diseases.

An objective in control of hospital infection is to expose patients to an environment at least as free from microbial hazard as that which they would find outside hospital.

Treatment

The clinical results of microbial contamination are influenced by details of treatment — favourably by correct surgical or medical procedures and chemotherapy, but adversely (as already mentioned) by treatment with immunosuppressive drugs or steroids.

Sources and routes of infection (see Fig. 1.1)

Self-infection of an operation wound may be due to bacteria causing infection (e.g. boils), or carried by the patient, without symptoms, on his skin or in his nose (mostly staphylococci, but occasionally streptococci), in his mouth (especially streptococci), in his intestines (especially coliform bacilli, *Bacteroides* spp., gas gangrene and tetanus bacilli). Endogenous infection with *Bacteroides* spp. and coliform bacilli is especially important in the lower intestinal tract, but the upper intestine and stomach may be heavily colonized by these bacteria in patients with gastric carcinoma and other pathological states.

4

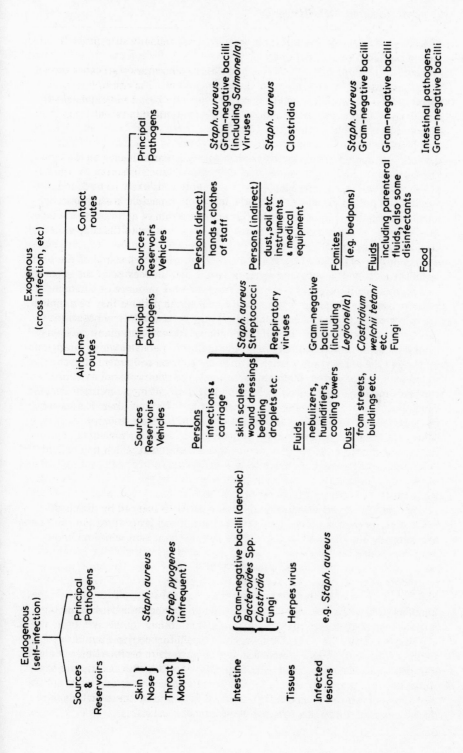

Cross-infection with some of these organisms may occur from other patients or members of staff by *contact* or by *airborne* routes. Infection may be transferred on hands or clothing of staff, visitors or ambulant patients, on unsterile objects or in fluids used in treatment, in food, etc.; members of staff (nurses, physiotherapists, doctors) who attend to many patients are likely to transfer infective organisms from one patient to another; visitors who attend one patient present a smaller hazard, though they may transfer their own micro-organisms. A foetus may be infected from the mother (e.g. with cytomegalovirus) *in utero* or on delivery (e.g. with *Neisseria gonorrhoeae*). Airborne transfer may occur through the dispersal of minute skin scales that are continuously shed from the surface of the body and often carry staphylococci; minute droplets dispersed from the mouth are a potential source of airborne infection, especially with respiratory infections. Epidemic infections arise through the presence of a case of the infectious disease or of a carrier of the causal organism in the ward, theatre or other place in the hospital where a number of patients may be exposed to contamination; the route or routes of transfer vary, depending on the survival of the organisms outside the body and other factors. Infection may occur also through contamination with organisms acquired from inanimate sources, e.g. Gram-negative bacilli in fluids, or tetanus bacilli on inadequately sterilized equipment. Insect vectors (e.g. cockroaches, ants, flies) may convey infective organisms to patients or to sterilized equipment. Legionnaire's disease appears to be acquired from the inanimate environment only; though rare, it is potentially dangerous.

Though the relative importance of different sources and routes can rarely be stated with any precision, there are certain patterns which are relevant to the choice of methods for controlling hospital infection. Of the sources, those in which bacteria are multiplying (e.g. patients with infectious disease and septic wounds, but also healthy surfaces of the body and contaminated solutions) are, in general, more important than dry objects or surfaces on which organisms may survive but cannot multiply (described above as 'reservoirs'); infected patients and septic wounds are more likely to be a dangerous source than healthy surfaces of the body, because the bacteria in the former can be assumed to be virulent, while those on healthy surfaces may often be avirulent. Vehicles which can convey the pathogenic organisms directly to the patient's susceptible sites (e.g. fluids used for aseptic procedures, surgical instruments, food, the hands of nurses handling newborn babies) are more likely to cause infection than sources or reservoirs which do not come in contact with such sites or with the patient. Some of the latter (e.g. floors, walls, furniture) are of very little importance unless incorrect procedures (e.g. sweeping with a broom) are used. The larger the number of stages of contact transfer from a source or reservoir, the smaller the numbers of bacteria that will reach the patients. Contact transfer is more important than airborne transfer for organisms that do not survive well under dry conditions outside the body. Gram-negative bacilli (e.g. typhoid and dysentery bacilli and *Ps. aeruginosa*), which have this characteristic because they are highly sensitive to drying, are more capable than Gram-positive cocci of survival in water, and are, therefore, more likely to be transferred in a fluid vector; a sufficient number, however, survive the effects of drying for them to be transmissible on the hands of nurses, doctors and other human contacts.

6

Principles of control of infection

Patients are protected against infection in hospital by a system of methods, including surgical asepsis and hospital hygiene, the purpose of which can be summarized under three headings: (1) to remove the sources and reservoirs of infection (or, more usually, to remove disease-producing microbes from potential sources or reservoirs of infection); this includes treatment of infected patients as well as sterilizing, disinfection and cleaning of contaminated materials and surfaces; (2) to block the routes of transfer of bacteria from these sources and reservoirs to uninfected patients, which include isolation of infected and susceptible patients, barrier nursing, aseptic operation and 'no touch' dressing techniques; and (3) to enhance the patient's resistance to infection — e.g. during operations, by careful handling of tissues and removal of slough and foreign bodies; also by enhancing the general defences, as by control of diabetes, reinforcement of immunity to tetanus, and the use of antibiotic prophylaxis if and when this is indicated.

Methods advocated for the control of surgical infection can be classified under four headings: (1) *established methods*, for which good evidence is available; (2) *provisionally established methods*, for which there is some evidence; (3) *rational methods*, which are consistent with our knowledge of bacteria, but which cannot be evaluated by experiments (e.g. avoidance of 'clutter' in operating rooms); and (4) *'rituals'* — methods which have been shown by experiment or observation to have no value or even to be harmful. From a large amount of research carried out in recent years we know that much infection can be prevented and some lives can be saved by applying certain methods of controlling infection. At the same time there is, in many hospitals, a continuing incidence of endemic infection at levels which are similar to those reported many years ago. This may be due, in part, to more adventurous surgery and medicine, and to the presence of more patients who are highly susceptible to infection; but there is evidence, too, of erratic and unstandardized aseptic methods which probably contribute a large share to the incidence of cross-infection. In a number of British hospitals there has recently been a decline in the incidence of staphylococcal cross-infection and of antibiotic-resistant *Staph. aureus* (Parker *et al.*, 1974; Rosendal *et al.*, 1977; Ayliffe *et al.*, 1979; Phillips, 1979); there has also been a fall in the incidence of invasive and fatal *Ps. aeruginosa* infections in patients with severe burns. These changes, echoing a reduction thirty years ago in the importance of *Strep. pyogenes* as a wound pathogen, are evidence of a widespread improvement in the control of hospital infection. The focus of attention is shifting, to some extent, from general problems of cross-infection to the control of endogenous infection in colorectal surgery and in patients with diminished antimicrobial resistance, to problems of sterilization of difficult pieces of equipment and to containment of dangerous communicable diseases. But cross-infection is still common in many places (e.g. in developing countries numerous patients with burns die of *Ps. aeruginosa* infection), and the neglect of proven measures of hygiene and asepsis can lead to a resurgence of infection; this happened in some centres when protection of neonates with hexachlorophane was abandoned some years ago on the discovery of its potential neurotoxic effects. With the fall in prevalence of staphylococcal infection there has been a relative increase in infection with certain Gram-negative organisms (notably *Klebsiella* spp. and, in some centres, *Serratia* and *Providencia*). Such organisms are of special importance as a cause of urinary tract infection, which is found to be the commonest form of hospital-acquired infection in many hospitals. There is an increasing awareness of the importance of the personal factor in preventing hospital infection, and of the need of a proper understanding of the facts by all members of the hospital staff. Although the subject is complex and involves many disciplines, the basic ideas are simple, and many of the details of asepsis can be made easier by forms of standardization based on evidence of effectiveness and practicability.

Training

It is important that all members of hospital staff and all involved in the design of hospitals should have some knowledge of the facts and problems of cross-infection and understand the principles and methods of controlling infection. Appropriate training should be provided for medical and nursing staff; pharmacists; technicians, biochemists and other laboratory workers; physiotherapists, radiographers and physicists; catering staff; domestic staff and porters; administrators and secretaries; engineers and architects. Because of the wide variation in background and the fact that many persons who join the hospital staff in specialized, ancillary and paramedical roles have had no previous instruction on control of infection, it is necessary that separate, special courses on the subject should be arranged for different categories of staff.

Training can be classified under five main headings: (1) basic training, as part of medical, nursing or other vocational curricula; (2) induction courses for new entrants into hospital staff; (3) refresher courses for doctors, nurses and others, at intervals of several years, to refresh their knowledge and bring it up to date; (4) special courses for Infection Control Nurses and others specializing in hospital infection; (5) meetings, courses or symposia on particular procedures or aspects of hospital infection and its control.

Training facilities already exist in hospitals and at colleges of further education for some grades of hospital staff. More comprehensive and standardized courses are being launched by the Control of Infection Panel of the Joint Board of Clinical Nursing Studies. Clinical microbiologists, infection control nurses and nursing instructors have, as one of their commitments, the instruction of doctors and nurses on control of infection. Other members of staff who have attended special courses will be requested to pass on the main information they have received at such courses to members of staff working in the same field at their own hospitals; this can best be done in set talks followed up by informal explanations and discussions.

It is important that training courses should be designed to equip the student not only with *knowledge and skills*, but also with *attitudes* which are relevant to the control of infection in hospital.

Contents of this handbook

Each section of the book is devoted to one major subdivision of the subject, though inevitably there are many overlaps and cross-references. *Section A* presents an outline of the ways in which hospitals can obtain information on the incidence of infection and organize methods of control. *Section B* describes the methods by which micro-organisms can be destroyed in, or removed from, potential sources of infection. *Section C* is mainly concerned with methods of preventing the transfer of disease-producing micro-organisms to patients in hospital wards and operating theatres. Enhancement of the patients' resistance by immunization and chemotherapy is the subject of *Section D*. *Section E* consists of a short chapter on the care of hospital staff, considered from the angle of infection hazards and their control. In *Section F* the special problems and requirements of intensive care units, maternity hospitals and certain other departments are considered. *Section G* deals with diseases which present special hazards and problems of control. A list of books and papers for further reading and reference is provided at the end of the handbook. At the end of individual chapters there are a few references, mainly about recent developments or techniques mentioned in the text.

In surveying the wide range of alternative methods we have based our selection on the available evidence and taken into consideration practicability and cost as well as proven effectiveness or rationality. We have also excluded useless and potentially harmful rituals.

It is widely recognized that there should be more standardization to replace the excessive variety of procedures which are still in common use. At the same time some flexibility, with a choice of alternative methods, is needed to meet unforeseen difficulties, such as allergy to an antiseptic or mechanical failure of some equipment. There should be administrative machinery to change procedures when this is found to be desirable in the light of new knowledge. It is also important that 'high risk' patients should receive more intensive protection than the basic requirements for ordinary patients.

References

Ayliffe, G. A. J., Lilly, H. A. and Lowbury, E. J. L. (1979), Decline of the hospital staphylococcus? Incidence of multi-resistant *Staph. aureus* in three Birmingham hospitals. *Lancet*, i, 53.

Parker, M. T., Asheshov, E. H., Hewitt, J. H., Nakhla, L. S. and Brock, B. M. (1974), Endemic staphylococcal infections in hospitals. *Ann. N.Y. Acad. Sci.*, 236, 466.

Phillips, I. (1979), Antibiotic policies, in *Recent Advances in Infection*, 1 (eds D. Reeves and A. Geddes), Churchill Livingstone, Edinburgh, p. 151.

Rosendal, K., Jesson, O., Bentzon, M. W. and Bülow, R. (1977), Antibiotic policy and spread of *Staphylococcus aureus* strains in Danish hospitals, 1969–1974. *Acta path. microbiol. Scand.*, 85, 143.

Administration, Surveillance and Responsibility

CHAPTER TWO

Administration and Responsibility

In many hospitals the incidence of infection is unknown, and techniques of ascertainment or surveillance (i.e. discovery and recording) of infection are often not used. Infection records, when kept by the ward staff, are often inaccurate, and it is unusual for measures of control based on these records to be carried out. Surveillance has been defined as 'the continuing scrutiny of all aspects of a disease that are pertinent to effective control' (Benenson, 1975). Surveillance of infection in hospital is necessary for the following reasons:

(a) to recognize, by any unusual level or change in level of incidence, the existing or impending spread of an outbreak, and to identify the appearance of any particularly hazardous organism;
(b) to judge the desirability of introducing special measures to control an outbreak, or threatened outbreak, and to assess the efficacy of such measures;
(c) to assess the efficacy of the regular preventive measures in use in the hospital.

Of major importance is early recognition of an impending outbreak, or of possible hazards, such as contaminated incubators, which might be followed by infection.

It is the responsibility of the Health Authority to ensure that adequate arrangements are made to control hospital infection. These arrangements should include the setting up of a Control of Infection Committee and the appointment of a Control of Infection Officer and Nurse. The Health Authority should be responsible for implementing recommendations of the Officer or Committee. It is the responsibility of all members of staff to inform the Infection Control Officer or Nurse of potential hazards of infection. Without this information the team cannot be fully effective. Over and above the official responsibilities of the Health Authority and the Infection Control Team is the personal care and responsibility of the Clinician in Charge.

Infection Control Team

The team consists of members of the staff with a special interest in and knowledge of infection control in hospital. The head of the team will be the Infection Control Officer; it will include the Microbiologist (who will usually also be the Infection Control Officer), Infection Control Nurses, and a member of the scientific or technical staff with responsibilities in infection control. Although most of the problems occur within hospital, the present administrative structure

13

also involves the community. The Medical Officer for Environmental Health should be co-opted on to the team if community problems are being considered or an outbreak of a particularly dangerous infection has occurred for which he has legal responsibilities, such as Lassa fever. The team is responsible for investigations of outbreaks or other problems, and for giving advice, making day-to-day decisions and evaluating methods, policies and products involved in the control of infection. The particular duties of the Infection Control Nurse are described below in more detail. The team should meet at least weekly.

Infection Control Officer

The individual holding this appointment should be a senior member of the medical staff with ready access to committees and sufficient authority to command respect. He should have a special interest and training in hospital infection, and should be aware of recent developments in the subject. He should be appointed by the Health Authority in consultation with the medical staff. The Microbiologist is usually the logical choice, as he is suitably qualified and in an ideal position to keep the record system under constant scrutiny. The functions of the Infection Control Officer in conjunction with the other members of the team are to assess risks of infection, to advise on preventive measures and to check their efficacy in all parts of the hospital, including catering, laundry and Central Sterile Supply Department (CSSD), in domestic, pharmaceutical and engineering departments, as well as clinical and other areas. Information and advice may be given by him informally or at meetings of the Medical Staff Committee, Control of Infection Committee or District or Hospital Management Teams. However, if any immediate action is required the Infection Control Officer or Chairman of the Infection Control Committee should be empowered to take whatever steps may be necessary without prior reference to the Control of Infection Committee.

Infection Control Nurse

The Infection Control Officer usually has commitments which prevent regular visits to wards and theatres and do not allow him personally to carry out many of the day-to-day duties of the team, such as recording of infections and ensuring that procedures are satisfactorily performed. At least one Infection Control Nurse or other suitable person should be appointed to assist with these duties in every large hospital (or district). If a nurse is appointed she should be state registered, preferably with surgical, paediatric or infectious diseases experience; experience as a ward or theatre sister or as nurse tutor would be an advantage, but is not essential. Of much greater importance is an agreeable personality and an ability to deal tactfully with all grades of staff.

It is recommended that newly appointed nurses attend for at least one week a centre in which there are a suitably experienced nurse and microbiologist. The principles of hospital microbiology and methods of collection of specimens should be taught in the microbiology laboratory of her own hospital. The acquisition of laboratory skills is not required. It is hoped that all nurses will complete the Joint Board of Clinical Nursing Studies Foundation Course (329). This will take one year, but most of that time the nurse will continue to work

14

in her own hospital. For nurses not attending this course, the Joint Board Short Course (910) is available after one year in post. An advanced course is also proposed. The attendance of the nurse at the Annual Conference of the Infection Control Nurses' Association should be considered as part of his/her training.

The nurse responsible for a District or Area should be graded as a Nursing Officer, but in larger areas a Senior Nursing Officer would be appropriate. Junior appointments would normally be graded as Sister. Grading should depend on area of responsibility and should be reviewed at appropriate intervals. Failure to provide a career structure leads to a wastage of trained experienced nurses.

The Infection Control Nurse is administratively responsible to the District Nursing Officer (or Divisional Nursing Officer) and technically responsible (or possibly seconded) to the Infection Control Officer or Microbiologist, who controls her day-to-day activities. The Infection Control Officer should be responsible for advising on attendance by the nurse at conferences, courses and other relevant meetings. If a person other than a nurse is appointed to take on these duties, he or she should be on the laboratory staff and may be described, for example, as 'Infection Control Microbiologist' or 'Scientific Officer'. It is preferable that such an appointment should be in addition to that of a nurse.

The functions of the Infection Control Nurse are described below. These cover the whole field of infection control and involve co-operation with all the departments mentioned in the section on the Control of Infection Committee, and also the Staff Medical Officer; the nurse is a member of, and shares responsibility with, the Infection Control Team. The Nurse should visit all wards regularly and discuss problems with staff. The laboratory should be visited every morning. Keeping of records should not be the main part of her duties. Instruction of nurses and other grades of staff in the practice of infection control is an important function.

The day-to-day tasks of an Infection Control Nurse might include:

(1) identifying as promptly as possible potential infection hazards in patients, staff or equipment;
(2) compiling records of infected patients from ward notifications, case notes, laboratory reports and information collected in routine visits and discussions;
(3) arranging prompt isolation of infected patients (in co-operation with the ward sister and consultant, who have initial responsibility), in accordance with hospital or area policy, and ensuring that there are adequate facilities for isolating patients. Introducing other measures as necessary to prevent the spread of infection or organisms highly resistant to antibiotics;
(4) checking by inspection that infection control and aseptic procedures are being carried out in accordance with hospital policy;
(5) liaison between laboratory and ward staff; informing heads of departments and giving advice on infection control problems;
(6) collaboration with occupational health staff in maintaining records of infection in medical, nursing, catering, domestic and other grades of staff; ensuring clearance specimens are taken before infected staff return to duty;

15

(7) collaboration with and advising community nurses on problems of infection;

(8) prompt information by telephone of notifiable diseases to the Medical Officer for Environmental Health; this is additional to the written notification by the clinician in charge of the patient;

(9) informing other hospitals, general practitioners and others concerned when infected patients are discharged from hospital or transferred elsewhere, and receiving relevant information from other hospitals or from the community where thought appropriate;

(10) participation in teaching and practical demonstrations of control of infection techniques to medical, nursing, auxiliary, domestic and other staff;

(11) informing the District Nursing Officer or Divisional Nursing Officer of practical problems and difficulties in carrying out routine procedures related to nursing aspects of infection control;

(12) attending relevant committees, which are usually Control of Infection and Nursing Procedures Committees, and

(13) conferring with the Sterile Supply Manager about certain infections in hospital (e.g. serum hepatitis).

The nurse will collaborate with other members of the team investigating outbreaks, carrying out surveys, monitoring special units, collecting microbiological samples, preparing reports for the Control of Infection Committee, clinicians and administrators, and assisting in research projects.

Control of Infection Committee

The Committee of a large general hospital should have representatives from all the major departments which may be concerned with control of infection, i.e. medical, nursing (administrative, ward, theatre, maternity and tutorial), occupational health, engineering, pharmacy, supplies, domestic, CSSD, microbiology and administration. It is also advantageous to invite the local Medical Officer for Environmental Health to be a member. A smaller or specialized hospital may appoint a much smaller committee, and, if a small committee is thought to be preferable in a large hospital, representatives of departments not represented on the committee should be co-opted whenever their interests are being discussed.

Meetings should be either two-monthly or quarterly in large hospitals with complex problems, and at least yearly in smaller hospitals where problems tend to arise sporadically. The committees should:

(1) discuss any problems brought to them by the Infection Control Officer, Nurse or other members of the committee;

(2) take responsibility for major decisions;

(3) be given monthly sepsis reports;

(4) arrange interdepartmental co-ordination and education of committee members in control of infection (it is, therefore, advantageous to have a representation of members with varying interests);

(5) introduce, maintain and, when necessary, modify policies (e.g. disinfectant, chemotherapy, isolation);

16

(6) make recommendations to other committees and departments on infection control techniques, and

(7) advise Health Authorities on all aspects of infection control.

Implementation

If the committee or team is to be effective, the results of investigations and records of infection must be sent to the relevant authorities and recommendations rapidly implemented, especially when the safety of patients or staff is involved. Although the Infection Control Officer has an overall advisory responsibility in the hospital, other members of the committee should ensure that recommendations within their own areas of responsibility are carried out as considered necessary by the committee. Heads of departments, e.g. catering and laundry, should be invited to attend committee meetings when problems concerning their own departments are discussed.

The Control of Infection Committee is often a subcommittee of the Medical Staff Committee, but most of the members are non-medical and many of its suggestions are not related to medical practice. It may be preferable for it to be a subcommittee of the District Management Team, or at least that the Chairman or Infection Control Officer or another elected member should have direct access to the District Management Team or its equivalent. All recommendations, instructions or procedures involving any aspect of infection in the hospital issued by the administration, other committees, Health and Safety Executives, or Medical Officer for Environmental Health should be referred for approval to the Control of Infection Committee.

Action at time of an outbreak of infection

When an outbreak occurs, e.g. from the sudden appearance or increasing incidence of one type of infection in a ward, immediate action is needed to prevent the further spread to patients and staff. This action will vary with the nature and severity of the infection, but certain general principles apply. The Control of Infection Officer must be notified, and should take immediate steps (e.g. isolation of suspected cases), in consultation with the Microbiologist, the Infection Control Nurse and clinicians whose patients are involved.

If the recommendations involve closing of wards or movement of more than an occasional patient or of staff, the Area or District and Nursing Administration should be immediately informed. In a major outbreak likely to involve the community or a dangerous infection, e.g. Lassa fever, the Medical Officer for Environmental Health has a legal responsibility and should immediately be informed (see Chapter 17). If screening of staff is likely to be required, the Occupational Health Department and Laboratory should be informed. If the outbreak involves staff, the Infection Control or Occupational Health Nurse should discuss the situation with heads of departments, e.g. kitchens, CSSD, laundry and domestic, to relieve anxieties and indicate any necessary procedures.

The following steps are appropriate:

(1) Assessment of the situation. Details of patients with infection, including

17

date of admission and of first symptoms and nature of disease, are noted.
Bacteriological samples are examined and pathogens are, when possible,
typed (or kept on suitable medium for typing) in the hospital or the Public
Health Laboratory.

(2) Isolation of infected patients. For appropriate methods see Chapter 9.

(3) Closure of ward or wards. This is rarely required, but may be necessary if
the outbreak is considered to be acute and if the infection involves a hazard
of severe illness or even death in some patients. The ward should be closed
to further admissions, and thoroughly cleaned after discharge of the last
patient before re-opening. Such a procedure may also apply to a theatre or
other affected area.

(4) Epidemiological survey. This will provide evidence of time and place where
infection was acquired, including enquiry for possible admission of patients
incubating infection.

(5) Surveillance of contacts. These may be incubating the disease and surveillance is sometimes necessary. This includes clinical surveillance and laboratory screening.

(6) Bacteriological search for source of infection. Examination of all staff and
patients for carriage to see if, for example, the same phage type of *Staph.
aureus* is isolated from all infections; search for the infective strain in the
inanimate environment (e.g. fluids if the organism is *Ps. aeruginosa* or
another Gram-negative bacillus; food, if the illness is gastro-enteritis or
dysentery).

(7) Survey of methods, equipment, buildings. Such a survey should include
dressing technique, theatre discipline, kitchen hygiene, for evidence of
lapses and the 'personal factor'; also for effectiveness of sterilizers, ventilation, disinfection, and protection against recontamination of sterilized
objects and solutions.

Check-lists of practices should be prepared for investigation of infection
arising in surgical wards, in maternity wards, in general medical wards and in
special departments, e.g. operating suites, kitchens, laundries, central sterile
supply departments (Williams, *et al.*, 1966).

Visits to patients

Infection may be brought into hospital by visitors, or transferred by them from
one patient to another, or acquired by them from infected patients. Though
visitors do not appear to play an important role in hospital infection, some precautions are required to meet recognized hazards.

Prospective visitors should be shown a notice warning them not to enter a
ward if they have a bad cold, a sore throat, diarrhoea, boils or other communicable diseases. Special precautions (gowns, restricted movement, no touch)
should be used if visitors must be admitted to patients with enhanced susceptibility to infection.

The notice should instruct the visitor to confine his visit to one patient. If
this instruction is observed, visits by healthy people (e.g. of mothers to children)

do not present any special hazard of cross-infection. It may be necessary to evict or exclude visitors from a ward if they disregard these instructions.

Visits by susceptible persons (especially children) to patients in isolation with highly communicable diseases should be prohibited. When visits must be allowed, the visitor to such patients should be instructed to take self-protective measures — wearing a gown and, if indicated, a filter type mask as defence against contact and airborne infection; he should refrain from touching the patient, his bed and his belongings. When contact is unavoidable (e.g. in mother's visits to small children) gloves may be worn; intimate contact should be avoided. Hands should be thoroughly washed on leaving the patient.

Legal responsibilities of patients, staff, visitors and hospital authorities in the control of hospital infection

The legal responsibilities of hospital authorities and staff, visitors and patients depend upon the application of general common law principles and some statute law to the particular circumstances of each case.

Under the Occupiers Liability Act 1957 hospital authorities must provide safe premises, so that if patients are admitted to wards or to hospitals where there is a known outbreak of infection the hospital authorities might be made responsible for the death of a patient or for permanent injury suffered by a patient as a result of such infection. Nursing and medical staff therefore have a duty to report at the earliest possible opportunity such infection when it is discovered, and the Control of Infection Officer or Committee must decide immediately what steps should be taken to prevent a spread of the infection. There is a further duty of the hospital authorities to ensure that no staff are employed at the hospital who may transmit serious infection to others; if it becomes known to the hospital authorities that a particular member of staff is a carrier of organisms that cause typhoid fever or other dangerous infectious diseases, then the hospital authorities must take steps either to terminate that person's employment or to deploy him where there can be no risk of infection to other members of the staff or patients. These restrictions must not be applied in the case of less dangerous and commonly non-virulent organisms, such as *Staph. aureus*, which are often carried by healthy persons; special precautions should, however, be taken when these less dangerous organisms cause an outbreak of clinical infection (see pp. 17, 234).

In the case of tuberculosis, tuberculin testing should be routinely carried out and BCG inoculations should be given where there is a possibility of nursing and other staff coming into contact with patients suffering from the disease. If this is not done the hospital may be sued by a nurse who contracts tuberculosis on the grounds that the hospital is not providing a safe system of work. Immunization against other diseases which can be prevented in this way should, in some circumstances, be offered; all nurses and other members of staff working in a smallpox hospital must be kept in a state of active immunity by vaccination (see pp. 212, 229).

A patient in a hospital cannot be held liable either for introducing infection or for spreading it in the hospital, but it is clear that the hospital authorities must take care, by all reasonable precautions, including some kind of isolation, if necessary, to prevent the spread of infection. Similarly, a claim against the hospital authorities in respect of infection caused by a member of the hospital staff either to another member of the staff or to a patient or visitor would be rational only if the hospital had known about it and had failed to take any appropriate action. If it is known that a visitor is suffering from an infection which he is likely to communicate to hospital staff or to patients, there might be a responsibility upon the hospital to stop the visiting, but the hospital authorities cannot really be held responsible for every infection which may be either caused or spread by a visitor. A hospital authority can be and has been held legally responsible when a patient was discharged from a hospital suffering from a specific infectious disease which he subsequently communicated to another person. In that case it was held that there was negligence on the part of the hospital authorities in discharging somebody into the community who was likely to infect other members of the community; such a patient should have been kept in hospital and isolated.

When patients become infected through some error in aseptic techniques or hospital hygiene, the hospital authorities may be held responsible. If for example it could be demonstrated that it was the accepted practice to sterilize certain containers, e.g. of saline solutions, and the hospital fails to sterilize and maintain sterility of the fluid in the bottle before distribution to patients, then the hospital authorities may be held liable if contamination has taken place at any time before it is actually used. On the other hand, if some practice is not universally adopted, e.g. to provide 'ultraclean' air systems for total hip replacement operations, and the hip becomes infected, it could be argued that the hospital authorities were not liable, as their failure to provide such enclosure did not constitute failure to provide a reasonable standard of care in the treatment of the patient in accordance with general practice in this country.

Health and Safety at Work Act (1974)

Under this Act responsibilities are placed upon Health Authorities to provide and maintain plant and systems of work that are, so far as is reasonably practicable, safe and without risks to health of employees; and to arrange for ensuring, as far as is reasonably practicable, safety and absence of risks to health of employees in connection with the use, handling, storage and transport of articles and substances. Safety representatives may be appointed by staff, and, if they require it, Health Authorities must establish safety committees under the Safety Representatives and Safety Committees Regulations, 1977. If this has not been done it should be done immediately, as there are additional responsibilities on Area Authorities under the Act towards patients so that they are not exposed to risks to their health and safety. The Department of Health and Social Security circular HC(78)30 states that in view of the liabilities imposed by the Act on Health Authorities and their employees, each Authority should establish a general structure of responsibility which makes it clear who is responsible for the discharge of particular aspects of the general duties imposed by the Act. It also states, however, that the role of the Control of Infection Committee and Officers recommended in a much earlier circular, RHB (51) 100, need not be affected. It also sets out the responsibilities of management to have advisers and safety officers for specialist departments, safety liaison officers and, where staff require them, safety committees.

The circular refers to the legal responsibilities of the Health Authorities as employers and controllers of premises, but National Health Service Authorities are considered to be Crown bodies, and although they are bound by the Health and Safety at Work Act (1974) no prosecution can be brought against them and no statutory notice is served upon them. The Health and Safety Executive has given an assurance that no National Health Service employee will be prosecuted in substitution for his Authority, and prosecution would be brought only in cases where they would have been brought against employees not covered by the Crown privilege, and where an employee has been given by his Authority a specific safety responsibility; failure to discharge this responsibility, where it was reasonably practicable for him to do so, could result in liability and possible prosecution.

The Health and Safety Executive has stated that, whilst it would be prepared to consider the systems in force in hospitals to provide health and safety at work for employees, it would not necessarily be bound by those systems if it is considered that they were in any way inadequate.

Under the Unfair Contract Terms Act, 1977, a supplier of any goods, which will include drugs, dressings, equipment etc., or a servicing contractor, can no longer disclaim liability for negligence in the supply of the goods, the making of the equipment or the servicing of the equipment if the patient dies or suffers personal injury.

Balance of risks of infection and cost-effectiveness of preventive measures

The application of the Health and Safety at Work Act to infection in hospitals may create problems which are not present in factories or in the general community. The interpretation of the Act in terms of infection in patients is uncertain, since it is not intended to interfere with the clinical responsibility of the medical staff. The interpretation 'as far as is reasonably practicable' is difficult to define. Hospitals are establishments for treating sick people, many of whom are admitted with an existing infection or will acquire an infection during their stay. The diagnosis of an infection may take several days and non-infective conditions can closely mimic infective. Susceptibility of the patient and techniques of treatment are important factors in the emergence of infection. Most hospital infections are unlikely to be transferred to staff, and the incidence of acquired infection is usually very low, particularly if the common upper respiratory infections are excluded. Although every effort is made to minimize risks, staff should accept that a high standard of personal hygiene is necessary. The spread of infection between patients or between patients and staff cannot be eliminated, but can be reduced by simple methods such as hand-washing. Expensive measures, which may involve uneconomic use of staff and resources, may achieve little more than these simple basic measures. All grades of hospital staff are responsible

21

for carrying out measures to reduce the likelihood of spread of infection, and this personal responsibility cannot be passed on to the employing authority. Some departments, such as intensive care or isolation units, may be potentially more hazardous than others due to the types of patient treated in them and the methods of treatment required. Such risks must be recognized by staff working in these units, and they often cannot be reduced without reducing patient care. All patients and equipment should be considered to be possibly infective, and special measures may be recommended by infection control staff for known transmissible infections. The increased risks of infection should also be recognized by visitors, and, where appropriate, visitors should be made aware of these possible hazards.

Decisions on measures required in a particular situation must be made in terms of possible benefit to patients, the benefit to the hospital community and the cost of the measures. Cost-benefit is obviously not a term to be lightly used when considering infection in patients or staff, but it is unfortunately a necessity. The occasional failure of soundly based, commonly accepted measures is not necessarily due to negligence. If legal or other authorities are critical without well-founded evidence, infection control staff are likely to adopt a defensive approach which is detrimental to patient care and to the health service as a whole. Some examples of difficult decisions for infection control staff will be described.

A common problem is the management of a chronic salmonella carrier, either a member of staff or a patient. Person-to-person spread of salmonella is rare except in infant nurseries. The staff carrier could still, with reasonable safety, return to work after the cessation of symptoms provided he does not handle food, drugs or babies and is conscientious in matters of personal hygiene. A patient can, with reasonable safety, be sent home or to convalescence while still excreting salmonella if he is otherwise fit to be discharged and provided with suitable instructions in personal hygiene. If spread of infection occurs in either of these situations the hospital could be held legally responsible, but any other course of action would have been unrealistic. Similarly, a member of the medical or nursing staff who is a known hepatitis B virus carrier should be allowed to continue work, provided he/she takes reasonable hygienic precautions; nevertheless, there is a small risk of transfer.

The inanimate environment is not a major factor in the spread of infection and structural alterations can be costly. A good surveillance system is likely to be more cost-effective in the prevention of infection than routine environmental monitoring or routine screening of faeces of catering staff or the noses of theatre staff; routine monitoring of air or surfaces in operating theatres or pharmacies is an example of a test method which is not related to the risk of infection. Screening of staff means keeping staff unnecessarily off duty without evidence that the organisms they carry are likely to infect others. A large proportion of the staff will, if screened, be found to carry *Staph. aureus* in their noses, and a much smaller proportion may be found to carry β-haemolytic streptococci in the throat or salmonella in the faeces; the *Staph. aureus* may be regarded as a normal component of the nasal flora in these people, and most of them are unlikely to cause clinical infection. Screening for nasal staphylococci is reasonable only

22

in an outbreak of staphylococcal infection, when carriers of the epidemic strain will be sought by phage typing, withdrawn from ward duty, given nasal anti-microbial treatment if this is thought desirable, and monitored for removal of the epidemic strain before returning to ward duty.

Measures to 'control' infection can be expensive and time-wasting for staff and patients and should not be introduced unless evidence of their potential value is available.

Notification of infectious diseases

Some diseases are notifiable by law to the Medical Officer for Environmental Health; the doctor who diagnoses the infection is responsible for the notification. There are some differences in the lists of diseases notifiable in England and Wales, in Scotland and in Northern Ireland (see Appendix 2.1).

Although there is no statutory obligation to notify the detection of symptom-free carriers of bacteria that cause notifiable disease, it is recommended that persistent carriers of typhoid bacilli and other salmonellae should be reported to the Medical Officer for Environmental Health.

Appendix 2.1 Diseases notifiable to the Medical Officer for Environmental Health in the United Kingdom

England and Wales

Acute encephalitis
Acute meningitis
Acute poliomyelitis
Anthrax
Cholera
Diphtheria
Dysentery
Food poisoning (all sources)
Infective jaundice
Lassa fever
Leprosy
Leptospirosis
Malaria
Marburg disease
Measles
Ophthalmia neonatorum
Paratyphoid fever
Plague
Rabies
Relapsing fever
Scarlet fever
Smallpox
Tetanus
Tuberculosis
Typhoid fever
Typhus
Whooping cough
Viral haemorhagic fever (e.g. Ebola fever)
Yellow fever

Under Section 152 of the Health Services and Public Health Act, 1968, some local authorities have ordered the notification of other diseases, including rubella; consult the Medical Officer for Environmental Health for the area about local orders.

Scotland

Anthrax
Cerebrospinal fever
*Chickenpox
Cholera
Continued fever
Diphtheria
Dysentery
Encephalitis lethargica
Erysipelas
Food poisoning
Infective jaundice
Lassa fever
Leprosy
Malaria
Marburg disease
Measles
Ophthalmia neonatorum

Paratyphoid fever A and B
Plague
Pneumonia (acute influenzal)
Pneumonia (acute primary)
*Pneumonia (not otherwise notifiable)
Poliomyelitis — paralytic and non-paralytic
Puerperal fever
Puerperal pyrexia
Rabies
Scarlet fever
Smallpox
Tuberculosis — respiratory and non-respiratory
Typhoid fever
Typhus
Viral haemorrhagic fever (e.g. Ebola fever)
Whooping cough

*These are not notifiable in some areas of Scotland.

Northern Ireland

Acute encephalitis
Acute meningitis
Anthrax
Cholera
Diphtheria
Dysentery
Food poisoning (all sources)
Gastro-enteritis (persons under
    2 years of age only)
Infective hepatitis
Measles
Paratyphoid fever

Plague
Poliomyelitis — paralytic and non-paralytic
Rabies
Relapsing fever
Scarlet fever
Smallpox
Tuberculosis — pulmonary and non-pulmonary
Typhoid fever
Typhus
Whooping cough
Yellow fever

In addition, the Medical Officer for Environmental Health should be informed of the occurrence of brucellosis, leptospirosis, ornithosis, psittacosis, Q-fever, rabies (and possibly ringworm and scabies) although these diseases are not statutorily notifiable.

References and Further Reading

Benenson, A. S. (1975), *Control of Communicable Disease in Man*, 12th edn, American Public Health Association, Washington.
Gardner, A. M. N., Stamp, M., Bowgen, J. A. and Moore, B. (1962), The infection control sister: a new member of the infection control team. *Lancet*, i, 365.

Department of Health and Social Security (1974), *Health Services Management, Health and Safety at Work etc. Act*, Health Circular HC(78)30, HMSO, London.

Department of Health and Social Security (Oct. 1951), *Nursing Techniques — Prevention of Cross Infection*, Health Circular RHB(51)100, HMSO, London.

Ministry of Health (1959), *Staphylococcal Infections in Hospitals*, HMSO, London.

Occupiers Liability Act (1957), HMSO, London.

Unfair Contract Terms Act (1977), HMSO, London.

Williams, R. E. O., Blowers, R., Garrod, L. P. and Shooter, R. A. (1966), *Hospital Infection: Causes and Prevention*, 2nd edn, Lloyd Luke, London.

CHAPTER THREE

Surveillance, Records and Reports

Surveillance and record-keeping are not an end in themselves, but an instrument for measuring the effectiveness of an infection control programme and for giving early indication of outbreaks of infection or problem areas. The most useful records are those which fulfil these functions without infringing on other equally important aspects of the infection control programme.

Methods of surveillance of infection in patients

Various types of surveillance and methods of keeping records are used in different hospitals. Some examples are described below:

(1) **Ward record books**, filled in by ward staff (Sister or Clinician). This method has usually failed in the past and is not recommended.

(2) **Daily scrutiny of laboratory records** by laboratory staff. This method is simple and requires no extra staff or elaborate recording methods. Impending outbreaks can often be detected at an early stage. The incidence of clinical infection cannot be calculated and the usefulness of the method depends on taking bacteriological samples from all suspected cases of infection; closed infections, from which bacteriological samples cannot be obtained, will be missed if laboratory records are the only method of surveillance.

(3) **Wound infection cards.** This involves the completion by the Ward Sister or Clinician of a card containing the clinical information and sending it to the laboratory (see Appendix 3.1) with the sample for bacteriological examination. Cards are kept by the Microbiologist and assessed either by him or by the Control of Infection Officer or Nurse. This method has some of the deficiencies of method 2, but much more clinical information is available and infection rates can be calculated. The total number of operations, from which infection rates are calculated, can be obtained from operating theatre record books.

(4) **Laboratory records and routine visits to the wards.** An Infection Control Nurse examines the laboratory records every morning and completes the necessary information on the infected patient by visiting the ward. By frequent visits to the wards she can also encourage the ward staff to send samples from all patients with suspected infection and detect clinical

26

infections which have not had bacteriological investigation. In addition, the Ward Sister might also be encouraged to keep a daily note of any information on infection or related problems. This can be examined by the Infection Control Nurse if the Ward Sister is busy at the time of a visit.

(5) Inclusion of infection records in patients' notes. A simple system applicable to computerized patients' notes might be useful. This form is filled out for all patients on discharge from hospital (Appendix 3.2); though by itself it is inadequate for immediate control action, it ensures that all patients in the hospital are included in figures of incidence. Instruction for ward or clinical staff in use of the form is necessary if these results are to be of any value.

(6) Cross-sectional or prevalence surveys. If for any reason the maintenance of a continuous record is not possible, a discontinuous record can be kept; 'cross-sectional' (or 'prevalence') surveys of infection could be carried out at intervals (e.g. twice yearly) as follows. During a period of a few weeks, all patients in the hospital are assessed by the Control of Infection Officer or Infection Control Nurse. Records are prepared from an examination of patients' records, temperature charts, treatment cards (for antibiotic treatment), Kardex systems and from questions to Ward Sister on any possible acquired infection in the ward; from the data obtained, the incidence of infection in the hospital during a short time period is estimated. This method alone is not adequate as a source of information required for immediate control action, but it will provide some useful information on the incidence of infection for a Control of Infection Officer with little time to spare and would allow the Infection Control Nurse more time to carry out duties other than record keeping. Cross-sectional surveys may also be made in individual wards, and if associated with bacteriological sampling of patients they will provide additional useful information on the incidence of unsuspected infections or carriers.

Surveillance of infection in staff

Surveillance of infection amongst members of staff, in close co-operation with the Occupational Health Department, is also important. This includes enteric and other community-acquired infections, septic lesions, carriage of multiresistant *Staph. aureus*, and hospital-acquired infections (see Chapter 14).

Treatment and management of these infections can usually be decided in discussion between the Control of Infection Officer and the Occupational Health (or Staff) Medical Officer.

Detection of staphylococcal carriers

As approximately 30% of healthy people are nasal carriers of *Staph. aureus* and as there is no accepted laboratory test for virulence of the organism, routine nasal swabbing of staff in wards and operating theatres is rarely indicated. Routine nasal swabs from staff may be required in specialized units for the treatment of susceptible patients, during outbreaks of infection and as a follow-up after treatment of a carrier on the staff. If an identifiable strain of known virulence or a strain with unusual resistance to antibiotics is responsible for an outbreak of infection, routine nasal swabbing may be required for a limited time as part of a programme to eradicate the organisms from the unit. It is of greater importance to exclude staff with skin lesions or sepsis from wards or theatres than to spend time unnecessarily on the routine examination of nose swabs.

Detection of carriers of Group A β-haemolytic streptococci *(Streptococcus pyogenes)*

The incidence of puerperal infection caused by Group A β-haemolytic streptococci (formerly the major hazard) is now so low that routine nose and throat swabbing is no longer obligatory in maternity units. Swabs *must* be taken from staff and patients when an infection occurs in the unit (see Chapter 2, p. 17 and Chapter 9, p. 153).

Detection of faecal carriers of *Salmonella* or *Shigella* spp

Experience has shown that it is impracticable to demand bacteriological examination of faeces of food-handling staff; this measure is not recommended, unless specifically indicated by past history or recent visits to areas where enteric infections are endemic (see p. 175 and p. 230).

Routine monitoring of environment and equipment

Environment

Unless there is an outbreak of infection, routine bacteriological sampling of floors, walls, surfaces and air is rarely indicated. If sampling is done, quantitative or semi-quantitative techniques should be used. Results should be reported as numbers of organisms per unit area or volume. Random swabbing of areas of unspecified size will give results which are not comparable with each other or with previous results and are difficult to interpret. The non-quantitative isolation even of known pathogens may also be misleading. Selective and/or indicator media should be used for counting pathogens such as *Staphylococcus aureus* or *Clostridium welchii.* Standards for counts on surfaces are rarely valid; numbers of organisms on a surface vary according to the amount of recontamination from the air, and on floors also from shoes and trolleys. However, counting organisms on a surface may be useful for teaching and research purposes. The number of organisms in the air of wards or theatres depends mainly on the number of people in the room and their activity, and on the air flow (air changes per hour), which is rarely standardized except in operating theatres. Routine checking of air flow in a ventilated area is a more reliable guide to the efficiency of a ventilation system than bacteriological tests. Air sampling (settle-plates or slit-sampling) may be useful in recognizing the presence of staphylococcal dispersers in a ward or theatre and in testing individuals suspected of being dispersers. Contact plates from floors and other surfaces may similarly be used to detect dispersers.

Equipment

Routine monitoring of disinfection or sterilization processes is necessary. Physical or chemical measurement of the efficiency of the process is generally preferable to bacteriological assessment. The results of bacteriological tests are not available for 1 to 5 days depending on the organisms and the method of treatment. Sampling of treated equipment or fluids is of less value than process testing, since initial contamination may be low and a large proportion of samples may be sterile. If sampling of the treated product is required, tests should be made in laboratories skilled in this type of work and statistically valid results produced.

Sterilization or disinfection by heat is preferable to chemical methods and monitoring should, when possible, be carried out with correctly placed thermometers or thermocouples. Records of temperature and time should be obtained for every cycle. Initial bacteriological tests of the process may sometimes be useful and routine bacteriological monitoring may be necessary for some equipment when varying loads and materials are treated. Good and regular maintenance of equipment is as important as routine tests of efficiency.

Monitoring of sterilization processes is described in Chapters 4 and 5 (p. 45 and p. 58). Disinfection processes are often less well controlled. Heat disinfection of infant feeds, crockery, cutlery, laundry and bedpans, as well as pasteurization processes, should if possible be routinely controlled by temperature–time records. Initial bacteriological testing of the process is advisable, and in some instances, e.g. infant feeds and laundry, routine bacteriological tests are also advisable.

Disinfection by chemical methods also requires regular monitoring. Chemical tests of the process may sometimes be made, e.g. for presence and amount of hydrogen peroxide, formaldehyde and ethylene oxide. For most disinfectants regular bacteriological in-use testing is necessary, since disinfectants vary in stability and may be inactivated to a varying extent by materials; dilutions and time of application are less readily controlled than are heating methods. After chemical disinfection of certain special equipment, e.g. respiratory ventilators, it is advisable to confirm by bacteriological sampling that no pathogens can be found, but this is not necessary if the process is well controlled.

Collection of data

A number of possible methods of ascertainment are described and the choice depends on the type and size of hospital and availability of staff. It is recommended that as many as possible of the larger hospitals should keep records which will give a fairly accurate assessment of the incidence of hospital-acquired wound infection. Additional records may be kept, as described below.

An Infection Control Nurse or other suitable person will be required to carry out these duties. It is important that the nurse should not spend too much time on record keeping. If the nurse is employed in a large Health District, she may not be able to keep a detailed record of infections arising in all hospitals in the District, and some secretarial assistance may be required. The nurse should spend most of her time on the wards, seeing and discussing with ward staff the management of infected patients and carrying out any necessary epidemiological studies.

29

In hospitals without an Infection Control Nurse, method 2 (see p. 26) should be used, preferably with an additional annual prevalence survey (e.g. by a visiting Infection Control Nurse). A senior or chief technician could be responsible for reporting possible infections to the Control of Infection Officer and could keep a record of infected wounds. A regionally-based team which includes a micro-biologist, nurse and technicians experienced in infection control could provide additional support to the Infection Control Nurses and could ensure that pre-valence surveys are done yearly or twice a year in hospitals that do not yet have an Infection Control Nurse in post.

Wound Infection

Records must be kept with reasonable accuracy, particularly if comparisons are to be made between different periods of time in one hospital or between differ-ent hospitals. Standardization of basic information is necessary; in addition to name, age, sex, ward etc., some information on wound or operation should be recorded. (Collection of the following information, though allowing for some differences in interpretation, should help to standardize infection rates.)

(1) Type of operation, and whether drained or not
Operations are further classified as:
  (a) Clean — an operation not transecting gastro-intestinal, genito-urinary or tracheobronchial systems and not performed in the vicinity of any apparent inflammatory reaction (e.g. hernia repair).
  (b) Clean-contaminated — an operation transecting one of the above sys-tems where bacterial contamination could occur but evidence of defi-nite contamination is not available (e.g. operations on stomach or gall-bladder).
  (c) Contaminated — an operation transecting systems where bacteria are known to be present (and usually abundant), or in the vicinity of appar-ent inflammatory reactions (e.g. operations on colon, mouth or per-forated appendix).

(2) Presence or absence of pus

(3) Sepsis and degree of severity
  (a) Mild sepsis — small or superficial area of inflammation with minimal discharge.
  (b) Moderate sepsis — superficial inflammation of whole wound (or over one third) with a serous or small amount of purulent discharge, or a deeper infection involving a small area (one third or less) usually with a purulent discharge.
  (c) Severe sepsis — a deep, purulent infection, with or without sinuses or fistulae, or widespread cellulitis, or wound breakdown with an obvious inflammatory reaction and pus.

(4) Organisms and antibiotic sensitivities
30

(5) Other information

This can be collected as required by the individual hospital: e.g. operating theatre, surgeon, antibiotic treatment, probable origin of infection, time of dressing of wound, etc.

Probable place of infection

It would be advantageous to know where the infection was acquired and the following points may be helpful.

(1) Infection acquired in operating theatre

Deep infection in clean, undrained wound at any time. Infection occurring within three days of operation, or prior to first dressing in a clean wound. Supporting evidence — pyrexia, staphylococcus of type not isolated from any patient in the ward; staphylococcus of same type isolated from member of operating staff and not present in ward.

(2) Infection acquired in ward

Superficial infection in wound (usually drained), occurring after first dressing. Culture initially negative. Deep infection may develop later in a drained wound. Supporting evidence — staphylococcus of same type isolated from other patients or members of the staff in the ward.

(3) Place of acquisition of infection not known

Superficial infection in any wound after first dressing; evidence in favour of theatre or ward infection not available from bacteriology.

(4) Infection acquired from patient's own bacterial flora

These include infections due to *Staph. albus* or *Staph. aureus* that was present in patient's nose prior to, or at time of, surgery. Resistant strains may have been acquired by the patient's nose or skin in the ward before the operation. Infections due to antibiotic-sensitive Gram-negative bacilli, usually *Escherichia coli* and *Bacteroides* spp.

Other acquired infection

Other acquired infections may be included in the routine records, but the relevance of this information to control of infection, except in the case of urinary tract infection, is rather doubtful because it is often impossible to tell whether the infection is acquired in hospital; e.g. laboratory records of sputum examinations are rarely helpful in determining the incidence of acquired chest infection. Hospital-acquired or 'associated' infection is assessed mainly from clinical information and an agreed definition must be used for each site of infection. This is especially important in prevalence surveys. However, surveillance is recommended for all infections in maternity, neonatal and special units, and, in all wards, for enteric and other communicable infections, bacteraemia, and the presence of multiresistant organisms, e.g. methicillin or fucidin-resistant *Staph. aureus* or gentamicin-resistant *Klebsiella* spp. or *Ps. aeruginosa*.

Processing of data

Methods of recording information

For day-to-day recording and control of infection, a board showing all the wards in the hospital can be kept in the office of the Control of Infection Officer or Nurse. Coloured flags indicate the location of infections, the colours and shapes of the flags representing different organisms, phage-types or sites of infection. Although such a board can give an immediate visual impression of the current state of infection in the hospital, it is difficult to keep the record up to date.

Since much of the information collected at the present time is wasted, a method of recording which can be adapted for transfer to punch cards or computer tape is recommended. Analysis by computer would reduce the time spent by Infection Control staff in individual hospitals. Appendix 3.3 shows an example of such a card. Information can now be fed directly into a computer.

Another convenient record is the 'Kardex' (or a similar) system (Appendix 3.4). This system is particularly suitable for use with, or transfer to, a desk-top computer terminal.

Wound infection rate

The wound infection rate must be defined if comparisons are to be made within a hospital or between hospitals. A list of all operations performed may be obtained from the operating theatre and should be classified into clean, contaminated or clean-contaminated. A meaningful single overall infection rate for all types of wound is not possible, since the likelihood of infection differs in each of these categories. It is useful also to record the severity of infection in each type of wound, the presence or absence of pus and whether the wound was drained or not drained. A reasonable assessment of the incidence of wound infection can be made only if all these factors are considered. The infection rate should be based on clinical and not bacteriological findings. Only operations in which there has been a breach in the skin should be included in the assessment; endoscopies, manipulations and examinations under anaesthesia, vaginal operations and also incisions of abscesses should not be included in the total operations at risk for acquired infection. Cystoscopies should be considered separately as there are certain special problems concerned with the sterilization or disinfection of the instruments used. Infection following cystoscopy is important but should not be included under wound infections.

The report on incidence of sepsis should be considered at least monthly by the Infection Control Officer and distributed at intervals to the clinicians (quarterly). If the information is suitable for computer analysis, infection returns are likely to be produced with greater regularity and the intervals between reports might be reduced to one week and possibly even one day. Similar computer or punch-card processing of bacteriological findings, including antibiotic sensitivities, may give information on organisms prevalent in the hospital; it may also possibly reveal unnoticed cross-infection, particularly infections other than those of operation wounds. Information on current antibiotic resistance patterns will also assist in selection of antibiotics for treatment before a bacteriological report is available.

Early discharges present some difficulties in compiling accurate wound infection rates, since patients may be discharged before infection becomes apparent. General practitioners, the Community Nursing Service and Out-patient Departments may be able to supply information on these patients.

Presentation of reports

Information on the incidence of infection, the prevalent organisms in lesions and their antibiotic sensitivity patterns should be provided for medical, nursing and other hospital staff at monthly or at least quarterly intervals. Reports should be simple and preferably expressed graphically so that the current situation in wards or in theatre can be rapidly assessed. Overall rates of wound infection are of limited value and should be subdivided into clean, clean-contaminated and contaminated as previously described. The infection rate in clean undrained wounds is useful as a measure of acquired infection in the operating theatre and the total operations in each category can usually be obtained from the operating theatre. Since it is time-consuming to collect the total operations, it may be sufficient to report the numbers of infections in each category, provided the numbers of operations are reasonably constant.

Reports on other infections, e.g. urological, can be provided if requested or following a particular investigation. A useful way of expressing all these records is by updating an existing graph of infection rates and sending out the updated record. This can easily be done in a computerized system.

In addition to wound infection rates for the hospital, individual results may be provided for a surgeon on his own operations. This type of confidential report may indicate problems of cross-infection requiring further investigation or allay anxiety when several infected patients are present in one ward but there is no evidence of cross-infection.

Cross-sectional surveys, which include swabs from noses and lesions of patients and staff, of individual wards or units may sometimes be of value in assessing the extent of cross-infection. The ward staff are always interested in studies made on their wards and particularly in the results from their own nasal swabs. Reports should always be sent to the ward concerned, following a bacteriological survey. Since antibiotic therapy for individual patients is often required before the results of sensitivity tests are available, the medical staff should be provided with information on prevalent pathogens and their sensitivity patterns in the hospital (see Chapter 12).

Appendix 3.1 Infection Record (sent to laboratory with specimen) — 1

WOUND INFECTION

This card to be completed and returned to Department of Bacteriology

Full Name . . . .

Under Care of. . . . .   Diagnosis . . . .

Folder No: . . . .   Age. . . . .

Hospital. . . . .   Ward. . . . .

Type of
operation
performed . . . .   Theatre . . . .

Name of Surgeon performing operation . . . .

Severity of infected   Mild . . . . . .   Classification Clean . . . .
lesions: of operation:

                   Moderate . . .   Clean/
                                                contaminated . . . . .

                   Severe . . . . .   Contaminated. . . . .

Has wound been dressed in ward?   Number of days
                              since operation . . . .
             Yes/No? . . . .

                              Have antibiotics been given (specify)

Probable origin of infection: Theatre . . . .

                                Ward. . . . .

                                N/K . . . .

Date . . . .   Signature . . . .

Appendix 3.2 Infection Record (completed on discharge) — 2

Individual Patient Reporting Form

INFECTION REPORT

1. Does patient have any infection?   Yes ( )   No ( )

2. Did infection develop after admission? Yes ( )   No ( )

   Date infection developed ....

A. Type of infection:

   ☐ Respiratory   ☐ Postoperative wound   ☐ Urinary

   ☐ Gastro-intestinal ☐ Blood   ☐ Eye   ☐ Skin

   ☐ Other ....

B. Predominant organism(s) ....

                        Reported by....................

                        Date..........................

Appendix 3.3 Infection Record (for Infection Control Officer) — 3

HOSPITAL ☐☐

SEX ☐

WARD ☐☐

THEATRE ☐

OPERATION ☐☐☐

CLASS ☐

DRAIN ☐

INFECTION TYPE ☐☐☐

ONSET (DAYS) ☐☐

SEVERITY ☐

PUS ☐

SPECIALITY ☐☐

DELAY IN DISCHARGE ☐

SITE ORG. SENSITIVITY
☐ ☐ ☐☐☐☐☐☐
☐ ☐ ☐☐☐☐☐☐
☐ ☐ ☐☐☐☐☐☐

UNIT NO. ☐☐☐☐☐

ADMISSION DATE ☐☐☐☐☐

OPERATION DATE ☐☐☐☐☐

DISCHARGE DATE ☐☐☐☐☐

BACTERIOLOGY

SURNAME   WARD   UNIT NO.

FIRST NAME(S)   CONSULTANT

ADDRESS   DATE OF BIRTH

DATE OF ADMISSION

COMMENTS

☐☐

Appendix 3.4 Example of Kardex Record

Ward Date specimen	Patient	Month and year Date of birth	Date of admission	Consultant	Operation/ diagnosis	Date of operation	Type	Organism	Antibiotic resistance	Comments
1/1 W/S	John Smith	1.1.01	1.1	RS	Varicose ulcers	—	—	*Strep.* Gp A	Sens	Present on admission
10/1 W/S	John Jones	10.10.10	1.1	RS	Appendi- cectomy	6.1	C/C	*Bacteroides*	Sens	
25/1 W/S	John Doe	2.2.22	20.1	RS	Lumbar sympathectomy	23.1	Clean	*Staph. aureus*	PT	Phage type 80/81 drained

Abbreviations
W/S: Wound swab
Sens: Sensitive to all antibiotics tested
C/C: Clean/Contaminated
P: Penicillin-resistant
T: Tetracycline-resistant

References and Further Reading

Brachman, P. S. and Eickhoff, T. C. (eds) (1971), papers on surveillance In: *Nosocomical Infections*, American Hospital Association, pp. 272–97.

Henningsen, E. J. (1963), Administration and surveillance, In: *Infection in Hospitals* (ed. R. E. O. Williams and R. A. Shooter), Blackwell Scientific Publications, Oxford, p. 323.

National Research Council (1964), Postoperative wound infections, *Ann. Surg.*, 160, Suppl. No. 2.

Public Health Laboratory Service (1960), Incidence of surgical wound infection in England and Wales, *Lancet*, ii, 659.

Sterilization, Disinfection and Cleaning

CHAPTER FOUR

Sterilization and Physical Disinfection

Microbial contaminants can be removed by cleaning with a detergent and water, or destroyed by sterilization or disinfection. Cleaning followed by drying of surfaces other than those of the body can be almost as effective as the use of a disinfectant.

Sterilization means treatment which achieves the complete killing or removal of all types of micro-organisms, including the spores of tetanus and gas gangrene bacilli which are resistant to most disinfectants and more resistant to heat than non-sporing micro-organisms. *Disinfection* means treatment which reduces the numbers of vegetative micro-organisms (e.g. staphylococci, salmonellae, viruses) to safe or relatively safe levels. A *disinfectant* is a chemical compound which can destroy vegetative micro-organisms; the word *antiseptic* is often used for disinfectants which are applied to the skin or to living tissues, but since the purpose of antiseptics is to disinfect (one speaks of 'skin disinfection'), the word antiseptic might seem superfluous; it is, however, useful as an indication that the compound can be safely applied to tissues. The word *sterilant* has sometimes been used for the small range of chemical compounds (ethylene oxide, formaldehyde and glutaraldehyde) which, under controlled conditions, can kill sporing bacteria. All items to be sterilized should be physically cleaned before they are subjected to a standard sterilizing process. Methods of sterilization and physical disinfection are shown in Appendix 4.2.

All surgical instruments, dressings and other objects or solutions which are introduced into traumatic or operation wounds or by injection must be provided sterile (i.e. sterilized and adequately protected against subsequent contamination). The same applies, in general, to materials introduced into other areas normally sterile, though disinfection by 'pasteurizing' (see below) or boiling, which destroys vegetative bacteria, is accepted as adequate for cystoscopes and some other endoscopes that cannot tolerate heat sterilization. However, there is a possibility of clostridial infection arising after operations on the genito-urinary tract, and manufacturers should be encouraged to develop equipment able to withstand autoclaving.

Methods of sterilization

Sterilization can be achieved by moist heat at raised atmospheric pressure, by dry heat at normal pressure, by ionizing radiations (gamma radiation or electron beams), by 'sterilants' such as ethylene oxide and glutaraldehyde, or by filtration. It can also be obtained by steam and formaldehyde at sub-atmospheric pressure. If the article to be sterilized is not damaged by heat, heat sterilizing methods should always be used in preference to other methods, because they are more reliable and can be more effectively monitored.

Heat sterilization and disinfection

Heat sterilization depends on the temperature to which articles are exposed and on the time of exposure; the higher the temperature, the shorter the time required for sterilization. Two factors must be taken into account in deciding the time of exposure: (1) *the penetration time*, i.e. the time required for the least accessible part of the load to reach the selected sterilizing ('holding') temperature; and (2) *the holding time*, i.e. the period of exposure to the selected sterilizing temperature. These times will vary with different types of load.

Dry heat is less effective than moist heat and therefore requires a higher temperature and longer time at that temperature.

(1) Dry heat

Red heat from a Bunsen burner is of value in the laboratory, but is not suitable for sterilizing surgical instruments: the 'flaming' of a scalpel, dipped in spirit, is not satisfactory. For sterilization of certain hospital supplies the hot air oven is appropriate.

There are two main types of hot air sterilizers:

(a) The fan oven — Heat is produced by electric elements in the walls of the oven and a fan circulates the hot air evenly. The oven works at 160° C with a holding time of 60 min, and with a total cycle time of 2–2.5 h. It can be used for mixed loads of glass and metal instruments and also some sharp instruments used in ophthalmic surgery. Fats, oils and powders which are impervious to steam are also sterilized by this method. The main disadvantage is the long cycle time. All hot air ovens should be fitted with a door lock and a temperature chart recorder (mandatory requirements in England: DHSS-HTM10, 1980). Ovens without a fan are unsatisfactory.

(b) The conveyor oven — The conveyor oven was formerly popular for sterile syringe services, but since the general introduction of disposable syringes the method has been little used. The articles to be sterilized pass slowly along a conveyor system under an infra-red heat source. The oven works at 180° C with a holding time of 7.5 min.

(2) Moist heat

Steam or water boiling at atmospheric pressure, and at a temperature of 100° C, will not sterilize, but exposure at this temperature for 5–10 min or pasteurization at 75° C for at least 10 min may be sufficient treatment of some endoscopes and specula for which disinfection is generally considered adequate.

To ensure the destruction of bacterial spores by moist heat, a temperature above 100° C is required. In the autoclave (or pressure steam sterilizer), the boiling point of water and the temperature of the steam produced are raised in proportion to the increase in pressure. At a pressure of 15 lb/in^2 (103 kPa) above atmospheric pressure the boiling point of water is 121° C and at a pressure of 32 lb/in^2 (220.8 kPa) the boiling point is 134° C. Steam at these temperatures will sterilize objects in 15 min and 3 min respectively.

To sterilize effectively, steam must come into direct contact with the surfaces to be sterilized. The latent heat which is given out when steam condenses to water increases the sterilizing efficiency of steam, but this occurs only if the steam is not superheated — i.e. raised to a temperature higher than that at which water boils under the pressure present in the autoclave. It is essential to remove all air from the autoclave; this can be done by admitting steam into the upper part of the chamber, from which it will descend, pushing the air through an outlet in the floor of the chamber. This 'downward displacement' method is suitable for unwrapped instruments, bowls and bottled fluids. Air can also be effectively removed by the use of a high vacuum pump before the admission of steam; the high vacuum autoclave should be used for sterilization of porous loads (packs). Improved removal of air can be obtained by the use of pulsed steam (i.e. alternating vacuum with steam injection for 5 to 8 pulses); this method is especially useful when a small load is being sterilized in a large autoclave. Removal of steam and drying of the load in a high vacuum autoclave is achieved by drawing a vacuum after the release of pressure. The complete cycle for a high vacuum autoclave is approximately twenty minutes.

Ionizing radiation

These methods are not suitable for use in hospitals, but are used commercially. The process may damage some plastic materials and advice should always be sought before reprocessing any item. Equipment made of or containing metal, polythene, paper, wool, cotton, polyvinyl chloride, nylon, terylene and polystyrene are usually unaffected. Rubber varies in its response, but butyl and chlorinated rubber are not suitable for sterilization by these methods. Electron beams (β-particles from a linear accelerator) or gamma radiation (from cobalt-60, at a dosage of 2.5 Mrad (25000 Gy) is used. This dosage gives good penetration and leaves no residual radioactivity. Units used for radiotherapy in hospital are not suitable for sterilization purposes.

Chemical methods

(1) Ethylene oxide

Heat-sensitive articles may be sterilized by ethylene oxide gas. The temperature of the process is usually 55° C, and the ethylene oxide is commonly mixed with an inert gas, e.g. freon or carbon dioxide, to reduce risks of explosion. Since dried organisms show increased resistance to the gas, pre-humidification may be advisable. The relative humidity of the process should be controlled at least within the range of 50–60%. The high gas pressure may also damage flexible fibreoptic endoscopes on repeated processing (see

43

p. 87). The effectiveness of the gas as a sterilizing agent may be influenced by other factors, such as the presence of salt crystals and packaging. All materials must be scrupulously clean and packed under clean conditions. Paper and polypropylene or polyethylene film bags are suitable, but nylon film must not be used. Whichever material is used, a double wrap is necessary and film should be sealed by welding or with ethylene oxide sensitive tape. Ethylene oxide and its residues are toxic and irritant, and materials exposed to it should be thoroughly aired for up to seven days. The period of quarantine can be reduced by the use of a correctly designed heated and ventilated cabinet. The sterilizing process must be controlled by spore tests. It is obvious from the requirements described that ethylene oxide should be used only in certain centres, and the process should be well controlled, with trained operators and good microbiological facilities. Its use in the health service is limited to a few items (see p. 86), and machines should not be installed in small departments or individual units (e.g. operating theatres, cardiology or endoscopy units) where adequate control of the process is not possible. Irradiated articles should not be subsequently treated with ethylene oxide unless known to be safe after such treatment.

(2) Glutaraldehyde (see p. 67)

Immersion of equipment in a fluid is generally a less reliable method of sterilization (or disinfection) than exposure to heat or to ethylene oxide, and it has the disadvantage that thorough rinsing is necessary after processing (see p. 87). Glutaraldehyde when used in a 2% solution can be relied upon to sterilize in 10 h, but for practical purposes 3 h should provide an adequate sporicidal effect. Treatment for 10–20 min will only disinfect.

(3) Low temperature steam and formaldehyde (Alder et al., 1966)

This is an alternative method to ethylene oxide and may be preferable, as a prolonged airing period is not required. Although its sporicidal activity is less than that of steam at high temperature, there is a high probability of sterilization if conditions are strictly controlled. Most machines operate at a temperature of 71–75° C, and 1–3 h are required for a sterilizing process. A pulsed vacuum of 50 Torr is generally required to ensure adequate penetration, removal of formaldehyde, and drying of equipment. Steam is usually pulsed, but the best conditions for admitting formaldehyde and its optimal concentration have not been defined. Although it is not yet possible to define an optimal process, commissioning and routine testing methods are available which, if satisfactory, should ensure a high probability of sterilization. Many machines at present manufactured do not reach the required standard without some modification and require considerable attention from skilled engineers and microbiologists. The problems include excessive condensation, poor temperature control, variable formaldehyde concentrations in the chamber, and inadequate removal of residual formaldehyde or paraformaldehyde at the end of the cycle. Variability of temperature and formaldehyde concentration tend to be less in smaller machines, and improved design, such as the inclusion of a complete heated jacket, may be necessary. As some of the equipment processed is expensive, it is particularly important that a high temperature cut-out mechanism is fitted. This is usually set at a maximum of 80° C.

Disinfection by low temperature steam. Most of the difficulties with low temperature steam and formaldehyde sterilizers are concerned with the use of formaldehyde. Low temperature steam without formaldehyde is a disinfection process and 10 min at 71–75° C will meet most requirements in the hospital service. An advantage over chemical disinfection is that equipment is dry at the end of processing, and may be wrapped. There is also no problem of residual disinfectant. Routine microbiological tests are required for the use of low temperature steam and formaldehyde, but not for low temperature steam alone. A daily chamber leak test is required for both processes.

Dual purpose autoclaves, i.e. for use at both high and low temperatures, are not recommended by the Department of Health. Nevertheless, there is still a requirement for such a machine which is reliable, not too difficult to maintain, and with a mechanism to ensure that heat-sensitive items are not overheated; a well-trained operator, with clear instruction on the use of the two cycles, would be required.

Tests for effectiveness of sterilization

Autoclaves: steam at high temperature (porous loads)

On commissioning a new sterilizer and at regular three-monthly intervals the chamber temperature and steam penetration should be checked with standard thermocouples (DHSS, 1980). The temperature and pressure records for each cycle should be examined; a Bowie-Dick test and a chamber leak test should be carried out daily on all high vacuum autoclaves (see Appendix 4.1). Although a weekly leak test is sometimes suggested, a daily test is preferable. These tests may be supplemented with indicator systems, e.g. Browne's tubes and indicator tape, which should be stored under manufacturer's recommended condition and not used if out of date. It must be recognized that these indicator tests provide evidence of physical conditions required for sterilization, not of sterilization. Spore tests are not recommended for routine use, but may be of use in checking packaging or objects where penetration may be in doubt. They should also be used if there is any suspicion of infection occurring due to failure of an autoclave. Although often variable, spores strips containing approximately 10^6 *Bacillus stearothermophilus* produced by a recognized method and well controlled should be reasonably reliable.

Bottled fluid autoclaves

Detailed commissioning and regular testing of loads with multiple thermocouples are required. Charts should record temperature from a thermocouple in the load, as well as from the chamber drain. These charts must be compared with master charts of that particular load made during commissioning (DHSS, 1980).

45

Hot air sterilizers

These are tested by thermocouples; Browne's tubes are also used as indicators.
A chart recorder is required.

Ethylene oxide

A spore-strip (aluminium foil) containing 10^6 *Bacillus subtilis* var. *globigii* should
be included in every load initially, but this may be reduced when repeated testing shows the process to be reliable. Tests should also be made on new items
which may present problems of cleaning or gas penetration. Ethylene oxide indicators are useful for supplementing spore tests, but should not replace them.

Low temperature steam and formaldehyde (HEI 95/80)

On commissioning, tests should be made for steam penetration and air tightness
of the chamber (see BS 3970 Part 1, and DHSS 1980). If formaldehyde is used,
tests should be made with *B. stearothermophilus* spore strips, containing approximately 10^6 spores. Spore tests should detect penetration of formaldehyde in a
test piece related to the complexity of the instrument to be sterilized, e.g. a
metal helix (Line and Pickerill, 1973), and even distribution of the gas throughout the chamber. Routine tests should include a daily vacuum leak test and
insertion of a spore-strip in a test piece, initially in each cycle. The frequency of
spore tests could be reduced when repeated tests have indicated a reliable cycle
and if supplemented with a suitable process indicator in the test piece. Spores
should be incubated in at least 15 ml of tryptone soya broth without indicator
in an incubator at $56°$ C for at least 5 days, or for 14 days in commissioning and
routine maintenance tests.

As with other autoclaves, commissioning and maintenance tests should include electrical and other checks such as the high temperature cut-out.

Advice from sterilization engineers and microbiologists should be sought
when contemplating the purchase of new equipment to ensure that it will do the
job required of it and that it is known to be satisfactory.

Appendix 4.1 Autoclave Tests

1. Bowie–Dick autoclave tape test for high vacuum autoclaves*

The principle is very simple. A standard test pack is made up from huckaback
towels. In the centre is placed a piece of paper to which has been fixed a cross
of approved autoclave tape which has been stored according to the manufacturer's recommendations. This tape shows a colour change when exposed to
steam. The test pack is now autoclaved in the usual way. *If all the air has been
removed* the steam will penetrate rapidly and completely and the tape will show
a uniform colour change. *If all the air has not been removed*, when steam is admitted for the sterilizing stage the air will be forced into the centre of the pack,

*DHSS, 1980 and BS 3970 Part 1, 1966. Amendment No. 1.

where it will collect as a 'bubble'. The tape will not change colour in the region of the bubble because it has not been exposed to steam and this will show up when the paper with the tape cross is removed at the end of the run (see Fig. 4.1).

If the test is to be a reliable guide to the safe working of the sterilizer it must be carried out exactly as described.

Performance of the test

Up to 36 huckaback towels, 36 in x 24 in, complying with BS 1781 TL.5 are required. The towels should be washed before being used for the first time, and whenever they are soiled or discoloured.

Between tests they should be unfolded and hung out to air for at least an hour.

Each towel should be folded into eight thicknesses and placed one above the other to form a stack 10-11 inches high. The exact number of towels needed will depend on how often they have been used, but 25-36 may be needed to attain the recommended weight of 4.7 to 5 kg. A piece of paper, approximately 12 in x 12 in, to which approved autoclave tape has been applied in the form of a St. Andrew's cross, is placed in the middle of the stack; greaseproof or waxed paper should not be used. The stack may be placed in a dressing casket (such as that described in BS 3281) or in a box made of cardboard or metal, so long as it is not air-tight. If preferred, the stack can be wrapped, in fabric or paper, or

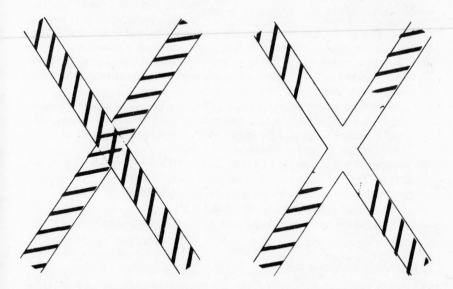

Fig. 4.1 The Bowie-Dick Test. A satisfactory result (left) shows an even colour change (dark stripes) along the strips of tape. A failed test (right) shows no change of colour in the central area.

it can be secured with tape. All that matters is that the towels should stay in position when the test pack is handled.

The test pack must be placed in the sterilizer by itself and subjected to a standard sterilizing cycle. The 'holding' or 'sterilizing' time must not be more than 3.5 min if a temperature of 134° C (273° F) is being used. If the automatic cycle is set for a longer holding time this must be cut short, for purposes of the test, to 3.5 min at 134° C by using the manual control. Should there be any doubt about how to do this the engineer should be asked for advice.

Reading the test

When the cycle is finished the pack should be taken out and the paper with the tape cross should be examined.

After a satisfactory run the tape will show a colour change *which is the same at the centre as at the edges* (Fig. 4.1).

If the tape at the centre is paler than it is at the edges it means that there was a bubble of air there and that the sterilizer was not working properly. If this happens the matter should be reported at once (Fig. 4.2).

The paper with its tape cross from each test can be marked with the date and other particulars and kept for reference.

The towels should be aired and folded ready for the next test.

Comments

Unless the test is carried out exactly as described it may not be truly reliable. In particular the following points should be noted:

(a) The more air there is to remove, the more exacting will be the test — that is why the test pack is used by itself in an otherwise empty chamber.

(b) The exact colour change shown by the processed tape may depend on the storage conditions. The important thing is whether the same colour change occurs at the centre and the edges.

(c) The contrast in colour change from centre to edge will be reduced to an unreadable level if long 'holding' periods are used. That is why the holding period must not exceed 3.5 min at 134° C. Even an extra minute or two may seriously affect a comparison of results.

(d) Because of this it is important to realize that if a sterilizer fails to pass the Bowie-Dick test as described, it cannot be made safe merely by increasing the holding time until a uniform colour change is produced. Such a sterilizer is in urgent need of skilled attention.

(e) The test should be viewed in parallel with results of the chamber leak rate test (daily).

2. Chamber leak rate test

This test is only applicable to high or low temperature high vacuum autoclaves, and it should be performed daily. There are two reasons why air leaking into the autoclave is unacceptable: these are (a) the presence of air prevents penetration of the load by steam, and (b) the air will not have passed through the bacteria-retentive filter and therefore there is a potential risk of recontaminating the load.

The test involves the drawing of a vacuum in the autoclave chamber, followed by the closure of all valves leading to the chamber, stopping the vacuum drawing system and observation of the chamber pressure for a timed period. The manufacturer's instructions should be followed and, in case of doubt, the advice of the sterilizer engineer should be sought.

A period of approximately five minutes should be allowed after the vacuum pump has stopped for the full closure of valves and for stabilization of conditions within the chamber. An absolute pressure gauge reading should then be recorded and a period of 10 min timed. After this period has elapsed the absolute pressure gauge reading should again be recorded. Considerable care and knowledge must be applied in the interpretation of the results (DHSS, 1980).

A leak rate of 10 mmHg in 10 min after stabilization is the maximum which should normally be permitted for a porous load sterilizer and a leak rate of 6 mmHg over a 10-min period for low temperature steam/formaldehyde autoclaves. Both the maximum leak rate and maximum vacuum level which gives an indication of the performance capability of the air removal system should be recorded in the sterilizer log book.

The leak rate test and the Bowie–Dick tape test for porous load sterilizers are complementary tests. A sterilizer which fails to meet the requirements of either of these tests must not be used until the fault(s) has been rectified and the sterilizer satisfies both of these tests.

Appendix 4.2 Methods of sterilization and physical

Category	Operating conditions (temperature and time for sterilizing)	Application
1 *Steam — DD*		
a. Laboratory autoclave	121° C/15′	cultures, media, glass
b. Instrument sterilizer	126° C/10′ 134° C/3.5′	unwrapped instruments and bowls
c. Bottle sterilizer	121° C/15′ 126° C/10′ 115° C/30′	bottled fluids
2 *Steam — HVHT* Porous loads	134° C/3–3.5′	dressings, rubber, wrapped
3 *Steam — HVLT*		
a. Without formalin	73° C/10′	heat-sensitive materials, fabrics, plastics, rubber
b. With formalin	73° C/1–3 h	endoscopes, electrical equipment
4 *Hot water* Pasteurizer	75° C/10′	endoscopes, specula
5 *Hot air*		
a. Fan oven	160° C/60′	glass, metal instruments
b. Conveyor oven	180° C/7.5′	
6 *Ethylene oxide*	20–60° C 1–6 atm P 200–1000 mg/ℓ 10–90% EtO	heat-sensitive materials fabrics, plastic, endoscopes, electrical equipment
7 *Liquid chemical agents* Glutaraldehyde	2% buffered solution	instruments, rubber, plastics

HVHT — high vacuum high temperature
HVLT — high vacuum low temperature
 DD — downward displacement

(Modified version of a table by Dr J. S. Kelsey (1964) to whom acknowledgements are due)

disinfection of equipment and supplies in hospital

Tests	Process time (approximately)	Notes
Thermocouples Browne's tubes	20–60 min	May be vertical or horizontal. See BS 2646
Thermocouples Browne's tubes	5–15 min	See BS 3970 Part 3
Browne's tubes and temp record thermocouples	2–12 h	If fitted with rapid cooling device process time can be reduced to one half or one third. See BS 3920 Part 2
Thermocouples Bowie-Dick and temp record, vacuum leak	20–25 min	See BS 3970 Part 1
Temp. and vegetative organisms	15–30 min	Low temperature steam — disinfects only
Temp. leak test Test piece with spores and thermocouples	1–3 h	Low temperature steam + formalin should sterilize
Thermometer	10–15 min	Disinfects only
Browne's tubes and thermocouples	2–4 h 30 min	Mixed loads possible (BS 3421) Homogeneous loads only
Spores	2–24 h	Various processes in use. Only suitable where constant and skilled bacteriological control is available — mainly industrial
Spores Kelsey-Sykes capacity test	3 h for sterilization 10 min for disinfection	An expensive chemical disinfectant which will sterilize

References and Further Reading

Alder, V. G., Brown, A. M. and Gillespie, W. A. (1966), Disinfection of heat-sensitive material by low-temperature steam and formaldehyde. *J. clin. Path.*, 19, 83.

Bowie, J. H., Kelsey, J. C. and Thompson, D. R. (1963), Bowie and Dick auto-clave tape test. *Lancet*, 1, 586.

British Standards Institution (1966), BS 3970 Part 1 *Sterilizers for porous loads.* Amendment AMD 304, August 1969.

British Standards Institution (1966), BS 3970 Part 2 *Sterilizers for bottled fluids.*

British Standards Institution, BS 3970 Part 3 (in draft).

British Standards Institution (1955), BS 2646 *Copper laboratory autoclave.* Amendment PD 5771, 1966.

British Standards Institution (1966), BS 3421 *Performance of electrically heated sterilizing ovens.*

British Standards Institution (1967), BS 1781 *Linen textiles for use by government departments, hospitals and local authorities.*

Department of Health and Social Security (1980), *Hospital Technical Memorandum* (HMT) No. 10. *Pressure steam sterilizers.* HMSO London.

Health Equipment Information (HEI) 95/80. Departmental Advice on some Aspects of Disinfection and Sterilization, 1980, DHSS.

Kelsey, J. S. (1964), Sterilization and disinfection techniques and equipment, In: *Proc. Hospital and Health Management Summer Conference*, Aug. 1964.

Line, S. J. and Pickerill, J. K. (1973), Testing a steam–formaldehyde sterilizer for gas penetration efficiency. *J. clin. Path.*, 26, 716.

Rubbo, S. O. and Gardner, J. F. (1965), *A Review of Sterilization and Disinfection.* Lloyd Luke, London.

Russell, A. D., Ayliffe, G. A. J. and Hugo, W. B. (eds) (1981), *Principles and Practice of Disinfection, Preservation and Sterilization*, Blackwell Scientific Publications, Oxford (in press).

Sykes, G. (1965), *Disinfection and Sterilization*, 2nd edn, Spon, London.

CHAPTER FIVE

Central Sterile Supply

Introduction

Centralization of production packs for aseptic techniques and of sterilization processes has a number of advantages. Nursing time is saved, aseptic techniques are safer and can be standardized throughout a hospital, area or region, and to some extent nationally. Sterilization processes are more effectively controlled and consequently safer. Reduction in cross-infection may also have occurred, but this is hard to demonstrate. The scope of sterile supply services has changed considerably during the time they have been in operation. They have taken over a greater variety of materials for processing, while disposables now replace some of the items which were once the main source of work in central sterile supply departments. Changes continue to take place, and local enthusiasms lead to departments being developed along different lines.

The functions of the central sterile supply services are:

(1) supply of sterile materials for dressings and procedures carried out in wards and departments (including X-ray and Cardiology);
(2) supply of operating theatres with the necessary sterile instruments and linen;
(3) disinfection or sterilization of medical and nursing equipment such as ventilators, oxygen tents and baby incubators;
(4) selection and distribution of single-use sterile supplies, such as catheters, suction tubing and syringes.

The provision of sterile fluids is the responsibility of the pharmacist, although occasionally sterile water for the operating theatre may be supplied by the CSSD.

Some of the abbreviations used for different types of sterile supply departments are:

CSSD — a department assembling, producing and distributing sterilized packs (Central Sterile Supply Department). The term is used also to describe collectively all types of sterile supply departments, including the Medical Equipment Cleaning Section (see below).
TSSU — A department dealing with the sterilization requirements of theatres only (Theatre Sterile Supply Unit).
HSDU — A department providing the full range of sterile supplies and distributing them within a hospital. The department services wards and theatres

and also undertakes decontamination of medical equipment (Hospital Sterilizing and Disinfecting Unit).

The HSDU should be the local headquarters of all the sterile supplies for a district general hospital. It should also have the responsibility for supplying smaller units in the area. This could become a diminishing responsibility as facilities are increasingly concentrated in a new district general hospital. Raw materials and disposable items such as catheters and standard dressing packs should be supplied to the HSDU in accordance with the Regional Supplies policy and advice from the Department of Health. CSSDs should be regarded as future HSDUs in almost all cases.

Administrative arrangements and supply policy

A sterile supply service provides sterile materials for many areas of the hospital, ranging from those used in routine ward procedures such as blood taking and wound dressings, to the provision of sophisticated items such as theatre operating sets or ventilators. It may also be called upon to provide sterile fluids or to decontaminate medical and nursing equipment.

Certain of the items required in a hospital will be obtained from a commercial source, e.g. pre-sterilized single use items, such as syringes, needles, catheters and drip sets. Current supply arrangements for these items are usually made on a regional basis, after local discussion and advice from the Department of Health. There is, however, need for constant vigilance to make sure that items are as described and functionally satisfactory. Competitive prices can only be considered in the light of safety and functional suitability of the product. There is no directive by the Department of Health or the Regional Health Authorities as to which materials are to be used, but recommendations on sterile packs and methods of sterilization are available.

Commonly used packs

Some items can be assembled in individual industrial therapy and local occupational therapy units, provided that the premises and supervision are adequate. The remaining packs which require more skill in assembling or contain special instruments are assembled in HSDUs or CSSDs. The sterilization of items produced in sheltered workshop conditions is preferably centralized in a department designed for this purpose. Those packs, which can be made at industrial occupational therapy units, are the following (present recommendations on packs are presented in the Cunliffe Report):

(1) Dressing packs – including sterile forceps.
(2) Supplementary packs of various types (cotton wool balls etc.)
    The contents of three basic dressing packs are given in Appendix 8.1 (p. 120).

Packs may also be made for procedures which do not require sterile materials, although they require disinfection after use. These include packs for oral toilet, ear toilet and colonic lavage.

All the returnable items could be returned for cleaning, reassembly and processing to central 'factories', but there is much in favour of having the more complex packs dealt with locally in an existing CSSD. Sharp instruments such as scissors will still need to be dealt with locally in the HSDU.

Sets of instruments and special local requirements

Sets of theatre instruments and procedure sets used in wards and departments are usually dealt with by the HSDU.

Domiciliary supplies

Many hospitals provide dressings for domiciliary services for early-discharge surgical patients by arrangements with general practitioners in the area of the hospital. Other items, such as perineal repair packs, obstetric forceps and paracentesis abdominis sets, are also provided when necessary. A more formal supply would not be possible without alteration of the National Health Service regulations, but all the requirements of the domiciliary services can probably be met by a relatively small variety of standard packs, and production of these should be allowed for in the capacity of HSDUs.

Organization of work in HSDU

The siting of a sterile supply unit in the hospital presents some difficulty. On the one hand it needs to be near to the main users, i.e. the wards and operating theatres, and on the other hand it must be accessible to delivery vans bringing bulky materials for processing and distribution. The department should be all at one level and must have a carefully planned work flow. Most departments are designed to supply 2000 beds excluding psychiatric, in an area of 8000 ft^2. The main areas in a department are the store for receiving unsterile supplies, the preparation area, sterilizing area and sterile store. The major equipment cleaning area and instrument workshop are usually separate from the main work flow. There are normally three separate doors: (a) for receiving unsterile materials, (b) for receiving materials returned from wards, theatres and departments, and (c) for supplying sterile materials.

The number of staff required for a full service to 2000 beds is approximately 30, comprising manager, sterile supply assistants, sterilizing attendants and porters. The basic equipment includes high pressure sterilizers, hot air ovens, a low temperature steam formaldehyde sterilizer, drying ovens, washing machines, ultrasonic cleaners and heat-sealing machines. It is not practical to detail requirements, as these vary locally and are well established in most hospitals. The requirements of a Medical Equipment Cleaning Section are discussed below.

Presentation of packs to the user

The paper used is in accordance with the specification of the DHSS. Generally, the contents of all dressing packs, supplementary dressing items and other soft dressing materials are packed in gussetted bags of an appropriate size to facilitate the aseptic removal of the contents; the bags may be of the heat-seal type or turn-over top which are secured with heat-sensitive (autoclave) tape. The heat-seal type usually has an indicator panel to define whether or not the contents have passed through a sterilizing process. Multiples of these packs will be packed in a thin cardboard outer box which serves both as the outer barrier and as a dispenser. Once empty this is expendable.

Procedure packs and special sets are wrapped in two separate layers of paper or two layers of paper and one of linen and finally placed into a bag of appropriate size before sterilization. This bag acts as a dust barrier.

Pre-set trays for operating rooms will have a minimum of three wraps, preferably one of linen and two of paper. A large bag is used as a dust cover during transport; a plastic bag may be used for this purpose if the tray has been allowed to cool. This is removed before entry to the clinical area. Packs of linen drapes, gowns etc., will be packed in a similar fashion. Supplementary dressings for operating rooms, bundles of radio-opaque materials etc., will have two separate wrappers and may be supplied in light cardboard dispenser-type boxes.

Central sterile supplies to operating theatres

Instruments are usually returned in a plastic bag on their tray directly from theatre to the HSDU, while theatre linen is processed in the hospital laundry before arriving in the HSDU.

On arrival in the Unit, the instruments are checked numerically before washing in an automatic washer-drier, and then a more thorough check is made for serviceability before packing for resterilization.

The type of packing used varies, but two main types of instrument tray are satisfactory. In the first method the tray is not included inside the pack but is overlaid with a linen drape, the instruments set out on the drape followed by radio-opaque swabs, patient drapes etc.; the outer drape is then folded to enclose the instruments and other contents of the pack. The tray itself is made of an alloy and is not perforated. The folds of the enclosing drape are made so as to allow aseptic opening of the pack in the theatre area. The complete assembly is wrapped in crepe paper and preferably placed inside an appropriate paper (e.g. 'Kraft' paper) bag which acts as a dust cover during transit and storage.

In the second method the tray is enclosed in the drape with instruments set out directly on top of the tray. In this case the tray should be perforated or have open, unwelded corners. After folding the drape around the tray, the instruments and the other contents of the pack, the additional paper covers are applied.

Paper wrappings of the approved patterns are a better bacteriological protection than linen and are preferred to all linen wrappings.

Sterilization of theatre materials is usually performed in a high vacuum autoclave with adequate mechanical monitoring of the sterilization process, a heat-sensitive seal on the packs to indicate that the pack has been through the process and a batch number. After sterilization the packs are returned to the theatre (DHSS, 1980).

Theatre linen

Theatre linen, i.e. drapes, gowns, and towels, requires inspection. The folding of drapes and gowns varies with local practice, but the method used must allow aseptic opening. A suitable method for surgeons' gowns is to turn the gown inside out and fold into three; the top end is then turned down a short way and the gown rolled from below upwards. To open the gown the top fold is grasped and the gown allowed to unroll towards the floor and gowning can then take place, the surgeon touching only the inside surface of the gown.

A typical linen pack would contain a split abdominal sheet, four towels (each 1 m^2), two skin towels and bundles of radio-opaque swabs, wrapped in a layer of crepe paper and put in an appropriate paper (e.g. 'Kraft' paper) bag before heat sealing. Gowns are usually packed separately, using a similar technique. Sterilization is best performed in a high vacuum autoclave with a holding time of 3 min at 134° C.

Medical equipment cleaning section (MECS)

It is suggested that an area of about 800 ft^2 (74 m^2) should be made available for the disinfection (and in some instances sterilization) of clinical machinery such as ventilators, incubators and suction apparatus. It is helpful to have this section contained within the boundaries of the HSDU.

The area may also be used as a store to accommodate such items as steam tents and kettles, suction apparatus, incubators, humidifiers and ripple beds. It is useful to have such equipment stored centrally and available in a serviceable condition.

The basic requirements of an MECS may be summarized as follows:

(1) 700–800 ft^2 (65–74 m^2) near to main user, especially ICU theatre.
(2) Solid floor with adequate drainage. An area of approximately 2 m^2, with sides sloping to a centre drain, is useful for the washing of larger items of equipment.
(3) Adequate electrical socket outlets (13 amp).
(4) Oxygen or compressed air outlets at 60 lb/in^2 (414 kPa) pressure.
(5) A bench, 10 ft (3.05 m) long, 36 in (91.4 cm) high, 18 in (45.7 cm) deep with storage shelving below.
(6) Wooden shelving for general storage.
(7) Two large sinks 4 ft (1.22 m) by 15 in (38.1 cm) by 10 in (25.4 cm) deep for washing and soaking larger items of equipment.
(8) A drying cabinet for endotracheal tubes, anaesthetic sundries, tubing etc.
(9) A high pressure water gun rinser (mains water supply required).
(10) A downward displacement instrument-type autoclave for sterilizing such items as suction bottles or parts from incubators. This equipment is not necessary if the HSDU autoclave is readily available. Alternatively, a low temperature steam formaldehyde sterilizer should be available.
(11) A washing machine heating to at least 70° C, although of doubtful value, may have some uses.
(12) A sluice hopper for the emptying of suction bottles etc.

(13) Air extraction unit to exhaust to atmosphere (for removal of formaldehyde and other noxious vapours).

At the present time the duties of personnel working in the Medical Equipment Cleaning Section fall outside the duties outlined in the job description for CSSD assistants (there has not been a revision of duties for personnel covering all the duties of HSDU).

Therefore, two levels of staff are employed in the HSDU, one for the CSSD and TSSU elements and one for the Medical Equipment Cleaning activities (Medical Equipment Attendant).

On-site training will be necessary and the number of staff employed will be dependent upon the section's work load; the HSDU manager will normally be responsible for this work.

The cleaning and disinfecting of anaesthetic equipment and respiratory ventilators is described in Chapter 7.

Control of sterilizing equipment

The care of an autoclave should be included in a planned maintenance programme. The following simply routine tasks must be carried out daily on each porous load sterilizer before any load is passed through the machine for sterilization. (See also Chapter 4, and DHSS, 1980.)

(1) The interior of the chamber must be cleaned using a clean mop retained for this purpose.
(2) Tests for penetration by steam and for removal of air with autoclave tape (Bowie–Dick test) (see Appendix 4.1).
(3) A test for air leaks when appropriate measuring instruments have been fitted to the machine. (See Appendix 4.1.)
(4) All dials and chart recorders must be visually checked to determine correct temperature and pressures in each sterilizing cycle.

These tasks must be carried out by the sterilizing attendant and the results recorded in a log book for each sterilizer. The tape test sheet and recording charts must be shown to the Manager or his deputy; interpretation of the tests may be the responsibility of the sterilizing attendant, but should there be any doubt as to the machine's efficiency, the Manager should be informed immediately, and it is he who will decide whether or not the sterilizer should be used.

Sterilization and packing of heat-sensitive materials

Reusable items should, whenever possible, be capable of surviving high pressure steam sterilization or dry heat. Items not capable of heat sterilization may have to be used in some fields and for these there are several methods available (ethylene oxide, low temperature steam and formaldehyde, glutaraldehyde — see Chapter 4), depending on the temperature to which the item can be exposed without suffering damage (see Chapter 7).

Distribution and storage of CSSD materials

Sterile materials are brought to the patient from a variety of sources; hospital-prepared CSSD materials directly from the department, sterile pharmaceuticals from the Pharmacy, factory-prepared packs and syringes often from general hospital stores. In addition to this, certain specially ordered instruments, apparatus or inserts may come directly from manufacturers to the department using them. There is danger in too haphazard a distribution network for sterile materials, because they may become damaged in storage or in transit or become contaminated from unsatisfactory surroundings or trolleys. As far as possible, all sterile materials should be stored together and distributed together by trained sterile supply assistants and under experienced supervisors. There will be exceptions to this policy, such as intravenous fluids, bottled sterile water and other pharmaceuticals which are the responsibility of the hospital pharmacist.

Transporting and distribution of sterile supplies within the hospital is carried out by HSDU staff using a specifically built trolley. If it is necessary to distribute basic dressings from a centralized production unit by way of the general stores, the materials should be enclosed in a dispenser-transport box impervious to bacterial contamination. A special area can be set aside in a general stores complex as a distribution centre. Distribution of sterile supplies to other hospitals will present a different problem. Providing the HSDU is of adequate size, a vehicle solely for this purpose is desirable and would almost certainly be completely occupied with this work. The vehicle need not necessarily be purpose-built or specially adapted. It must be accepted that normal inter-hospital transport will be used for conveying sterile supplies to small outlying units where weekly visits are made. However, where transport is used for many purposes, steps should be taken to prevent contamination of sterile supplies. Distribution of commercially produced sterile supplies from the HSDU sterile store should be made on a weekly basis, to allow the Manager to assess the quality and quantity of supplies required.

The 'shelf life' of packs (i.e. the time they remain sterile) should be indefinite, if they have been correctly sterilized and stored. However, it is advisable to use packs in the same order as they are prepared. Packs must be stored in an area free from moisture, dust and insects. Packs should not be handled with moist or even slightly damp hands, or placed on any damp surface. They must be examined for damage before use. Any packet that is even slightly damp must be discarded as 'non-sterile'.

Storage of sterile packs

'Open-type' dispensers should be discouraged as they are cumbersome and are exposed to contamination. Purpose-built shelving should be made available in operating suites and other areas for the accommodation of pre-set operation trays, gown packs and supplementary boxed items.

Return of equipment from wards and departments

Instruments which have been used for routine ward dressings — dissecting forceps, scissors, sinus forceps — should be discarded immediately after use into

59

a polypropylene container containing a suitable and appropriately diluted disinfectant-detergent solution (see Chapter 7). The container should have a screw lid. The instruments are left to soak overnight during which time deposits will be removed. An alternative method is collection of instruments in paper bags; but when this method is used it is more difficult to remove deposits.

Polypropylene hollow ware

Polypropylene hollow ware should be rinsed under running water and placed in a container for collection by HSDU staff. Polypropylene ware includes jugs, receivers, bladder wash-out sets and such items.

Special procedure sets

After use these should be rinsed under running water, returned to the tray or receptacle in which they were originally presented and placed in the container for collection. Dry disposable equipment and linen items should be discarded in the ward or theatre into suitable receptacles.

Pre-set trays

Instruments from operating rooms should, after use, be checked for numerical accuracy, returned neatly to the tray and collected. Bowl sets used for the operation should be rinsed and placed for collection. Cleaning in theatres or wards leads to loss of equipment and it is best to return the sets complete. All disposable equipment, linen or paper drapes should be discarded in the clinical area.

Responsibility, hygiene and training

The Manager of a sterile supply department is a technical manager within the administrative organization, but is medically responsible to the Consultant Microbiologist. He or she has the responsibility for assessing the efficiency of sterilization procedures, for organizing the supply and the distribution of all sterilized products.

The Microbiologist is responsible for assessing the safety of cleaning, disinfection and sterilization procedures in relation to staff and patients. He should visit occasionally, and at his discretion, the sterilizing and packing assembly areas, inspect the sterile store accommodation and assess the methods of distribution for risks of recontamination of sterilized materials and risks of infection from contaminated materials. He or another authorized competent person should also inspect records and charts of sterilizing machines and carry out bacteriological tests if indicated.

Transfer of infection in sterile supply service

The only area of a CSSD where infection is likely to be transmitted to staff is the reception and cleaning area for used instruments and equipment. A survey, however, has shown that, if simple routine precautions are observed, any infection hazard is minimal. To achieve this standard it is not generally necessary to autoclave instruments prior to handling by CSSD staff; if this is done, it becomes extremely difficult to remove blood, mucus etc., by normal cleaning methods. Staff working in this section should wear rubber gloves and plastic aprons when checking and sorting returned materials. Any septic lesions must be reported to the Manager. There must be adequate provision for hand washing. Ward and Theatre Sisters should inform the Manager of any special hazard, e.g. hepatitis, tuberculosis or salmonellosis, when equipment is returned, so that appropriate precautions (e.g. autoclaving or immersion in glutaraldehyde before washing) may be taken. Instruments with such contamination should be transported in sealed plastic bags labelled BIO-HAZARD. If an infection problem occurs, the Manager should consult a member of the Infection Control Team (see Chapters 13 and 18 for immunization procedures).

Personal hygiene and training of assistants working in CSSDs

Simple instructions on the care of the skin, especially of hands, should be given to all assistants. Since the work in the reception and cleaning areas involves the use of large amounts of water with added detergents, the use of skin barrier creams should be encouraged; creams should be available in suitably sized containers which can be replaced daily. Long flowing hair should be well retained. Long painted finger nails should be discouraged. If a finger is pricked or skin broken during the handling of potentially contaminated items, the member of staff should stop work immediately, encourage bleeding as much as possible, apply a sterilized, water-proof dressing and report to the CSSD Manager or Deputy. CSSD staff should be given some instruction in simple microbiology, care of instruments, packaging methods, and principles of sterilization and disinfection.

Training of medical and nursing staff in sterile supply activities

Nursing and medical staff should be trained in the correct procedures for opening sterile packs. The fewer the persons opening sterile packs, the smaller will be the risk of contamination; for this reason medical staff, when performing ward procedures such as lumbar puncture or intravenous cut down and chest catheter insertion, should arrange the contents of the sterile pack themselves, the nurse or assistant having previously opened the packet. Arranging the sterile equipment with Cheatle's forceps has become an obsolete technique, as is the 'laying-up' of trolleys for surgical ward procedures. Medical and nursing staff alike must receive training in the techniques of handling equipment from CSSDs. Adequate training must also be given to all personnel in operating theatres who are likely to be involved in the opening of sterile packs, whether processed in the CSSD or obtained commercially.

Future developments

Techniques and materials are constantly changing and sterile supply services are changing with them. To keep in touch with developments, the Manager of the unit should be a member of the Control of Infection Committee, Nursing Procedure Committee and Theatre Users' Committee. Although at present the supply of packs is based mainly on production by the Health Service, this could change if cheap and acceptable standard packs were produced commercially. This has already happened with syringes and needles.

References and Further Reading

Bowie, J. H., Gillingham, F. J., Campbell, I. D. and Gordon, A. R. (1963), Hospital sterile supplies: Edinburgh pre-set tray system, *Lancet*, ii, 1322.

Cunliffe Report (1977), Report of the Steering Committee on *Standardisation of Supplies from CSSDs*. See DHSS Health Circular HC(78)43.

Department of Health and Social Security (1980), *Hospital Technical Memorandum*, No. 10.

National Health Service (1977), *Standardisation of Supplies from Central Sterile Supply Departments*. Interim Report of the Steering Committee.

Nuffield Provincial Hospitals Trust (1963), *Central Sterile Supply: Principles and Practice*. Oxford University Press, London.

Weymes, C. (1965), A Central Sterile Supply Service for a group of hospitals. *Brit. Hosp. J. Soc. Serv. Rev.*, 75, 1493.

CHAPTER SIX

Disinfection (1) Types of Chemical Disinfectant and Formulation of Policy for Disinfection

A Public Health Laboratory Service Committee (1965) has advised that hospitals and possibly Regions should produce a rational policy for the use of disinfectants (including antiseptics). Most hospitals have done so, but it is still possible to find inappropriate disinfectants being used at inadequate concentrations. Expensive or ineffective disinfectants are still in use when cheaper or more effective agents are available, or when a disinfectant is not required at all. There remains a need for some degree of regional, if not national, standardization; a sound disinfectant policy should considerably increase the cost effectiveness of disinfection in hospitals.

Types of Chemical Disinfectants

Phenolics

Phenols and cresols are usually derived from the distillation of coal tar, but mixtures of synthetic phenols may be used. Chlorinated fractions and petroleum residues may also be added.

(1) Black and white fluids

These are crude coal tar derivatives. Black fluids (e.g. Jeyes fluid) are solubilized in soap and tend to be toxic and irritant to the skin. White fluids (e.g. Izal) are emulsified suspensions and tend to precipitate on surfaces, making subsequent cleaning more difficult. These disinfectants, especially white fluids, are sometimes used for environmental disinfection in hospitals, but have largely been replaced by clear soluble phenolics.

(2) Clear soluble phenolics (e.g. 'Stericol', 'Hycolin', 'Clearsol')

Like other phenolics, these compounds are active against a wide range of bacteria, including *Pseudomonas aeruginosa* and tubercle bacilli. They are fungicidal, kill some viruses, but show no useful activity against bacterial spores. They are relatively cheap and not readily inactivated by organic matter. Uses are mainly confined to environmental disinfection, since they are too corrosive or toxic to be applied to the skin. These and other

63

phenolics should not be used in food preparation areas or on equipment likely to contact mucous membranes. 'Sudol' is an effective and reliable compound often used in postmortem rooms, but is too corrosive for routine use.

(3) Chloroxylenols (e.g. 'Dettol', 'Ibcol')

These are non-irritant but are readily inactivated by organic matter and hard water (see Public Health Laboratory Service, 1965) and high concentrations are required (2.5%–5%). Addition of a chelating agent (EDTA) increases the activity of chloroxylenols against Gram-negative bacilli; however, these compounds are not recommended for routine hospital use.

Pine oil disinfectants

These compounds are non-toxic and non-irritant, but are relatively inactive against many organisms, in particular *Pseudomonas aeruginosa*. They should not be used as disinfectants in hospitals.

Halogens (compounds or solutions releasing chlorine, bromine, or iodine)

(1) Hypochlorites

These are cheap and effective disinfectants which act by release of available chlorine. Solutions are unstable at use-dilutions, are readily inactivated by organic matter (e.g. pus, dirt, blood etc.) and may damage certain materials, e.g. plastics, some metals and fabrics. Hypochlorites are not compatible with some detergents, and should not be mixed with acids, since the free chlorine produced may be harmful, particularly in a confined space. Hypochlorite solutions may be stabilized with alkalis or sodium chloride. Hypochlorite disinfectants are particularly useful for food preparation areas, but may also have other uses in the hospital environment. They are active against viruses, and are recommended for use where special hazards of viral hepatitis exist. Buffered solutions are active against bacterial spores (Death and Coates, 1979). Preparations include:

(a) Strong alkaline solutions (e.g. 'Chloros', 'Domestos', 'Sterite') containing approximately 10% available chlorine. The concentrated solutions are corrosive. Dilute solutions (e.g. 1:100) should be used with a compatible detergent and will only reliably disinfect clean surfaces.

(b) Hypochlorite solutions containing 1% available chlorine and stabilized with sodium chloride (e.g. 'Milton' or a preparation of comparable properties). These solutions are usually diluted 1:80 for the disinfection of infant feeding bottles. The low chlorine content is inactivated by very small amounts of organic matter and in-use solutions have a narrow margin of safety.

(c) Hypochlorite/hypobromite powders (e.g. 'Septonite', 'Diversol BX'). Solutions of the powders (0.5–1.0%) are used in the same way as other hypochlorite preparations, and are rather less corrosive. The powder may be used for cleaning baths and sinks where an abrasive preparation is not desirable.

(d) Hypochlorite tablets (e.g. 'Multichlor'). Tablets are stable and a convenient method of storing and dispensing hypochlorites, but the prepared solutions deteriorate quickly. The cost of preparing solutions with a low concentration (e.g. 200 ppm available chlorine) is comparable to that of liquid preparations, but the use of tablets is an expensive method for preparing high concentrations (e.g. 10 000 ppm available chlorine).

(e) Abrasive powders containing hypochlorites (e.g. hospital scouring powder, 'Vim', 'Ajax' etc.).

(f) Non-abrasive powders (e.g. 'Countdown') containing hypochlorites are now usually preferred to abrasive powders for cleaning and disinfecting hospital baths and sinks.

(2) Iodine and Iodophors

A 1% solution of iodine in 70% alcohol is an effective pre-operative skin antiseptic. Skin reactions may occur in some individuals: for this reason 0.5% alcoholic chlorhexidine is usually preferred.

Iodophors are complexes of iodine and 'solubilizers' which are claimed to possess the same activity as iodine, but are non-irritant and do not stain the skin. Iodophors are mainly used for hand disinfection, e.g. povidone-iodine ('Betadine', 'Disadine') detergent preparations or 'surgical scrubs', and are effective for this purpose. Alcoholic preparations are suitable for pre-operative preparation of the skin at the operation site. Some iodophors may also be used for disinfection of the environment, but they are expensive and cannot be recommended for general disinfection in hospital. Iodine is the only antiseptic which has been shown to have a useful sporicidal action on the skin; when applied as an iodophor it can be left on the skin long enough to remove most spores (see Chapter 7). Buffered hypochlorite may also prove to be effectively sporicidal on skin, but this still awaits assessment.

Quaternary ammonium compounds: e.g. benzalkonium chloride (e.g. 'Roccal', 'Zephiran', 'Marinol') and cetrimide ('Cetavlon')

These are relatively non-toxic antibacterial compounds with detergent properties; they are active against Gram-positive organisms but much less active against Gram-negative bacilli and are readily inactivated by soap, anionic detergents and organic matter. Quaternary ammonium compounds at higher dilutions inhibit the growth of organisms (i.e. they are 'bacteristatic') but do not necessarily kill them (i.e. they do not show a 'bactericidal' effect). For this reason their effectiveness has often been exaggerated. Their use in hospital is limited because of their narrow spectrum of activity, but they may be useful for cleansing dirty wounds (e.g. cetrimide). Apart from possible uses in food preparation areas, quaternary ammonium compounds should not be used for environmental disinfection. Contamination of a weak solution with Gram-negative bacilli is a possible hazard which can be prevented by avoidance of cork closures or of 'topping-up' stock bottles.

Chlorhexidine ('Hibitane')

This useful skin antiseptic is highly active against vegetative Gram-positive organisms, but less active against Gram-negative bacilli. It is relatively non-toxic but is inactivated by soaps. Its use in hospital should be restricted as much as possible to procedures involving contact with skin or mucous membranes; it is too expensive for environmental use. If it is used at all for disinfection of inanimate objects, the concentration should not be less than 0.2%.

'*Hibiscrub*' is a detergent solution containing chlorhexidine at 4%. It has been found highly effective in disinfection of the hands. 1% Chlorhexidine powder is sometimes used as a prophylactic application to the umbilicus of neonates.

'*Savlon*' is a mixture of chlorhexidine and cetrimide. The hospital concentrate contains 15% cetrimide and 1.5% chlorhexidine. Since chlorhexidine is the more active antibacterial component of the mixture, the chlorhexidine in 'Savlon' is likely to be too weak when use-dilutions are made on the ward (1:100 is commonly used for cleaning). 'Savlon' is expensive; if used, it should be reserved for clinical procedures and not used for environmental disinfection.

'Hibisol' is a 2.5% solution of chlorhexidine gluconate in 70% isopropyl alcohol, for disinfection of clean, intact skin.

Hexachlorophane

This compound is highly active against Gram-positive organisms but less active against Gram-negative. It is relatively insoluble in water, but can be incorporated in soap or detergent solutions without loss of activity. These solutions are prone to contamination with Gram-negative bacteria unless a preservative is included in the formulation. Potentially neurotoxic levels can be obtained if emulsions or other preparations of hexachlorophane are repeatedly and extensively applied to the body surface of babies (Kensit, 1975; Goutières and Aicardi, 1977). This product, though very effective, is now rarely used for skin disinfection in hospitals, and can be obtained for use only on medical advice. Toxic levels are not approached when a hexchlorophane dusting powder is used on the umbilical stump of neonates, and this method, which has been found highly effective in the control of staphylococcal infection, may still be considered to have a role in hospital practice.

Alcohols

70% Ethyl alcohol (ethanol) is an effective and rapidly acting disinfectant and antiseptic with the additional advantage that it leaves surfaces dry, but it has poor penetrative powers and should only be used on clean surfaces. The recommended concentration (70%) is optimal *in vitro* for killing organisms, and is more effective than absolute alcohol; on the skin, higher concentrations (95%) have been found as effective as 70% alcohol, presumably because the alcohol is diluted by surface moisture of the skin; the higher concentration has the advantage of allowing more rapid drying. Alcohol may be used for the rapid disinfection of smooth surfaces, e.g. trolley tops. It is commonly used for skin disinfection (e.g. without additives for treating skin prior to injection). Alcohol with the addition of 1% glycerine or other suitable emollients is an effective agent for the rapid disinfection of physically clean hands. The addition of other bactericides to alcohol does not appreciably increase its immediate effect as a skin antiseptic, but on repeated use it may lead to lower equilibrium levels of bacteria on the skin, and non-volatile antiseptics (e.g. chlorhexidine) have a residual antiseptic action on the skin. There is some doubt about the efficiency of alcohol in killing tubercle bacilli and certain viruses. 60% Isopropyl-alcohol, which is less volatile than ethanol, can be used as an alternative; it is slightly more effective than ethanol on the skin.

Aldehydes: formaldehyde and glutaraldehyde ('Cidex')

Though formaldehyde is required for the fumigation of rooms after smallpox, and may sterilize if used with sub-atmospheric steam, solutions of formaldehyde are too irritant for use as general disinfectants. Glutaraldehyde is preferred to formaldehyde; both will also kill vegetative organisms, including tubercle bacilli. Aldehydes are more active against spores than other commonly used chemical agents with the exception of ethylene oxide and buffered hypochlorites (Babb, Bradley and Ayliffe, 1980). Glutaraldehyde may be irritant and can cause sensitization. Alkaline solutions such as 'Cidex' require activation; once activated they remain stable for only one–two weeks. To ensure sporicidal activity, an exposure period of at least three hours is required. Acid solutions of glutaraldehyde may not require activation, but usually have a slower sporicidal effect; sporicidal activity can be improved by use at a temperature of 50-60° C; alkaline glutaraldehyde is inactivated at these temperatures.

Ampholytic compounds (e.g. 'Tego')

These compounds combine detergent and antibacterial properties. They are similar to the quaternary ammonium compounds and may be of value in the food industry, but are expensive; there are few indications for their use in hospitals.

Other antimicrobial compounds

Many other antimicrobial compounds have been used. Among these are the acridine and triphenyl methane (crystal violet and brilliant green) dyes, which were at one time widely used as antiseptics for skin and for wounds.

'Irgasan DP300' has recently been introduced as a substitute for hexachlorophane in antiseptic soaps, and a 2% liquid soap containing the compound is shown to have considerable effect on repeated use. Silver nitrate and other silver compounds (e.g. silver sulphadiazine) have a valuable place as topical antiseptics in prophylaxis against infection of burns. 8-Hydroxy quinoline has been found effective as a fungicide. Mercurial compounds have poor bactericidal powers, but they are strongly bacteristatic; phenyl mercuric nitrate has been used as an effective preservative for ophthalmic solutions. Hydrogen peroxide has a useful role in the disinfection of certain types of respiratory ventilator. Peracetic acid, a highly unstable compound, has been used as a disinfectant for some types of equipment (e.g. isolators). Further details on some of these agents are given in sections devoted to the applications mentioned.

The formulation of a policy for environmental disinfection

The general principles for formulation of a policy are summarized below (see Kelsey and Maurer, 1972). The Hospital Infection Control Committee should decide on a type of disinfectant policy; this requires consultation between the Microbiologist, Infection Control Officer and/or Nurse, Pharmacist, Supplies Officer and representatives of medical, nursing and domestic staff. Demands for disinfectants come from many departments of the hospital and there are many sources of supply. All requests for disinfectant should be approved by the hospital pharmacist who can check if they are in agreement with the hospital policy.

Principles

(a) List all the purposes for which disinfectants are used, then check requisitions and orders to ensure list is complete.

(b) Eliminate the use of chemical disinfectants when heat can be reasonably used as an alternative, when sterilization is required, where thorough cleaning alone is adequate, or where disposable equipment can be economically used. There should be few remaining uses for disinfectant fluids.

(c) Select the smallest possible number of disinfectants for the remaining uses.

(d) Arrange for the distribution of disinfectants chosen at the correct use-dilution or supply equipment for measuring disinfectants at the site of use.

(e) All potential users of disinfectant should receive adequate instruction in their use. Instruction should include:

    (i) The correct disinfectant and concentration to be used for each task.

    (ii) The shelf-life of the disinfectant at the concentration supplied, the type of container to be used and the frequency with which the solution should be changed in use.

    (iii) Substances or materials which will react with or neutralize the disinfectant.

    (iv) Personal safety measures, e.g. should rubber gloves be worn, how can the product be safely opened and mixed, what action is required if the product comes in contact with the skin or eye?

(f) The policy should be monitored to ensure that it is and continues to be effective. In-use tests and chemical estimations of concentration may be required.

Selection of disinfectants

(1) Antimicrobial properties

Where compatible with other requirements, disinfectants used should be bactericidal rather than bacteristatic, active against a whole spectrum of microbes and not readily inactivated. The manufacturer can supply information on activity, but independent tests are also required. The improved Capacity Test (Kelsey and Maurer, 1974) should be used to calculate the use dilutions. Rideal–Walker or Chick–Martin tests are not applicable to hospital disinfection. The capacity test should be carried out only by a laboratory experienced in its use.

(2) Other properties

The properties of the disinfectants chosen should be considered in terms of acceptability as well as antibacterial activity. Toxicity and corrosiveness should be assessed by the pharmacist with the aid of relevant information obtained from manufacturers. Acceptability and cleaning properties should be assessed by the domestic superintendent. Cost is clearly important and a regional contract for one or two generally acceptable disinfectants should considerably reduce costs. A trial period of possibly three months might be introduced and an assessment of all relevant factors should be made before the policy is permanently introduced.

Recommended disinfectants and use-dilutions (disinfectant policy)

A phenolic and a hypochlorite disinfectant should be sufficient for most environmental hospital requirements.

A clear soluble phenolic disinfectant (e.g. 'Stericol', 'Hycolin', 'Clearsol') should be chosen as the disinfectant for routine use (see Appendix 7.2). There is little to choose between these compounds in terms of effectiveness at the recommended use-dilutions. 'Sudol' and 'Izal' are also effective and may be chosen, but have the disadvantages already mentioned. For most purposes the concentration required for light contamination will be adequate; it provides a reasonable margin of safety and should be used unless otherwise indicated. The strong concentrations should be used for heavily contaminated areas or if contamination with tubercle bacilli is likely (disinfection by heat or use of disposables is particularly important for dealing with contamination by tubercle bacilli). Phenolics are not usually suitable for use against viruses.

Hypochlorites have the disadvantages and advantages already mentioned. They may be incorporated in a powder (abrasive or non-abrasive) for cleaning baths, toilets, wash-basins. Hypochlorite solutions (0.1% available chlorine) may be used for disinfecting clean surfaces and, when necessary, for food preparation areas. Hypochlorites (0.1 to 0.5% available chlorine) should be used if disinfection of virus-contaminated material is required. (Disinfection by heat or use of disposables are particularly important if the hepatitis virus is involved; see Chapters 18 and 19).

A list of recommended disinfectants is shown in Appendix 7.2 (at the end of

Chapter 7); one of the phenolics and one hypochlorite disinfectant should be chosen for all environmental disinfection in the hospital. A compatible detergent should be added to the disinfectant unless one is already present in the formulation. Narrow spectrum or expensive disinfectants mainly used for clinical purposes are not included in the list for general environmental use, but may sometimes be required for special equipment. Glutaraldehyde should be available for disinfection of metal objects heavily contaminated with hepatitis B virus.

Dilution and distribution of disinfectants

Inadequate concentration is the commonest cause of failure of a disinfectant to kill organisms, and survival of contaminants in the disinfectant is unlikely if it is at the recommended use-dilution. It is, therefore, preferable for the Pharmacist to supply departments with containers of disinfectant already prepared at the correct use-dilution. Containers should have the date of issue and the date after which the disinfectant should not be used (e.g. one week after issue); they should be clearly labelled 'do not dilute', 'use undiluted' or labelled with a similar instruction. Containers should be thoroughly washed and preferably disinfected by heat before refilling. If heating is not possible, thorough drying after washing should be adequate as this will kill most of the bacteria likely to be present. Corks should not be used; containers should have glass or plastic closures which can be easily cleaned.

The main disadvantage of this method of dispensing is the transport of large quantities of fluid (mainly water), particularly if large amounts of disinfectants are used. The alternative method is to supply undiluted disinfectant to the department and dilutions are prepared when required. A suitable and relatively fool-proof measuring system is required both for disinfectant and water. A measuring device attached to the container is commonly used, but unless staff are well trained, dilutions will be inaccurate. A measured amount of undiluted disinfectant in a bottle or sachet is an alternative. In both of these methods, the water must also be measured. The strong disinfectant solution requires careful handling to avoid damage to the skin or the eyes of the operator.

Training and staff instruction

Whichever system of supplying disinfectants is used, all personnel handling or using them should be adequately trained and supervised (see principle (e) above).

In-use tests

Since disinfectants are used under a variety of conditions, it is essential to test their effectiveness under actual conditions of use. Contamination of a disinfectant solution is a particular hazard, and 'in-use' tests (Kelsey and Maurer, 1972) should be carried out when a new disinfectant or different concentration of an existing disinfectant is introduced. Repeat tests should be carried out occasionally to ensure that no changes in the recommended policy have occurred or that resistant bacterial strains are not selected. If the cleanliness of the equipment

70

immersed in the disinfectant is uncertain (e.g. mops and brushes), the surface should also be examined by a microbiological surface sampling technique (e.g. cotton-wool swabs).

Review of policy

This should be considered annually. Defects of the current system should be noted and changes introduced where necessary.

References and Further Reading

Babb, J. R., Bradley, C. R. and Ayliffe, G. A. J. (1980), Sporicidal activity of glutaraldehyde and hypochlorite, and other factors influencing their selection for the treatment of medical equipment. *J. hosp. Infect.*, 1, 63.

Death, J. E. and Coates, D. (1979), Effect of pH on sporicidal and microbiocidal activity of buffered mixtures of alcohol and sodium hypochlorite. *J. clin. Path.*, 32, 148.

Goutières, F. and Aicardi, J. (1977), Accidental percutaneous hexachlorophane intoxication in children. *Brit. med. J.*, iii, 663.

Kelsey, J. C. and Maurer, I. M. (1972), *The Use of Chemical Disinfectants in Hospitals*. PHLS Monograph Series, No. 2.

Kelsey, J. C. and Maurer, I. M. (1974), An improved Kelsey–Sykes test for disinfectants. *Pharm. J.*, 213, 528.

Kensit, J. G. (1975), Hexachlorophane toxicity and effectiveness in prevention of sepsis in neonatal units. *J. antimicrob. Chemother.*, 1, 263.

Public Health Laboratory Service (PHLS) (1965), Report of Committee on Testing and Evaluation of Disinfectants. *Br. med. J.*, i, 408.

Russell, A. D., Hugo, W. B. and Ayliffe, G. A. J. (eds) (1980), *Principles and Practice of Disinfection, Preservation and Sterilization*. Blackwell Scientific Publications, Oxford (in press).

CHAPTER SEVEN

Disinfection (2) Cleaning and Disinfection Procedures

Cleaning and disinfection of skin and mucous membranes

Principles

The bacteria present on healthy skin have been classified as follows:

(a) resident organisms that colonize the skin and are mostly harmless, though in some people they include pathogenic staphylococci (*Staphylococcus aureus*);

(b) transient organisms — i.e. microbes that happen to be deposited on the skin but do not multiply there.

Most of the transient bacteria (e.g. bacterial cultures spread on the skin for tests of disinfection) can be removed by a thorough wash with soap and water, and against these contaminants a thorough wash with soap and water may be almost as effective as disinfection. The resident bacteria, on the other hand, are mostly left on the skin after washing with soap and water, but can be reduced to very small numbers by disinfection. Some naturally acquired bacteria that do not multiply on the skin (e.g. gas gangrene bacilli present through faecal contamination of the buttocks) may resemble the resident flora in their persistence after washing with soap and water. Transient bacteria rubbed on to the skin are more persistent on washing, though not on disinfection, than those laid on the skin without friction.

Large numbers of bacteria are found as residents of the mucous membrane in the mouth, nose and vagina, but different organisms predominate in different sites; disinfection by antiseptics which are not irritant or damaging to the tissues has a limited though potentially useful effect. The urethra normally has a few commensal bacteria, but is liable to become contaminated on passage of catheters or other instruments; disinfection of the urethra before instrumentation is one of the important components of prophylaxis against infection of the urinary tract. The conjunctiva also has few bacteria, but these may include *Staph. aureus* (see Chapters 15 and 16).

Cleansing and disinfection of hands

Washing with soap (or another detergent) and running water helps to remove the dead skin scales and the bacteria present on them. For the removal and killing of resident bacteria, washing with an antiseptic detergent preparation is effective — e.g. 4% chlorhexidine detergent solution ('Hibiscrub'), a povidone-iodine (iodophor) detergent preparation (e.g. 'Betadine' surgical scrub), a 3% hexachlorophane liquid soap (e.g. 'Ster-Zac') or detergent cream (e.g. 'Phisohex') or a 2% 'Irgasan DP300' detergent preparation (e.g. 'Zalclense'). The immediate effects of a single disinfection with hexachlorophane or Irgasan DP300 preparation are poor. To obtain the best results (i.e. a cumulative reduction to a low equilibrium level from successive disinfections) the antiseptic detergent preparation should be used for all handwashing during work hours (or at least three handwashes a day); the manufacturer's instructions should be followed. Before the first operation of the list it is advisable, though not essential, to use a brush, so that loosely adherent epithelial squames can be more effectively removed; the under surface of the nail edge should also be cleansed with a scraper.

An alternative and even more effective method of disinfecting the hands for removal of resident and transient organisms is to rub the whole surface of hands and forearms vigorously with two successive 5 ml amounts of 0.5% chlorhexidine and 1% glycerol in ethanol within the range 70–95%; water should not be poured on to the hands during the procedure and the alcohol should be allowed to dry on the skin while rubbing. Aqueous 0.5% chlorhexidine rubbed on for two minutes followed by rinsing and drying with a towel is also effective, though less so than the alcoholic solution; (a cursory swabbing of the hands with gauze soaked in alcohol is much less effective). These methods could be used before the second and later operations in a list; a detergent wash is, however, probably advisable before the first operation, and necessary when the hands become contaminated with blood, plaster or adherent materials.

For ward staff in 'high infection risk' areas the main hazard is from transient organisms, which may be picked up while the nurse is attending to an infected patient and promptly handed on to an uninfected patient. Alcohol with or without chlorhexidine rubbed on to the hands until they are dry, as described above, has been found more effective in removing these transient organisms than washing with an antiseptic detergent preparation and water; the latter may be little more effective, if at all, against superficial transients than soap and water.

For removal of some viruses (e.g. hepatitis B virus in blood) a solution of hypochlorite may be more effective than the routine skin antiseptics, should it be required.

For wards in which there is no special risk of hospital infection, ordinary bar soap is probably adequate, but repeated use of a 2% hexachlorophane bar soap (if available), or a 0.75% 'Irgasan' bar soap (e.g. 'Derl') can be expected to reduce the occasional hazard arising through heavy hand carriage of *Staph. aureus*.

Cleansing and disinfection of operation sites

A rapid reduction of skin flora is required in pre-operative preparation of operation sites. For this purpose, a quick-acting antiseptic is essential. In comparative studies on several recommended alternatives the one found most effective has been 0.5% chlorhexidine in 70% ethyl alcohol; (1% iodine in alcohol was found to be as effective, but it causes skin reactions in some people). Hexachlorophane or Irgasan which act slowly, are quite unsuitable for this purpose. The antiseptic should for most operations be applied on a sterile gauze swab, with friction, over and well beyond the operation site for three or four minutes; application with a gloved hand is more effective than gauze; the skin should have been washed previously with soap and water and dried with a sterile towel. If a gloved hand is used as the applicator of antiseptic, a second glove should be worn by the surgeon over his operating glove and removed when the preparation of the operation site is completed (Lowbury and Lilly, 1975).

To obtain a higher degree of disinfection (e.g. in patients with exceptional susceptibility to infection) the operation site should be cleansed and disinfected in the ward on the day before the operation, as well as in the operating room; two or three treatments may be given for optimum effect, and the site should be covered, after each such preparation, with a sterile towel. For these treatments before the day of operation, 'Hibiscrub' or a hexachlorophane liquid soap, both of which have residual activity after rinsing and drying the skin, are effective, but the preparation in the operating room must be with a quick-acting alcoholic antiseptic (e.g. 0.5% chlorhexidine in 70% ethyl alcohol). Alcoholic chlorhexidine, rubbed on until the skin is dry (see above), can reduce the numbers of resident bacteria on a single application to levels approaching the low equilibrium obtainable on repeated application.

Before operations on hands with ingrained dirt (e.g. in gardeners), or operations on the leg in patients with poor arterial supply (e.g. amputations for diabetic gangrene of the foot), a compress soaked in povidone-iodine (e.g. 'Betadine' or 'Disadine') solutions applied to the operation site for 30 min will greatly reduce the numbers of spores of gas gangrene bacilli that present a special hazard in such patients; ordinary methods of disinfection are inactive against bacterial spores, but washing with detergents, grease-solvent jellies (e.g. 'Swarfega', 'Dirty Paws') when necessary and ethyl alcohol helps to remove physically the dirt and dead skin scales on which these organisms are carried.

Cleansing and disinfection of mucous membranes

Repeated application (three or four times a day) of a cream containing neomycin (0.5%) and chlorhexidine (0.1%) ('Naseptin') to the inside of the nostrils has been shown to eliminate pathogenic staphylococci from a fairly large proportion of persistent carriers of these bacteria. *Streptococcus pyogenes* can usually be cleared from the throat by a course of penicillin (injected or given by mouth, but not by local application). Alcohol has been found to have little disinfectant activity on the mucous membrane of the mouth because of the dilution by saliva; aqueous solutions of iodine or of an iodophor, or possibly chlorhexidine preparations, are effective and these should probably be used, rather than alcoholic iodine solutions, for pre-operative disinfection of mucous membranes. Treatment of the vaginal mucosa with obstetric creams containing chlorhexidine or chloroxylenol is considered to have little disinfectant action. Povidone-iodine in a vaginal douche (25 ml of the 10% solution in 500 ml sterile water) has been recommended, and its effect may be enhanced by instillation of povidone-iodine vaginal gel (5 g) for more prolonged action.

74

Cleaning and disinfection of the ward environment

Ward surfaces that have been well cleaned and allowed to dry do not require disinfection except in special circumstances, in particular when contaminated with known pathogens (e.g. by spillage of pus or faeces). A clean hospital environment is necessary to provide a background for the required standards of hygiene and asepsis and to maintain patients' confidence. Cleaning materials such as mops and the water used for cleaning can be a source of contamination and should be removed from the patients' environment as soon as possible when not in use. The equipment should be cleaned and dried after each use and may require periodic disinfection, preferably by heat. Single-use disposable wipes should be used for surface cleaning in an isolation room, and cleaning equipment must not be transferred to another room unless it has been thoroughly cleaned. Chemical disinfectants should only be used as part of an approved policy, and if used they should be accurately diluted to the correct strength and promptly disposed of after use.

Duties and responsibilities of domestic staff

The Domestic Manager is responsible for all domestic staff and should ensure that they are adequately trained and supervised. Routine cleaning of the environment, including floors, toilets, baths, wash basins, beds, locker tops and other furniture, should be the responsibility of the domestic service in all wards and departments. Domestic staff specially trained and aware of possible infection hazards should be available to clean and, if necessary, disinfect the rooms occupied by infected patients. The cleaning procedures in use should be agreed with the infection control staff, and should include a list of the contents of the room to be cleaned or disinfected, methods for disposal of waste material, and methods of disinfection of cleaning equipment. Nursing and other departmental staff should, wherever possible, be relieved of cleaning tasks. Surfaces or equipment contaminated with potentially infectious material require immediate attention. Nurses should continue to clean or disinfect these items when trained domestic staff are not available. If there is an unusual infection risk associated with the presence of a particular patient, e.g. in cleaning blood spillage from a hepatitis patient, the ward sister should ensure that the domestic staff are aware of that risk. It may be considered that the task could be performed more safely by a trained nurse.

Cleaning should be carried out in a planned manner and cleaning schedules should be drawn up for each area to include all equipment, fixtures and fittings. New items should be added to schedules as commissioned. Schedules should be sufficiently detailed to specify method, frequency, timing where relevant, the equipment to be used, where equipment is to be stored and how it is to be cleaned.

The responsibility for carrying out each task and the supervisory responsibility should be indicated. This should include the maintenance of paper towel cabinets and soap or dispensers and replacement of cleaning materials and linen.

The schedules should be discussed and agreed with representatives of all

75

grades of staff concerned, e.g. medical, nursing, domestic and infection control. All staff in the department should be aware of the procedures in operation.

Floors

Good cleaning techniques are usually adequate and routine use of disinfectants is not required. Possible exceptions include ultra-clean units and hospitals for mental or subnormal patients where soilage is frequent; disinfectants should be used when contamination with infected material has occurred, e.g. in isolation rooms in infectious disease units. Cleaning a surface with soap or detergent and water alone removes approximately 80% of organisms, disinfectants remove or kill 90-99% of organisms (Ayliffe, Collins and Lowbury, 1966). Recontamination of the floor of a busy ward from the air and from trolleys and shoes is rapid, irrespective of whether a disinfectant is used or not. In general wards, the bacteriological advantages of using a disinfectant rather than detergent and water, or a wet rather than a recommended method of dry cleaning, are marginal. (For carpets, see p. 119).

(1) Dry cleaning

Brooms redisperse dust and bacteria from the floor into the air and should not be used in patient areas. Floors should be cleaned daily with a vacuum cleaner fitted with an efficient filter. The exhaust should be directed away from the floor. Vacuum cleaners should have an inner paper bag which is discarded daily and staff should be trained to remove it safely without dispersing clouds of dust into the air. Filters should be inspected at intervals and changed when visibly dirty, or after three months' use.

An oiled mop or a mop made of a dust-attracting material (e.g. nylon) may be used in addition to a vacuum cleaner, but is a less efficient alternative. Non-impregnated dry mops (apart from dust-attracting types) should not be used for sweeping. Oiled or dust-attracting mops, unless disposable, should be cleaned and processed when obviously dirty and in any case should not be used for more than two days. A suitable procedure would be to wash nylon mop-heads in the hospital laundry and issue clean mops to the wards each day.

(2) Wet cleaning

Ward floors should be wet-cleaned when necessary, using detergent and water with a mop or suitable scrubbing machine. Annexes such as sluice rooms, toilets and bathrooms, require wet cleaning at least once daily. Water used for wet mopping should be changed frequently to prevent a build-up of bacteria in the bucket. A two-compartment bucket may be used with advantage, the clean water drawn from one side and the mop wrung out in the other, or two buckets mounted on a wheeled stand may be used in the same manner. Disinfectants are not necessary unless contamination with material from a known source of infection has occurred.

Gram-negative bacilli will grow rapidly overnight if kept in a moist condition (e.g. in mops), but die if allowed to dry. Mops cannot be adequately

76

dried in a ward, so disinfection of the mop is necessary in areas where high-risk patients are treated and in operating theatres. Sterilization or disinfection in a central area by heat, either by autoclaving or by high temperature washing, or the use of a disposable mop head would be desirable in all areas. If possible, the mop should be thoroughly washed in clean water and allowed to dry with the mop-head upwards and supported in a stand. If it is necessary to disinfect mops chemically, because heat disinfection is not available, the mop should be rinsed and then soaked in a 1% solution of hypochlorite bleach (0.1% available chlorine) for 30 min, rinsed again and stored to dry. A clear soluble phenolic may be used as an alternative to bleach. Since the materials used in the manufacture of some mops may inactivate the disinfectant, the bacteriological efficiency of the method should be checked. After use, the mops and buckets should be cleaned, the bucket dried and stored inverted.

The brushes and pads of scrubbing machines should be detachable, and should be removed and thoroughly washed and dried after each use. Brushes and pads used in operating theatres, special care and other high risk areas, should not be used elsewhere. The pads and brushes should be autoclaved at least weekly. If brushes or pads are transferred into or out of these areas, they should be autoclaved before use. If operating theatres, intensive care units or kitchens use scrubbing machines, each department should have its own machine, and models fitted with a tank should preferably not be used. Where scrubbing machines fitted with a tank are used, the tank should be emptied and the machine stored dry between uses. If it is not possible to drain the tank completely or to remove the tank and autoclave it, the machine is unsuitable for use in patient areas. Machines that cause excessive splashing from the brushes are unsuitable; splash guards should not be removed.

Walls and ceilings

Only very small numbers of bacteria can be isolated from clean, smooth, dry, intact wall surfaces. These surfaces are unlikely to be a significant infection hazard. Ceilings show an even smaller number of bacteria. The cleaning of walls and ceiling should be carried out sufficiently often to prevent the accumulation of visible dirt, but intervals between cleaning should not usually exceed twelve months in patient treatment areas. Disinfection is not required unless known contamination has occurred. Splashes of blood, urine or known contaminated material should be cleaned promptly. When cleaning walls, the surface should be left as dry as possible. Plaster exposed through damage to the paint of the wall surface cannot be effectively cleaned or disinfected, and may become heavily colonized with bacteria if it becomes moist (e.g. through condensation). Damaged wall surfaces should be promptly repaired with a fresh coat of paint or other wall finish.

Surfaces

Locker tops should be washed daily with detergent and water. Furniture should also be washed with detergent and water or damp-dusted with clean materials. Shelves and ledges should be damp-dusted weekly or more often if dust accumulates. Disinfection is not required, unless the surface is contaminated with infected material.

Baths, sinks and wash basins

Baths and wash basins should be cleaned at least daily by the domestic staff and after each use by the user. When a bath has been used by an infected patient, ward staff should ensure that it has been properly cleaned before it is re-used.

Detergent is adequate for routine cleaning. A mild scouring cream may occasionally be required to remove scum, but should not be used on fibreglass baths unless approved by the manufacturer. It may be necessary to disinfect baths after use by infected patients, or before use by patients with open wounds. A non-abrasive hypochlorite powder, e.g. 'Countdown', can be used for this purpose. Abrasive powders, e.g. 'Glitto', 'Vim', 'Ajax' etc., are effective, but they damage porcelain surfaces, and must never be used on fibreglass. Alternatively 'Domestos' or 'Chloros' 0.5% may be used with a detergent, but only if the detergent is known to be compatible. Sink outlets should be cleaned regularly, but it is unnecessary to attempt to disinfect sink traps or outlets.

Toilets and drains

Toilet seats should be cleaned at least once daily, and when visibly soiled. A detergent solution should be used for routine cleaning. Disinfection with a clear soluble phenolic may be required if the seat is obviously contaminated, or after use by patients with enteric or other relevant infections; if a phenolic is used, the seat should be rinsed with water and dried before use. Pouring disinfectant into lavatory pans or drains is unlikely to reduce infection risks.

Crockery and cutlery

Centralized arrangements for machine washing and drying of all crockery and cutlery is preferred to washing on individual wards. A washing machine with a final rinse temperature of 82° C in ward kitchens is a satisfactory alternative (see section on kitchen hygiene in Chapter 11) and is necessary in isolation wards.

Cleaning materials

Single-use wipes should, wherever possible, be used for cleaning surfaces (e.g. baths, sinks, bowls, mattresses, beds, furniture etc.). The use of disposable wipes for mopping up spillage from a known source of infection and for cleaning cubicles occupied by infected patients is of particular importance. If disposables are not available in other areas because of cost, the following alternative can be used:

(a) A nylon brush (e.g. 'Addis'), which can be quickly dried, may be used for cleaning baths. Cotton mops or bristle brushes become heavily contaminated and should not be used, even if stored in disinfectant.
(b) If non-disposable cloths are used for cleaning, these should be washed after use, preferably in washing machine heated to 75° C, and dried. Separate cloths should be used in the kitchen, ward area and the other ward annexes. A colour code might be used to distinguish the areas.
(c) Toilet brushes should be rinsed well in the flushing water of the lavatory pan; after shaking off excess water, they should be stored dry. Autoclaving weekly is worthwhile, if possible.

Sponges are difficult to disinfect and should not be used.

Central processing of cleaning equipment

A central area for the daily processing of mops and cleaning cloths (if used) is recommended. Mop-heads (cotton and nylon dry mops) may be enclosed in a cotton-bag and washed in a washing machine at a temperature of over 75° C for 10 min. Cloths may be similarly treated.

An autoclave would also be useful for daily treatment of brushes of floor-cleaning machines. Weekly treatment of toilet brushes and other equipment, e.g. buckets from special areas, is recommended. Heat-resistant equipment should be used if possible, and manufacturers should be encouraged to produce such equipment, e.g. a fluid tank and drain which are easily removable from a floor-washing machine.

Disinfection of rooms with formaldehyde gas

Formaldehyde disinfection is required for rooms that have been occupied by patients with smallpox, and may be required for Lassa fever and other dangerous exotic diseases. This method is not required or recommended for terminal disinfection of rooms occupied by patients with the normal range of infectious diseases or hospital-acquired infections.

The windows should be sealed and formaldehyde generated by addition of 150 g of potassium permanganate to 280 ml of formalin for every 1000 ft^3 (28.3 m^3) of the room volume. The ratio of formalin to potassium permanganate should be strictly adhered to. This reaction may produce a considerable amount of heat: a heat-resistant container must be used and the container should stand on a heat-resistant surface. Temperature and humidity should be 18° C and 60% respectively. To ensure adequate humidity it may be necessary to nebulize water into the air. After starting the generation of formaldehyde vapour, the door should be sealed and the room left unopened for 48 h.

Disinfection of non-medical equipment

Handwashing and shaving equipment

(1) Plastic wash bowls

The bowls should be thoroughly washed after use with a detergent and hot water, and dried. It is particularly important to remove any traces of fluid remaining in the bowl after cleaning, and the bowls should, if possible, be stored separately and inverted. It is desirable that each patient should have his own washing bowl and this should be terminally disinfected with a clear soluble phenolic before it is issued to the next patient. A convenient hanging basket for storage of washing bowls under the bed would be suitable.

(2) Nail-brushes

Since nail-brushes are frequently contaminated with Gram-negative bacilli even when stored in a disinfectant solution, their use in wards should be avoided except for special procedures. Nylon brushes kept in a dry state are less often contaminated than bristle-brushes. For all clinical procedures sterilized nail-brushes should be supplied by the CSSD singly wrapped.

(3) Soap dishes and dispensers

Soap dishes are rarely necessary, but if used should be washed and dried daily. The nozzle of liquid soap dispensers should be cleaned daily to remove residues, and the outside should be cleaned and dried. Topping-up should be avoided and the inside of containers should be cleaned and dried before re-filling. The channel and reservoir between the refill and nozzle require periodic cleaning in cartridge-type dispensers, and the surfaces in contact with the liquid soap also require periodic cleaning in pump-type dispensers. Liquid soaps used in hospitals should contain a preservative (e.g. 0.3% chlorocresol) to prevent the growth of bacteria.

(4) Razors

For pre-operative preparation, a disposable or autoclavable razor is preferred. Communal razors used by the hospital barber should be disinfected after each shave with 70% alcohol or a clear soluble phenolic for 5 min. If a phenolic disinfectant is used the razor should be well rinsed. Electric razor heads should be immersed in 70% alcohol for 5 min.

(5) Shaving brushes

Contaminated brushes used for pre-operative shaves have caused serious postoperative infections, and for that reason a shaving brush is best avoided. If the use of a brush is unavoidable, a separate prepacked sterile shaving brush should be used for each shave. Sterile gauze and a brushless shaving cream, or an antiseptic shaving foam is preferred. A brushless shaving cream or shaving foam should also be used by barbers for shaving patients, but if a brush is used it should be immersed in 70% alcohol for 5 min after each shave.

Beds, bedding, curtains and toys (see also Chapter 11)

(1) Bed frames

Beds should be washed with detergent solutions after discharge of patients. Wash with a solution of clear soluble phenolic if disinfection is required (after occupation of bed by infected patient).

(2) Mattresses and pillows

Since mattresses and pillows cannot be readily disinfected if they become contaminated, they should be enclosed completely in waterproof covers when in use. The pillow case should be placed over the waterproof cover with the open end at the opposite end to the opening of the waterproof cover. Cleaning the outside of the cover with detergent solution should provide adequate decontamination in most circumstances. Excessive wetting should be avoided; disposable wipes should be used and the cover should be allowed to dry thoroughly before re-use. The repeated use of phenolic disinfectants or some other agents such as silver nitrate may cause damage to plastic or coated nylon mattress covers or to rubber mattresses or rings. Chemical disinfection of these items should be avoided unless strictly necessary. When used the disinfectant should be rinsed off afterwards and the surfaces wiped dry. If the mattress or pillow becomes contaminated it may be possible to disinfect with low temperature steam or by steam under pressure if facilities are available, though not all types of mattress or pillow will withstand this treatment.

(3) Bedding

Bacteria accumulate rapidly in bedding; clean bedding may be heavily contaminated by *Staph. aureus* from a carrier or infected patient within several hours. Frequent changing is of limited value in controlling the spread of infection. Cleaning and disinfection of linen and of cotton blankets by laundry is described in Chapter 11 (see p. 172).

(a) **Blankets.** Cotton blankets should be used and changed on the discharge of a patient, after two weeks, or when contaminated with infected material.

(b) **Sheets** should be changed every two days (or more frequently if contaminated) and on discharge of the patient.

(c) **Bed-covers** should be changed weekly (or more often if visibly contaminated) and on discharge of the patient.

(4) Curtains

Contamination reaches a maximum in one or two days depending on the level of air contamination in the ward. Since frequent changing is impractical, curtains should be changed and washed when dirty, for aesthetic reasons, and at least every three to six months. When barrier-nursing in the ward is advised for a patient with severe staphylococcal infection, the curtains around the bed should be changed after the discharge of the patient.

81

Levels of contamination are not related to the type of material (e.g. Terylene, fibreglass, cotton) of which the curtain is made.

(5) Rubber sheets

These should now be replaced with plastic, which can be disinfected and re-used.

(6) Bed-cradles

These should be maintained in good condition. Disinfection is necessary only after use by an infected patient; then the cradle may be wiped over with a clear, soluble phenolic. It should be washed when dirty and stored in a clean area of the hospital.

(7) Toys

Disinfection is rarely necessary. If contaminated, solid toys may be wiped over with a clear, soluble phenolic which is then removed with water. Soft toys may be disinfected with formaldehyde or low temperature steam, but if grossly contaminated should preferably be destroyed.

Disinfection of surgical and medical equipment

Ampoules (see also Chapter 16 p. 277)

The neck should be cleaned with sterile cotton wool and 70% alcohol. Ampoules handled by scrubbed-up staff must be sterile; heat-stable solutions can be autoclaved in ampoules. The pharmacist's advice should be sought. Ampoules must not be stored in disinfectant solution because of the risk of possible seepage of the solution through invisible cracks into the ampoule.

Dressing-trolley tops

Clean with a paper wipe and 70% ethyl alcohol or a clear soluble phenolic and dry.

Instruments, bowls etc. for clinical procedures

These should be supplied in sterile packs by the CSSD (see Chapter 5 p. 53). In some circumstances, disinfection or sterilization on the ward may still be necessary. Autoclaves should be used rather than boiling 'sterilizers'. However, existing boiling 'sterilizers' should not be removed from a ward or department until the CSSD can supply all requirements, since boiling is usually preferable to chemical disinfection. In an emergency, clean instruments may be disinfected (but not sterilized) by placing in a clear soluble phenolic or 70% alcohol for 10 min. If a phenolic disinfectant is used, the instrument should be well rinsed after disinfection. Some instruments, e.g. specula, may be required in larger numbers than can be supplied by the CSSD; the use of a small autoclave is preferred to a boiler in the ward for these treatments.

Cheatles forceps are now infrequently used for aseptic techniques and their use is not recommended. If used, forceps and container should be autoclaved or boiled daily; forceps should stand in a clear soluble phenolic disinfectant which is replaced daily.

Soiled instruments should be transferred to a bucket containing a clear soluble phenolic and compatible detergent. Alternatively, instruments may be transferred to a paper or plastic bag, and the bag and instruments placed in a container without disinfectant for transfer to the CSSD.

Oral thermometers

It is preferable to store thermometers in a dry state; contamination with Gram-negative bacilli is frequent when thermometers are stored in individual containers of disinfectant. Contamination of individual thermometers is often due to irregular changing of disinfectant or to the use of an inappropriate solution, e.g. glycerine and thymol. Two methods for treating thermometers are described.

(1) Terminal disinfection

All thermometers are collected after the temperature round, wiped with a paper tissue and immersed together in a single container of freshly prepared disinfectant solution, e.g. a clear soluble phenolic or 70% ethanol, for a minimum of 10 min. The thermometers should then be removed from the solution, rinsed if a phenolic is used, dried and stored dry.

(2) Stored in individual dry container for each patient

Wipe the thermometer with 70% alcohol after each use and return to dry individual holder. The use of cotton wool or other absorbent padding at the bottom of the tube should be avoided if possible, but if used should be changed frequently. After discharge of the patient the thermometer and the holder should be removed, cleaned and disinfected as in the first method. The thermometer holder should be attached to the locker or the bed. If it is attached to the wall, there is a risk of the bed being moved and the thermometer subsequently being used by a different patient.

Rectal thermometers

A disposable sleeve will reduce contamination, and subsequent treatment is that of method 1 for oral thermometers. If a sleeve is not used, the Vaseline should be removed by wiping with 70% alcohol. The thermometer should then be immersed in a disinfectant with detergent properties and treated as in method 1 for oral thermometers.

Bedpans

The main hazard is the transfer of infection on the hands of staff; hands should be washed thoroughly after handling any bedpan that has not been properly disinfected after its previous use.

83

Non-infected patients

For patients who do not have enteric or urinary tract infection, or sepsis on buttocks or surrounding area, the following arrangements are appropriate:

(a) Non-disposable bedpans, and a bedpan washing machine with or without a heat disinfection cycle (e.g. models supplied by Dent and Hellyer, Stanbridge, Sterilizing Equipment Company Ltd., etc.). Those with a heat disinfection cycle are preferable.

(b) A disposable bedpan used with a macerator e.g. 'Sluicemaster' or 'Clinimatic' (see below).

(c) Empty bedpan into the sluice, wash thoroughly and allow to dry.

Infected patients

Non-disposable bedpans, and a bedpan washer with a heat disinfection cycle.

The final stage should raise the temperature of the surface of the bedpan to at least 80° C for one minute; this can be achieved by steam or hot water. The machine should be checked periodically to ensure that it reaches an adequate temperature. The heat conduction of metal bedpans is better than that of polypropylene, though polypropylene bedpans are often preferred by nursing staff. This is the preferred method for patients with infectious diseases and for burns wards, and possibly also for obstetric, paediatric and urological wards.

Disposable bedpans

This method is an acceptable alternative providing the macerator (or 'destructor') is well maintained and the drains are adequate. Drains are adequate for the installation of a destructor only if the horizontal course of soil pipes above ground floor level is not longer than 20 ft (7 m), and they should have an overall fall of 1 in 40: otherwise wards and operating theatres may be flooded with sewage. There was some leakage of aerosols around the lid of earlier models of destructors, but this has now been corrected by both major manufacturers. The destructor must be of a type which does not cause environmental contamination by aerosol (Gibson, 1973). The existing type of paper-pulp bedpan requires a non-disposable carrier to support it. This is undesirable because the carrier often becomes contaminated with faeces; nevertheless the risk of cross-infection by this route appears to be slight. Bedpan carriers should be thoroughly washed after use and, if visibly contaminated with faeces, disinfected by wiping the surface with a clear soluble phenolic. A disposable bedpan capable of supporting the weight of a patient without the use of a non-disposable carrier would be of value. Because of possible damage to macerators by dressings that might fall into bedpans, disposable bedpans are not suitable for use in burns units.

Other methods of disinfection

(a) Heat disinfection. Bedpans can be placed in boiling water for 10 min. This is rarely practical or necessary except possibly in an infectious diseases ward.

(b) **Chemical disinfection.** Bedpans should be totally immersed in a tank of clear soluble phenolic for 30 min after cleaning. Unless tanks are frequently emptied and cleaned, resistant Gram-negative bacilli may grow in the disinfectant solution. The use of tanks should, therefore, be avoided if possible. A less efficient method is to wipe the entire surface of the cleaned bedpan with a clear soluble phenolic. The ward bath is not a suitable container for disinfection of bedpans; a once weekly disinfection of bedpans is unlikely to prevent spread of infection.

Boiling or chemical disinfection of bedpans are procedures especially likely to cause contamination of the hands and clothing of the operator. Gloves and plastic aprons or gowns should be worn and disposable wipes should be used.

Commodes

Whenever possible the containers should be treated as bedpans. The seat should be cleaned at least daily and between patients and other surfaces at least weekly, with a detergent solution. If visible soiled with faeces, or if the commode is used by someone with an enteric infection, the seat should be cleaned with a clear soluble phenolic disinfectant. It should be rinsed and dried before re-use. Disposable wipes should be used for cleaning and the operator should wear disposable gloves and a plastic apron; hands should be washed even if gloves are worn.

Urinals

A urinal which has been washed but not disinfected should be treated as possibly contaminated, and the attendant should always wash the hands after handling. Routine disinfection, although preferable, is not necessarily required in general wards, other than urological, or after use by patients without an infection. Routine washing is carried out with a detergent solution followed by rinsing and thorough drying. Urinals in a urological or infectious diseases ward should be disinfected by heat, either in a bedpan washer with a steam cycle, or in a washing machine which rinses at $80°$ C or above. However, the use of a washing machine or pasteurizer for urinals should be encouraged in all wards. Disposable urinals are an alternative, but are disliked by many clinicians as they are opaque, and direct inspection of the urine is not possible. Chemical disinfection is possible by complete immersion in a solution of a clear soluble phenolic for 20–30 min, followed by rinsing and drying. Tanks of disinfectant should be avoided since they encourage the emergence of resistant strains which may contaminate all the bottles in the tank. Disinfectant solutions should be discarded after 12–24 hours' use. If a method of reliable heat disinfection is not available a separate labelled urinal should be supplied to any patient with an infection. The urinal is washed after each use and disinfected after discharge of the patient. Separate urinals for each patient should also be considered in urological and high risk wards if a method of heat disinfection is not available.

Sterilization and disinfection of special medical equipment

The forms of treatment required can be classified under two categories as follows (Ayliffe and Gibson, 1975):

Category A — Sterilization essential

Sterilized equipment is essential for all procedures involving a break in the skin or mucous membrane.

Category B — Sterilization preferred, but disinfection is usually adequate

Infection due to spore-bearing organisms is most unlikely to occur (if it ever does) through contact of contaminated equipment with intact mucous membranes. Disinfection is therefore usually adequate for equipment used in such procedures, though sterilization is always preferable, particularly where a normally sterile site is involved. Most of the equipment in this category requires decontamination only and is not used for aseptic procedures, but sterilization is preferable for these items, since all organisms, including viruses, are more reliably killed by sterilizing procedures than by methods of disinfection and the margin of safety is increased.

The manufacturer should state which methods of sterilization or disinfection can be used for any piece of equipment. Non-disposable equipment and materials in Category A should be able to withstand moist heat, preferably to 134° C; those in Category B to 70-80° C. If items are damaged or destroyed at these temperatures, and if they cannot be cleaned easily, they should not be bought. Blood monitoring equipment is difficult to clean and sterilize, and if this is not possible, the equipment can sometimes be satisfactorily protected from contamination. The use of filters, separating patient from machine, reduces the need for disinfection of respiratory ventilators.

Most of the items in Category A (e.g. surgical instruments, dressings, surgical drapes and gowns, parenteral fluids and water for aseptic techniques), can be sterilized by steam at high temperature. Dry heat is often used for sterilizing some instruments in eye-surgery and dental surgery, also glass syringes and powders. Disposable items, if their use involves contact with intact mucous membranes, should be sterilized by the manufacturer, since commercial techniques for sterilization (i.e. ethylene oxide and gamma radiation) are as easily carried out as disinfection. Inexpensive items which are difficult to clean should not be re-used, and all reprocessed equipment should be thoroughly cleaned before sterilization prior to use.

Endoscopes

The highest standard of sterilization or disinfection that is obtainable without damaging the instrument should be used. Before using any method it is advisable to consult the manufacturer and give them the exact details of the method you intend to use. This is particularly important if a new antibacterial or cleaning agent, temperature above room temperature, pressure above atmospheric, or exposure to a vacuum, is likely to be used. It should also be remembered that low temperature steam may reach 80° C and ethylene oxide 55° C with pressures up to 80 lbf/in² (552 kPa). Some of the disinfectants suggested for treating endoscopes are more corrosive than others. Automatic cleaning machines may not clean all parts of the endoscope and a double cycle may be necessary. If connections with a machine are loose, leakage may occur damaging fibre-bundles. The main problem with endoscopes is that the time available between patients is often insufficient for effective disinfection or sterilization. The method described for flexible fibreoptic gastroscopes (Category B) is more effective than cleaning alone and probably reduces the risk of infection to a low level. However, exposure to the disinfectant of all channels of the endoscope for 10–20 min is necessary to disinfect reliably.

These short treatments are inadequate for Category A endoscopes, although buffered hypochlorites which are sporicidal in a short time (e.g. 10 min) look promising for the future.

Endoscopes: Category A (arthroscopes, laparoscopes, ventriculoscopes, etc.)

Clean thoroughly and treat with ethylene oxide or low temperature steam and formaldehyde. Immersion in 2% glutaraldehyde for 3 h is commonly used, but is less reliable due to possible presence of air bubbles and recontamination on subsequent rinsing.

Endoscopes: Category B

(1) Flexible fibreoptic endoscopes (e.g. gastroscopes etc.)

    (a) *Treatment between patients.* Clean suction channel with brush, flush thoroughly with detergent followed by 2% glutaraldehyde for at least one to two minutes and finally rinse well. Clean and wipe the outside of the insertion tube with 2% glutaraldehyde, rinse and dry, or wipe with 70% alcohol. Clean and disinfect or preferably autoclave cleaning brush and biopsy forceps.

    (b) *Before and after sessions.* Thoroughly clean and disinfect according to manufacturer's instructions (including water bottle and its connections). Wear gloves when handling glutaraldehyde and check the suitability of the solution with the endoscope manufacturer. Do not use any other type of disinfectant, apart from (possibly) povidone-iodine. If contamination with tubercle bacilli, hepatitis virus, *Salmonella* spp. or agents of other infectious disease is known or suspected, carefully clean channels and insertion tube with glutaraldehyde mixed with a compatible detergent. Immerse insertion tube and fill channels with glutaraldehyde for at least 20 min. For additional safety, treatment with ethylene oxide may be desirable, avoiding pressures of over 20 lb/in² (138 kPa). Bronchoscopes with associated brush and biopsy forceps should be routinely immersed in 2% glutaraldehyde for 20 min between patients, since contamination by tubercle bacilli is more likely with a bronchoscope than with a gastroscope. Do not autoclave or use low temperature steam, with or without formaldehyde, on

'Olympus' flexible or any other endoscope unless agreement is obtained from the manufacturer.

(2) Rigid fibreoptic endoscopes, cystoscopes (Mitchell and Alder, 1975). Clostridial infection of the urinary tract is rare, but may occur after operations (e.g. prostatectomy); cytoscopes should if possible be sterilized by heat. Unfortunately, most cytoscopes available today are damaged by autoclaving and many may even be damaged by boiling. Cystoscopes (and all other endoscopes) should be dismantled and thoroughly cleaned prior to disinfection or sterilization. Disinfection by heat (low temperature steam) is preferable to chemical disinfection, but manufacturers should be consulted before any heating method is used.

(a) *Low temperature steam.* After dismantling and cleaning, place in a paper bag and seal. Treatment for 10 min at 71-75° C without formaldehyde will disinfect.

(b) *Pasteurization.* Immerse dismantled instrument in a thermostatically controlled bath of distilled water for 10 min at 75-80° C.

(c) *Chemical methods.* Cystoscopes should preferably be placed in the disinfectant in a vertical position to allow air bubbles to escape and the disinfectant to penetrate all parts of the instrument. The preferred method is immersion in 2% glutaraldehyde for 10-20 min. The instruments should be rinsed well before use. Spores are not killed unless the exposure time is increased to at least 2-3 h. Exposure to 0.5% chlorhexidine in 70% alcohol for 3 min will also disinfect, but a longer exposure should be avoided because it may damage the lens cement in some cystoscopes.

Respiratory and anaesthetic equipment (Category B)

This equipment should preferably be cleaned and disinfected in the Medical Equipment Cleaning Section (MECS) of a CSSD. Thorough washing, rinsing and drying should be adequate, but whenever possible most items should also be decontaminated by autoclaving at high or low temperatures. The life of the equipment may be considerably prolonged by using low temperature steam (71-75° C) instead of autoclaving at 121° C or 134° C. It is rational to provide every patient with a set of decontaminated equipment at operation, but this may not always be possible. Sessional or daily treatment of tubing and reservoir bag is a reasonably safe alternative. However, all patients should have a clean face mask and a decontaminated airway and endotracheal tube. Routine decontamination of anaesthetic machines is rarely possible or necessary, but treatment with gaseous formaldehyde may be required after use by an infected patient. Disposable face-masks, tubing and reservoir bags should be used on patients with a diagnosed or suspected transmissible infection (e.g. tuberculosis). If not disposable all items used on such patients should be autoclaved.

Airways — single-use or autoclave; if heat-labile, low temperature steam (LTS) or ethylene oxide.

Endotracheal tubes — autoclave; if heat-labile use LTS or ethylene oxide.

Reservoir bags — LTS; washing machine (at over 70°C); (glutaraldehyde; see note on p. 92).

Corrugated tubing — autoclave; if heat-labile, LTS, washing machine (running at over 70° C); (glutaraldehyde).

Face-masks and connections, laryngoscope blades — thorough washing and drying is usually sufficient. If used on known infected patients, treat with LTS or in washing machine (rinsing at over 70° C); (glutaraldehyde).

Oxygen masks — single-use.

Ambu bags — autoclave or LTS.

Tracheostomy tubes — single-use, autoclave or LTS.

Scavenging equipment — the tubing and bag close to the patient or the anaesthetic machine should be disposable or autoclavable. It should be regularly changed, e.g. weekly, and after use by an infected patient.

Suction equipment

In the absence of piped suction a separate machine should be available for each patient requiring suction, and it should be decontaminated before use by another patient. If piped suction is used, the tubing and trap bottle should be autoclaved; the return valve attached to the lid is usually not autoclavable and should be washed and dried, and preferably treated with LTS. If the suction bottle becomes more than about half full, foaming is likely and may contaminate the environment. It is preferable to empty the bottle regularly, but an antifoaming agent such as 'Fomatrol' can be added. Bacterial multiplication may occur in the aspirate if it is allowed to stand for long periods. Bottles should be emptied at least twice daily, or preferably more often, irrespective of the amount of fluid aspirated. The use of a disinfectant in the bottle may be responsible for excessive foaming, is often ineffective, and could be toxic to the patient. Avoid disinfectants if possible during suction, but if they are considered necessary, use a non-toxic agent such as chlorhexidine (fill 1/10 bottle with 0.5% chlorhexidine) rather than a phenolic disinfectant. If the contents are considered hazardous to staff, a clear soluble phenolic can be added to the aspirate before disposal. Add sufficient disinfectant to give a final concentration suitable for a 'dirty' situation, and leave for at least ten minutes. The bottle should be washed and dried before re-use. If a patient requires suction for more than 24 h, the bottle and tubing should be changed. When the machine is not in use, the bottle should be kept dry and the catheter should not be connected to it until it is required. The tubing and catheter should, if possible, be transparent.

Independent vacuum pumps (e.g. the 'Matburn') must have a bacterial filter between the reservoir bottle and the pump, to avoid the dispersal of bacteria from the pump effluent. When vacuum bottles, which are connected by a Schraeder connector, are uncoupled, there may be a sudden contamination of the air of the room from the socket outlet, due to a brief reverse gas flow. This can be prevented by interposing a bacterial filter in the line between the vacuum bottles and the Schraeder connector (see Chapter 9).

Respiratory ventilators

Many varieties of ventilator are available, but those with both expiratory and inspiratory circuits (e.g. Cape) are the most difficult to disinfect. Effective routine cleaning is not possible, so that prevention of gross contamination of the machine is necessary. This may be accomplished by:

(1) changing of tubing between machine and patient at least daily or more often if secretions are excessive. The incorporation of moisture traps in the tubing will be of further value, not only in preventing contamination of the machine but also in assessing when a change of tubing is necessary. The machine should be changed and disinfected at least twice weekly unless filters are fitted.
(2) Protection of the machine by insertion of bacterial filters in the inspiratory and expiratory limbs. Filters with a low resistance to gas flow are available (e.g. microflow) (Lumley *et al.*, 1976). Provided that the filters can be heated to prevent water in the expired air from condensing and increasing resistance, these have proved bacteriologically and mechanically satisfactory for two weeks. Certain types of siliconized filters (Mitchell and Gamble, 1973) are also bacteriologically satisfactory. Other filters with low resistance to gas flow even when wet are being introduced.

Disinfection of the ventilator (Lumley, 1976)

An autoclavable respiratory circuit which can be changed daily provides the best solution, and such machines are available; efficient filters would, however, be an adequate alternative and are required even if the circuit is autoclavable. Most methods of chemical disinfection suitable for ventilators will not work efficiently in the presence of organic matter, and none of the methods is entirely reliable. Of the methods available, nebulization with hydrogen peroxide (a modification of that described by Judd *et al.*, 1968) is chosen. The method is quick, the peroxide readily breaks down and is not toxic to patient or staff. If the ventilator is visibly contaminated, it must be stripped down and cleaned prior to disinfection. The method is described in Appendix 7.4 and should be followed exactly for machines with inspiratory and expiratory circuits. An alternative method of disinfection is by the use of formaldehyde (Benn, Dutton and Tully, 1973). This method can be used only on machines with closed circuits and great care is necessary to remove residual formaldehyde. If the patient is known or suspected to be suffering from pulmonary tuberculosis the use of the formaldehyde method is advisable.

90

Nebulized hydrogen peroxide may be used on machines with single circuits, though these may often be easily dismantled, washed and disinfected by heat or by 2% glutaraldehyde. Smaller machines may sometimes be treated with ethylene oxide or with LTS.

Humidifiers

Humidifiers in which water vapour (not an aerosol) is blown towards the patient, although sometimes contaminated, are not a serious infection hazard. The water may contaminate the hands of staff and humidifiers should be cleaned and dried between patients, or twice weekly. Disinfect by heat if possible, before refilling with freshly drawn tap water. Chlorhexidine in a final concentration of 0.1% may be used to prevent bacterial growth in the evaporator type of humidifier, but not the nebulizer type.

Contaminated nebulizers, which produce an aerosol, may be responsible for lung infections caused by Gram-negative bacilli, especially *Ps. aeruginosa*. Their use should be avoided unless they can be decontaminated by heat daily. If this is not possible, the container should be cleaned and dried daily. Water should be replaced and not topped up. If the nebulizing part of the machine is liable to damage by heat, it should be flushed through with 0.25% acetic acid or 0.1% chlorhexidine in an area away from the patient; occasional bacteriological tests should be made to ensure the nebulized air is not contaminated.

Infant incubators

These are frequently contaminated and often not adequately cleaned on the ward. After discharge of a patient, the inner surface of the incubator should be thoroughly cleaned with a paper wipe and detergent and dried (Gram-negative bacilli multiply in moist areas). Particular care is necessary with rubber seals, which should be removed and cleaned. Since adequate cleaning and drying is effective, disinfection is rarely necessary and may fail without preliminary cleaning of the incubator. If disinfection is required, the cleaned surfaces can be wiped with a freshly prepared hypochlorite solution (125 ppm available chlorine), rinsed and dried. Alternatively, surfaces can be sprayed or wiped with 70% ethyl alcohol. Since there is a fire hazard, this should be done outside or in a well-ventilated room, and the incubator must be properly aired before re-use. Formaldehyde cabinets are occasionally used, but are expensive. Since prior cleaning of the incubator is still necessary, the routine use of a cabinet is of rather doubtful value.

Oxygen tents

These should be washed and dried after each patient. Oxygen masks and tubing should be disposable. There is no evidence that piped medical gases become contaminated with bacteria.

Haemodialysis equipment

See Chapter 18.

Miscellaneous items

Many of these items, such as catheters, grafts and internal pace-makers, should be supplied in sterile packs by the manufacturers.

Catheters — (Category A) Single-use catheters are preferred; some expensive catheters, e.g. cardiac, may be sterilized with ethylene oxide provided the cleaning process is efficient.

Grafts — (Category A) Heart valves, arterial grafts, joints and other implants: autoclave; if heat-labile ethylene oxide; sterilization in hospital should not be necessary.

Cryoprobes — (Category A) Can sometimes be autoclaved, but if not, LTS/ formaldehyde or ethylene oxide.

Pace-makers (internal) — (Category A) Ethylene oxide.

Transducers — (Category A) Ethylene oxide, or LTS/formaldehyde if not damaged at 71° C.

Fibre-lights — (Category A) Ethylene oxide or LTS/formaldehyde.

Electrical leads — (if Category A) Autoclave, ethylene oxide or LTS/formaldehyde.

Large polypropylene syringes — (Category B) Autoclave.

Bladder and surgical drainage equipment (other than catheter) — (Category B) Single-use, autoclave, or LTS.

Stomach, rectal tubes etc. — (Category B) Single-use, autoclave or LTS.

Use of glutaraldehyde

If none of the other methods are suitable or available, immersion in 2% glutaraldehyde may be adequate although sometimes less reliable. Thorough rinsing is most important, particularly for respiratory equipment; glutaraldehyde can cause damage to the lung.

Category A items — 2% glutaraldehyde for at least 3 h.
Category B items — 2% glutaraldehyde for at least 10 min.
Special risk items (e.g. tuberculosis, hepatitis) (see endoscopes) — 2% glutaraldehyde for at least 20 min, preferably 1–2 h (heat treatment or ethylene oxide is advised). Some preparations of glutaraldehyde may be more corrosive than others and particular care is necessary if new preparations are used on expensive equipment.

Appendix 7.1 Summary of methods for cleaning and decontamination of equipment or environment

Heat
Autoclave if materials are not likely to be damaged by high temperatures, otherwise use low temperature steam or pasteurization.

Chemical disinfection
(A) Clear soluble phenolics at concentrations recommended for light contamination, unless otherwise specified; (B) hypochlorites (see p. 99 for concentration); (C) 2% glutaraldehyde; (D) alcohol (use either 70% ethyl or 60–70% isopropyl).

Equipment or Site	Routine or Preferred Method	Acceptable Alternative or Additional Recommendations	See page
Airways and endotracheal tubes	(1) Heat sterilize (2) Heat disinfect	(3) Chemical disinfection (C) For patients with tuberculosis use disposables or heat sterilize	88
Ampoules	Wipe neck with 70% alcohol	Do not immerse	82
Baths	*Non-infected patients* Wipe with detergent solution and rinse. Cream cleaner may be used for stain and scum removal	*Infected patients and patients with open wounds* Chemical disinfection (B) (a) Hypochlorite detergent solution (b) Non-abrasive hypochlorite powder, e.g. 'Countdown'	78
Bath water	Antiseptic bath additive not added as routine	For staphylococcal dispersers apply 'Hibiscrub' when bathing. For infected patients or during outbreaks add 'Steribath' or 'Savlon' to the water	118
Bedding	See section on laundering		172

Equipment Site	Routine or Preferred Method	Acceptable Alternative or Additional Recommendations	See page
Bed-frames	Wash with detergent and dry	After infected patient, disinfectant (A)	81
Bedpans	(1) Wash in machine with heat disinfection cycle or use disposables. Wash carriers for disposable pans after use	Patients with enteric infections If (1) is not possible, heat disinfection after emptying and washing, or chemical disinfection (A). Individual pan for infected patient.	83
Bowls (surgical)	Autoclave		82
Bowls (washing)	Wash and dry	For infected patients use individual bowls and disinfect on discharge (1) Heat disinfection (2) Chemical disinfection (A)	80
Carpets	Vacuum daily. Clean periodically by hot water extraction	For known contaminated spillage Chemical disinfection (A) leave 10 min then rinse and dry	119
Cheatle forceps	Do not use	If used, autoclave daily and store in fresh solutions of clear soluble phenolics	83
Crockery and cutlery	(1) Machine wash with rinse temperature above 80° C and dry in air (2) Hand wash by approved method	For patients with enteric infections or tuberculosis use disposables or heat disinfect.	78, 177
Cystoscopes	Clean thoroughly and disinfect by low temperature steam	Chemical disinfection (C)	88
Drains	Clean regularly	Chemical disinfection is not advised	78

Item	Method	Notes	Page
Endoscopes (gastroscopes, bronchoscopes, laparoscopes, arthroscopes)	see p. 87		87
Feeding bottles and teats	(1) Presterilized or terminally heat-treated feeds	(2) Use teats and bottles sterilized and packed by CSSD (3) Hypochlorite ('Milton') should only be used in small units where other methods are not available	247
Floors (dry cleaning)	(1) Vacuum clean (2) Dust-attracting dry mop	Do not use broom in patient areas	76
Floors (wet cleaning)	Wash with detergent solution. Disinfection not usually required.	Known contaminated and special areas, chemical disinfection (A)	76
Furniture and fittings	Damp dust with detergent solution	Known contaminated and special areas, damp dust with disinfectant (A)	78
Haemodyalisis equipment	see p. 311		311
Infant incubators	Wash with detergent and dry with disposable wipe	Infected patients — after cleaning wipe or spray with 70% alcohol or hypochlorite solution (125 parts/10^6)	
Instruments (surgical)	Heat	If contaminated instruments require handling before reprocessing, disinfection (A) (tubercle) or (C) (hepatitis virus)	91
Locker tops	See furniture		41
Mattresses	Water impermeable cover, wash with detergent solution and dry	Disinfect (A) if contaminated; do not disinfect unnecessarily as this damages the mattress	78
			81

Equipment Site	Routine or Preferred Method	Acceptable Alternative or Additional Recommendations	See page
Mops (dish)	Do not use	See p. 174	174
Mops (dry — dust-attracting)	Do not use for more than two days without reprocessing or washing	Vacuuming after each use may prolong effective life between processing or washing	78
Mops (wet)	Rinse after each use, wring and store dry. Autoclave periodically	If chemical disinfection is required, rinse in water, soak in 1% hypochlorite (0.1% available chlorine) 30 min, rinse and store dry	78
Nail brushes	Use only if essential	A sterile nail brush should be used for all clinical procedures	80, 166
Pillows	Treat as mattresses		81
Razors (safety and pen)	Disposable or autoclaved	Chemical disinfection (A) or (D)	80
Razors (electric)	Immerse head in 70% alcohol		80
Rooms (terminal cleaning or disinfection)	*Non-infected patients* Wash surfaces in detergent solution and allow to dry	*Infected patients* Wash surfaces in disinfectant (A) or hypochlorite (0.1% available chlorine) for viral hepatitis. Fogging not recommended	75, 79
Shaving brushes	Do not use for clinical shaving	Autoclave. Use brushless cream or shaving foam	80
Sputum container	Use disposable only	Non-disposable — should be emptied with care and autoclaved	116
Suction equipment	See p. 89		89, 163

Thermometers (oral)	(1) Collect after round, wipe clean and disinfect with (A) or (D) for 10 min, rinse (if phenolic), wipe, and store dry	(2) Individual thermometers wipe with 70% alcohol, store dry; terminally disinfect as (1)	83
Thermometers (rectal)	Clean with 70% alcohol and treat as above		83
Thermometers (electronic clinical)	(1) Use disposable sleeve (2) Wipe probe with 70% alcohol	Do not use without sleeve for oral or rectal temperatures or for patient with typhoid, tuberculosis etc.	
Toilet seats	Wash with detergent and dry	After use by infected patient or if grossly contaminated, chemical disinfection (A), rinse and dry	78
Tooth mugs	(1) Disposable	(2) If non-disposable, heat disinfection	119
Toys	Clean first but do not soak soft toys; if contaminated, disinfect (a) heat (b) chemical; wipe surface with 70% alcohol or disinfect (A)	Expensive or treasured toys may withstand low temperature steam or ethylene oxide; the latter needs long aeration. Heavily contaminated soft toys may have to be destroyed	82
Trolley tops	(1) Clean first then chemical disinfection by wiping or spraying with 70% alcohol	(2) Clean first then chemical disinfection (A) and wipe dry	112, 120
Tubing (anaesthetic or ventilator)	(a) Heat disinfection (b) wash thoroughly and disinfect (C)	For patients with tuberculosis (1) Use disposable tubing (2) Heat sterilization or disinfection	88, 90

Equipment Site	Routine or Preferred Method	Acceptable Alternative or Additional Recommendations	See page
Urinals	(1) Use washer with heat disinfection cycle or use disposables	(2) Chemical disinfection (A). If a tank is used it must be emptied, dried and refilled at least weekly	85
Ventilator (mechanical)	See p. 90		90, 101, 162
Wash basins	Clean with detergent. Use cream cleaner for stains, scum etc. Disinfection not normally required	Disinfection may be required if contaminated. Use Boycott's method or non-abrasive hypochlorite powder. Sink trap only requires disinfection if contaminated with known epidemic strain	78
X-ray equipment	Damp dust with detergent solution; switch off, do not over wet, allow to dry before use	Wipe with 70% alcohol to disinfect	272

Appendix 7.2 Disinfectants for environmental use

Disinfectant	Type*	Routine use dilution (%)	Approx.† Cost/ gallon use dilution (pence)	Strong concentration (%)	Manufacturer
'Stericol'	CSPD	1.0	2.4	2	Sterling Industries Ltd.
'Hycolin'	CSP	1.0	3.0	2	Wm. Pearson Ltd.
'Clearsol'	CSPD	0.625	1.9	1	Tenneco Organics Ltd.
'Sudol'	CSP	0.625	1.9	1	Tenneco Organics Ltd.
'Izal'	W	1.0	2.2	2	Sterling Industries Ltd.
'Chloros', 'Domestos', 'Sterite' or similar compounds	H	1.0 (approx. 0.1% available chlorine)	0.4	10 (approx. 1% available chlorine)	

*CSP — Clear soluble phenolic
 D — contains added detergent
 W — white fluid
 H — hypochlorite
†Trade price December 1979. Hospitals obtain bulk supplies at reduced cost by contract with manufacturers.

Appendix 7.3 Disinfectants ('antiseptics') for skin and mucous membrane (March 1980)

Disinfectant Preparation	Used for	Cost*	Quantity
Chlorhexidine gluconate 0.5% in 70% ethyl alcohol	Operation site	65p	500 ml
Iodine 1% in 70% ethyl alcohol	Operation site	10p	500 ml
Povidone-iodine 10% in 70% ethyl alcohol (Betadine Alcoholic Solution)	Operation site	60p	500 ml
Aqueous solution of povidone-iodine 10% (Betadine Aqueous Solution)	Mucous membrane	60p	500 ml
Aqueous solution of Lugol's 1% iodine	Mucous membrane	£1.64	500 ml
Ethyl alcohol (70%)	Skin before injection or venepuncture	18p	500 ml
Isopropyl alcohol (70%)		34p	500 ml
Chlorhexidine gluconate 0.5% aqueous	Hands (rinsing in isolation ward) or on operation site	30p	500 ml
Chlorhexidine gluconate (0.5%) in isopropyl alcohol ('Hibisol')	Hands of surgeon	98p	500 ml
Chlorhexidine gluconate ('Hibitane') 0.5% in 95% ethyl alcohol, with 1.0% glycerol	Hands of surgeon	60p	
Chlorhexidine 4% detergent solution ('Hibiscrub')	Hands of surgeon	£1.43	500 ml
Povidone-iodine 'surgical scrub'	Hands of surgeon	78p	500 ml
Hexachlorophane 3% detergent preparation	Hands of surgeon	£1.17	500 ml
Hexachlorophane powder	Skin and umbilical stump of neonates	£1.60	100 g
Neomycin 0.5% and chlorhexidine 1% cream ('Naseptin')	Removal of epidemic strain of staphylococcus from nose	17p	5 g

*The cost of disinfectants varies from region to region depending on regional contract prices, and in some instances from hospital to hospital if the use of a particular item is low.

Appendix 7.4 Disinfection of Cape Ventilator with hydrogen peroxide (see figure below)

Method

(1) Freshly prepared 20 volume hydrogen peroxide should be used each time. This should be made by diluting a 100 volume hydrogen peroxide solution 1:5 with sterile distilled water. Freshly drawn tap water may be used in areas supplied by a high quality soft mains water.

(2) A flow rate of 15 l/min is required to drive a suitable nebulizer (e.g. Ohio). The direct oxygen supply can be used if the pressure is sufficient; the valve on the top of the nebulizer is set at 60% to prevent build up of pressure and release of peroxide through safety valve.

(3) The ventilator should be switched on and adjusted so that respiratory volume is set at 1000 ml/respiration; the respiration rate is 25 rev/min and expiratory assistance control is set with the black spot exactly in the midway position between minimum and maximum. This is very important; failure to do this will cause a section of the expiratory circuit to remain unexposed to the aerosol. The oxygen inlet should be closed with a cap during decontamination.

The three drainage taps should be opened and left open with the machine working for 2 to 3 min, then closed and the drain tap cover door closed. This should remove moisture accumulated in use which may neutralize nebulized hydrogen peroxide.

(4) Hydrogen peroxide should be nebulized for 60 min with the nebulizer placed at point A (air intake) and the aerosol allowed to escape directly into the air at point B (inspiratory port). Potassium iodide indicator paper placed at point B should turn deep brown within five minutes of the process commencing.

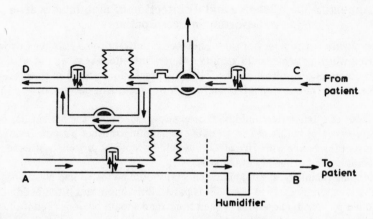

Cape Ventilator

101

(5) The nebulizer should then be removed and placed at point C (expiratory port) to allow aerosol to emerge at point D (air outlet). This should be similarly monitored with the potassium iodide indicator paper at point D. To save time, two nebulizers can be used at the same time.

(6) This system will not decontaminate the length of tubing from the valve block to the spirometer outlet. If a spirometer has been used and decontamination of this part of the circuit is required, an additional 10 min nebulization will be required on the expiratory side with the spirometer switch held in the 'in' position.

(7) The machine should be adequately aired after this process. Remove nebulizer, open the three drainage taps and allow the machine to run for 10 min; close the drainage taps and continue to pass air through the machine until peroxide can no longer be detected at points B and D and the spirometer outlet; a period of 2 to 4 h will be required. The three drainage taps should again be opened for 10 min at the end of the airing process. If the spirometer is involved, a period of at least 30 min venting will be required with the spirometer switch held in the 'in' position. Detection of residual peroxide vapour: if potassium iodide indicator strips held at points B and D and the spirometer outlets for 5 min do not show detectable brown discolouration the machine may be considered free of peroxide vapour.

(8) It is advisable, if not immediately required, to air the machine again on the following day with drain taps open for the first 5 min. Tests with potassium iodide indicator papers should be repeated and show a satisfactory level at the end of this test.

Note

Filter paper strips are prepared by immersion in a saturated solution of potassium iodide in distilled water and dried in a peroxide-free atmosphere.

Appendix 7.5 Cleaning and disinfection of ambulances after transporting infected patients

The inanimate environment of the ambulance is unlikely to be a source or reservoir from which patients could acquire ordinary infections (e.g. wound, skin, childhood infections). Provided the following precautions are taken there should be little risk of transferring infection to staff or subsequent occupants.

(1) Hands of attendants should be thoroughly washed after the patient has been removed, and before eating, smoking or handling another patient. Disinfection of the hands with 70% alcohol would be a useful procedure if washing facilities are not readily available.

(2) Bedding (blankets, sheets, pillow covers) should be sealed in a plastic bag and laundered before re-use. This is particularly important if the bedding is soiled by blood, excretions or secretions (and should be done even if the patient is not designated as infected).

(3) Spillage of blood, pus, excretions, vomit etc. should be promptly removed

with disposable wipes and a phenolic disinfectant. Discarded wipes should be sealed in a plastic bag and sent for incineration.

(4) The stretcher should also be wiped over with a phenolic disinfectant. Disposable gloves should be worn for cleaning, and a plastic apron may be worn to protect clothing. Hands should be washed even if gloves are worn.

(5) Respiratory resuscitation equipment should be returned to a hospital CSSD or Medical Equipment Cleaning Section for processing.

Additional procedures for special infections

When an ambulance is used for a specially designated infection it is advisable: to remove any equipment not considered necessary, e.g. spare stretcher; to seal equipment locker with adhesive tape (terminal cleaning of inside will not then be necessary); to seal clean blankets and bedding in a plastic bag and carry in cab and to seal box containing resuscitation equipment, so that if it is contaminated only the outside of the box will require cleaning or disinfection.

Diarrhoea and vomiting of unknown origin or gastro-intestinal infection

Bedpans, urinals, vomit bowls, etc. should be either washed in a bedpan washer with a steam disinfection cycle or washed in a phenolic disinfectant. Disposable cups should be used. If surfaces are extensively contaminated the ambulance should be taken out of service and all surfaces cleaned with a phenolic disinfectant. Surfaces should be dry before the ambulance is re-used.

Infectious or serum hepatitis

As above, but disinfect with 1% hypochlorite (containing 0.1% available chlorine).

Tuberculosis

As above. Sputum containers and wipes used for removing secretions from patient should be sealed in a plastic bag and incinerated.

Highly dangerous infections

Lassa fever and other viral haemorrhagic infections and small-pox: special precautions are required (see Chapter 17).

Immunization

Ambulance staff should be immunized against poliomyelitis, tetanus and tuberculosis (if tuberculin-negative).

References and Further Reading

Ayliffe, G. A. J., Collins, B. J. and Lowbury, E. J. L. (1966), Cleaning and disinfection of hospital floors. *Brit. med. J.*, ii, 442.
Ayliffe, G. A. J. and Gibson, G. L. (1975), Health and Social Services Journal, 15 March, p. 598.

Benn, R. A. V., Dutton, A. A. C. and Tully, M. (1973), Disinfection of mechanical ventilators: an investigation using formaldehyde in a Cape ventilator. *Anaesthesia*, 27, 265.

Gibson, G. L. (1973), A disposable bedpan system using an improved disposal unit and self-supporting bedpans. *J. clin. Path.*, 26, 925.

Judd, P. A., Tomlin, D. J., Whitby, J. L., Inglis, J. C. M. and Robinson, J. S. (1968), Disinfection of mechanical ventilators by ultrasonic nebulization. *Lancet*, ii, 1019.

Lowbury, E. J. L., Lilly, H. A. and Ayliffe, G. A. J. (1974), Pre-operative disinfection of surgeons' hands: use of alcoholic solutions and effects of gloves on skin flora. *Brit. med. J.*, iv, 369.

Lowbury, E. J. L. and Lilly, H. A. (1975), Gloved hand as applicator of antiseptic to operation sites. *Lancet*, ii, 153.

Lumley, I., Holdcroft, A., Gaya, H., Darlow, H. M. and Adams, D. J. (1976), Expiratory bacterial filters. *Lancet*, ii, 22.

Lumley, J. (1976), Decontamination of anaesthetic equipment and ventilators. *Br. J. Anaesth.*, 48, 3.

Maurer, I. M. (1978), *Hospital Hygiene* (2nd Edn). Edward Arnold, London.

Mitchell, N. J. and Gamble, D. R. (1973), Evaluation of the new 'Williams' anaesthetic filter. *Br. med. J.*, ii, 653.

Mitchell, J. P. and Alder, V. G. (1975), The disinfection of urological endoscopes. *Br. J. Urol.*, 47, 571.

Russell, A. D., Ayliffe, G. A. J. and Hugo, W. B. (eds) (1981), *Principles and Practice of Disinfection, Prevention and Sterilization*, Blackwell Scientific Publication, Oxford (in press).

Prevention of Spread of Infection

CHAPTER EIGHT

Prevention of Infection in Wards (1) Ward Procedure and Dressing Techniques

Introduction

This chapter and the next deal with the methods by which patients in hospital wards can be protected against micro-organisms from various sources, in particular from other patients, and transmitted by staff, by contaminated objects ('fomites') and by air. Surgical patients are exposed to special hazards of infection during the relatively short period of the operation, and the prevention of these hazards is the subject of Chapter 10. Infection may occur also in the ward, where the period of exposure of some unhealed wounds may be prolonged. A clean, closed wound is unlikely to become infected after 24 h following operation, and exposure for change of dressing is usually short, but the risk may be greater and more prolonged in some patients, especially those with drained or open wounds and with burns. Patients with septic lesions and other infective conditions will often be nursed in the same ward as patients who are at special risk of infection because of inadequate natural defences. The largest reservoir of infective micro-organisms is among patients, and the most important mode of transfer is by the staff who have contact with them. It is therefore important to ensure that adequate measures of protection are used.

Control of infection in wards, as in operating theatres, involves the application of the principles of aseptic technique and hygiene in the numerous details of patient care. It involves also the design, equipment and ventilation of the ward in such a way that patients may, when necessary, be placed in isolation, to prevent infection passing from them or to them. Research and experience have shown that good buildings, though important, are less vital to the prevention of infection than good aseptic and hygienic procedures; but patient isolation methods involve both structures and procedures. Isolation methods are discussed in Chapter 9. This chapter is concerned with the general principles of aseptic and hygienic technique which apply in all hospital wards; the requirements of special departments and some individual procedures are considered in Chapters 15 to 19. Examples of methods recommended for performing various aseptic procedures are presented in Appendix 8.1 (at the end of this chapter).

Ward structure and facilities

Spread of infection (particularly staphylococcal) is most likely to occur in large open wards. Wards should, therefore, be subdivided in units of four to six beds with complete separation from other areas and with adequate single rooms for isolation of infected patients. Although single rooms for 25% of patients have been recommended, a smaller number is probably sufficient (e.g. four single rooms for a 30-bedded adult ward), depending on whether a hospital isolation unit is available. Patients with communicable infections, including staphylococcal sepsis, if caused by an epidemic or highly resistant strain, should be given priority for isolation if single room accommodation is limited. To further reduce risks of cross-infection, bed centres should be at least eight feet apart and overcrowding with extra beds should be avoided. A day room for walking patients will also reduce the number of patients in the clinical area. Toilet facilities should be adequate and provided with handwashing basins. Since patients are today allowed out of bed much earlier than formerly, washing facilities should be considerably increased. Separate toilet and handwashing facilities should be available for the staff. Showers should be provided whenever possible, in addition to baths. Handwashing basins for the staff should be readily available in the clinical area and supplied with paper towels of good quality. Sluice rooms should be adequate in size with suitable storage space for bedpans, urinals and cupboards for urine testing and other equipment. Storage areas for cleaning equipment should be provided. Wards should be kept in a good state of repair and provided with readily cleanable surfaces.

Aseptic techniques

The terms *asepsis* and *aseptic technique* are used to describe methods which have been developed to prevent contamination of wounds or other susceptible sites (e.g. the urinary tract) in the operating theatre, the ward and other treatment areas, by ensuring that only sterile objects and fluids will make contact with these sites and that the risks of airborne contamination are minimized. When first introduced the term *asepsis* was used to mean the provision of heat-sterilized instruments and equipment in the operating theatre, to supersede *antisepsis* by immersion of instruments etc. in a phenolic solution as previously used by Lister. Today the word asepsis is not used in contrast with antisepsis, but includes antiseptic methods (e.g. skin disinfection) which are still required. Any procedure which involves penetration of the skin, exposure of wounds or instrumentation (except that of the gastro-intestinal tract) should be done with sterile materials (supplied by a CSSD, where that service exists). The details of aseptic technique must to some extent vary from hospital to hospital in relation to existing facilities such as the extent of services from a CSSD.

Masks

A distinction was formerly made between 'deflector' masks, which were impervious barriers protecting patients' wounds against the direct impaction of bacteria from the mouth, and 'filter' masks, which protected the wearer when exposed to hazard of airborne communicable disease. Modern types of mask are suitable for both purposes. The principal role of the mask is to protect the patient against organisms dispersed from the upper respiratory tract of the nurse or other attendant. Most of the bacteria dispersed on sneezing or talking come from the mouth and are normally harmless to wounds (though occasionally *Streptococcus pyogenes* and *Staphylococcus aureus* may be present in the mouth); *Staph. aureus* is commonly present in the nose, but the nose disperses very few bacteria into the air. *Staph. aureus* is commonly shed into the environment on skin scales and a mask will do little to reduce dissemination of these.

Experimental studies and trials have indicated that masks contribute little or nothing to the protection of patients in wards against infection, and their routine use for aseptic ward procedures, including postoperative dressings is, therefore, unnecessary.

If a mask is thought to be necessary, most of the commercially available types will reduce the risk of impaction of bacteria from the mouth and may be considered satisfactory. For the dressing of burns or extensive open wounds effective surgical masks are appropriate, as in operative surgery. When a mask is removed, it should not be worn again, but should, if necessary, be replaced by a fresh mask.

Protective clothing

Clothing may be of some importance in the contact transfer of *Staph. aureus.* The front of the apron is the area most often contaminated. It is, therefore, rational for the nurse to wear protective clothing while she carries out aseptic procedures, so as to prevent the transfer of bacteria from her uniform to the patients, and also to prevent contamination of her uniform. It is unnecessary to change the gown or apron between patients following routine procedures on uninfected patients (see also Chapter 9, p. 127 for procedure on infected patients).

Cotton is permeable to bacteria and moisture, and a water-repellent apron, impermeable to bacteria, would be more appropriate. A disposable plastic apron worn during dressings and other aseptic procedures is cheap and convenient, and the front can be disinfected by spraying with 70% alcohol following procedures on infected patients. There is little advantage in wearing a gown rather than a plastic apron because the nurse's shoulders and upper arms are unlikely to become contaminated in normal circumstances; however, if a gown is worn, the nurse's arms should be bare to the elbow.

Hands

The hands of nurses, doctors, physiotherapists and others who handle patients are probably the most important vehicles of cross-infection, and it is essential that effective methods should be used to minimize this hazard. There is evidence to suggest that nurses are often uncertain when a handwash is necessary, and that they regard the product used and the length of time of handwashing as more important than the technique. In tests of handwashing with a dye it was found that over half the nurses did not wash some part of the thumb, and many also

109

missed areas of the finger tips and palm (Taylor, 1978). These are the areas most likely to come into contact with patients and equipment and to transfer infection. Hands should be thoroughly washed on arrival for duty; before and after aseptic procedures or attending to infants; before attending to patients in protective isolation and after attending to patients in source isolation; after making the bed of an infected patient; after giving a bedpan, and after treating pressure areas. Where handwashing is difficult or inconvenient, clean, but not necessarily sterile, disposable gloves may be used; they should be used also for handling highly contaminated objects (e.g. drainage tubes, endotracheal tubes) or patients (e.g. those who are incontinent of faeces); for aseptic procedures sterile gloves or forceps should be used. Hands should be washed when gloves are removed after handling an infected patient or objects contaminated by patients with sepsis.

In the course of her work the nurse will touch many objects contaminated with staphylococci and other organisms capable of causing wound infection; she can easily transfer pathogenic organisms, which her hands have just picked up from an infected patient, to the next patient whom she visits in the ward. Such recently acquired contaminants are 'transient' bacteria which are not growing in the skin and which, unlike the 'resident' bacteria, can be greatly reduced in numbers by washing with soap and water; disinfection with 70% alcohol is more effective. Some of these bacteria which remain on the skin may become 'residents'. For most purposes in the ward a thorough wash with soap and water is adequate. It is important to ensure that all surfaces of hands and fingers are covered during the wash. Antimicrobial preparations (see Chapter 7) may be indicated in special units, e.g. intensive care, infectious diseases and special care baby units, and in general wards during an outbreak of infection. The use of 70% alcohol with an emollient, with or without an additional antimicrobial agent, is of particular value in wards lacking convenient handwashing facilities or during dressing or napkin-changing rounds. It is also more effective than the antimicrobial detergents. A suitable routine for a ward would be soap for general handwashing, with an alcoholic preparation available for special procedures.

Soap containers used on wards may be a source of contamination (see Chapter 7). Containers for bar soap should be easy to clean and regularly cleaned. Liquid soap dispensers should be regularly cleaned, maintained and refilled.

Wound dressings

Place for dressing procedures

The place where wounds are dressed will be determined by the structure of the ward and the availability of single rooms. If the design of the dressing room is poor and without mechanical ventilation (as in many hospitals at present), dressing all wounds in one small room increases the risk of infection by creating a high level of airborne contamination when the wounds are exposed. A single room, preferably with an extractor fan or other mechanical ventilation, should be used for source isolation of patients with infected wounds, priority being given to those infected or colonized by multiple-resistant strains of *Staph. aureus* or with open wounds (see Chapter 9). Dressings of small wounds may reasonably be changed at the bedside, if care is taken to avoid dispersal of bacteria from

110

dressings that are being removed; such procedures should cause little increase in airborne contamination by wound pathogens. For larger wounds and burns it is desirable to change dressings in a mechnically ventilated dressing room or theatre, if source isolation of the patient in a mechanically ventilated single room is impossible.

It may sometimes be preferable to change the dressing in the operating theatre. If a wound dressing or treatment room is considered necessary, it should be ventilated with eight or more air changes per hour (a burns dressing station should have twenty air changes per hour). The doors should be large enough for a bed to pass through. At least ten minutes should be allowed after use by an infected patient, and the cover on the couch (if used) should be changed. The ventilation system should be regularly checked by the engineers (e.g. at least six monthly). Even if the room is adequate in all respects, it may be impracticable and time-consuming to move some patients in their beds to a dressing station (e.g. those in traction beds). In addition, where team nursing or patient allocation is practised, one dressing room may be inadequate.

Since the cost of a correctly ventilated room is high and the evidence of its value (except for burns) is limited, it would seem to be rarely worthwhile incorporating a plenum-ventilated dressing room either in a new general ward or an old, open general surgical ward. However, a small treatment room with a limited ventilation system (e.g. extractor fans) may be useful for preparing trolleys and for carrying out minor procedures on walking patients. This system should be adequate if single rooms are available for patients with wounds infected by organisms likely to be transmitted in the air (e.g. antibiotic-resistant *Staph. aureus*).

Dressing materials

The functions of a dressing are to provide conditions which promote healing, to protect the wound against contamination which may lead to sepsis and consequent delay in healing, and to prevent the transfer of micro-organisms from an infected wound to other patients. Gauze swabs supplied in standard dressing packs are not the most suitable of dressing materials, as they tend to adhere to the wound and to become soaked through by exudate ('strike-through'). The healing process is thus disturbed, and once the dressing is soaked through there is no barrier to the passage of micro-organisms to or from the environment. For the dressing of burns, gauze dressings with antimicrobial creams have been found effective and not adherent.

Dressing materials vary in certain properties, e.g. absorbency, non-adhesion, semi-permeability, impermeability, which are relevant to their functional effectiveness. Clean, undrained wounds seldom require dressing if they can be adequately protected against contact and friction. Where a dressing is required, a material having properties appropriate to the nature of the wound should be selected. For discharging wounds, an occlusive, membranous dressing impervious to bacteria but permeable to water vapour (e.g. 'Opsite') may often be effective. A similar dressing may be applied to discharging lesions, such as varicose ulcers or bedsores, before operations, to protect the operation wound against contamination from these prolific sources of wound pathogens.

111

Dressing techniques

These are described in Appendix 8.1. They may require modification in the light of further studies or under special circumstances. Some general principles are considered here.

It is usual to recommend that ward cleaning should cease 30 min, and curtains should be drawn 10 min, before a dressing is started, but the evidence suggests that the recommended routine cleaning methods (see Chapter 7) do not significantly increase the numbers of airborne organisms. Certain other procedures may disperse much larger numbers of organisms into the air. These include bed-making, high dusting and changing curtains. It is often impractical to stipulate that all these activities must cease while dressings are in progress, particularly on wards where patient allocation or team nursing is practised, though it is clearly desirable that they should be avoided if possible and, if unavoidable, reduced to a minimum. It is more practical to ensure that these procedures do not take place in the immediate vicinity of the bed where the dressing is being done. To reduce opportunities for airborne contamination to a minimum, a wound should be exposed for the minimum time and dressings should be removed carefully and placed quickly in a bag and sealed; a large paper or plastic bag should be available for disposal of large dressings.

CSSD packs should be supplied in dispenser racks or boxes, stored in a preparation room and transferred to the dressing trolley when required. All instruments should be supplied by the CSSD and chemical disinfection before use should now be unnecessary. However, it may, on rare occasions, be necessary to disinfect a clean instrument (e.g. when there is a shortage of sterile supplies and the ward has no sterilizer); immersion in 0.5% alcoholic chlorhexidine for 5-10 min should then be adequate. It must be realized, however, that this is an emergency procedure, and the instrument, though probably free from staphylococci and other vegetative organisms, will not necessarily be sterile. The dressing trolley should be thoroughly cleaned at the beginning of a dressing round and the top may be disinfected, if this is thought necessary, with 70% alcohol or a clear soluble phenolic disinfectant. The top of the trolley must be dry before the sterilized paper pack is placed on it.

An aseptic or non-touch technique is important. Forceps are usually used, but sterile, disposable gloves (or a sterile plastic bag, enclosing a hand) could with advantage be used more often, particularly for removing large, contaminated dressings. The chance of dispersing organisms may be further reduced by inverting the glove (or plastic bag) over the dressing and discarding both together.

The dressing-pack should be opened carefully with washed hands as instructed. The paper working surface should lie flat on the trolley top and should never be flattened with the fingers. Forceps used for removal of stitches or for inserting safety-pins in drains should be capable of holding the sutures or the pin firmly; otherwise gloved fingers should be used.

Clean wounds (apart from burns and certain extensive traumatic wounds, q.v. in Chapter 15) should not be treated with antiseptics or antibiotics. Cleaning around a clean wound is rarely required, but sterile normal saline may be used if considered necessary. 'Savlon' (1%), a mixture of cetrimide with chlorhexidine, is a detergent preparation with some antiseptic activity (see Chapter 6) commonly

112

used for cleaning dirty wounds and burns. If an antiseptic is considered necessary, 0.2-0.5% aqueous chlorhexidine is suitable; a calcium hypochlorite solution with boric acid or with bicarbonate (e.g. 'Eusol') is commonly used for cleaning septic wounds.

If dressings on clean and dry wounds without drainage are thought to be necessary, they should be left until the stitches are removed unless there are signs of infection or leakage. These wounds are unlikely to become infected in the ward, and depending on surgical approval may be left after the first 24 hours without a covering dressing. Drained wounds should be covered with a dressing until the drainage wound is healed and dry. This may not be necessary with very small drains with a closed drainage system, e.g. Redivac, until after removal. Drains should not be used unless absolutely necessary and should be removed as quickly as possible. If required at all, drainage must be adequate and may, therefore, require large drains, but Redivac and other small tube drains are less likely to be associated with acquired infection. Contaminated wounds (e.g. after colectomy, abdomino-perineal excision of rectum, and operations on pelvic abscess), though initially infected with the patient's own sensitive organisms, may acquire antibiotic-resistant hospital strains if care is not taken with aseptic techniques. All discharging wounds should be adequately covered, and dressings must be changed immediately if they are soaked; organisms readily penetrate wet dressings.

Septic wounds and contaminated wounds (e.g. colostomy) should be dressed at the end of the dressing list. Sutures should be removed at the beginning of the list. The use of absorbable sutures may allow a patient to be sent home earlier; any procedure which reduces the patient's time in hospital, either pre- or postoperatively, will reduce the hazards of infection.

Injections

Although the risk of infection is small, cleaning of the skin with 70% ethyl or isopropyl alcohol before giving an injection is recommended for hospital patients. The alcohol should be rubbed vigorously on to the skin with a gauze or other swab.

Intravenous infusions

The rubber plug or diaphragm of the infusion container must be swabbed with 70% ethyl or isopropyl alcohol before the cannula is introduced or solutions are added. The setting up of intravenous infusions should be carried out with strict aseptic precautions; special attention should be paid to hand disinfection, and the skin of the infusion site should not be palpated after disinfection. The patient's skin and hands of the operator should be disinfected thoroughly with 70% ethyl or isopropyl alcohol, with or without added chlorhexidine. The wearing of masks is unnecessary, but a disposable plastic apron should be worn.

The infusion container should be inspected for faults, leaks or particulate contamination before connecting to the drip set, and if any of these are present it must be discarded. It is important to recognize that the fluid may remain clear

113

despite the presence of significant numbers of micro-organisms. Check that the cotton wool plug is present in the airway, and if wet at any time the plug should be changed. To prevent infection at the drip site, cover with a dry dressing and strap tubing to skin to prevent movement of cannula or needle. If an antibacterial agent is required, spray with povidone-iodine daily or on changing the dressing (though this is of uncertain value). The drip should be changed at least every 48 hours (and always after infusion of blood), and the cannula should be changed if possible after 2–3 days. The drip site should be inspected daily. If there are signs of phlebitis or infection the cannula should be removed; a swab from the site and the tip of the cannula should be sent to the laboratory. If indicated a blood culture should also be taken.

Therapeutic substances should be added to i.v. infusion containers only when absolutely necessary and must never be injected into glucose-containing or nutrient solutions or into blood or its products which are excellent culture media for bacteria. Intravenous fluids which remain unused after being connected to a drip set must be discarded and not re-used. It is often recommended, if a sterile drug has to be added to intravenous infusion fluids, that this should be done with strict asepsis in the pharmacy and not in the ward. Nevertheless, trained medical or nursing staff can often more conveniently carry out this procedure on the ward. Provided the fluid is used immediately, the risk of infection is small; most intravenous fluids will not support the growth of organisms commonly present in the air.

Hyperalimentation therapy

The administration of intravenous fluids containing protein hydrolysates, dextrose and other components such as vitamins and trace elements has increased in recent years. The risk of infection is particularly great because of the possible long period of treatment with a catheter in a central vein and the likelihood of bacterial or fungal growth in the fluid. Few organisms grow in normal saline or dextrose-saline but Gram-negative bacilli and especially yeasts are able to grow in the hyperalimentation fluid. Septicaemia is a common complication. Prevention of infection depends on scrupulous aseptic techniques both in inserting the cannula and in the subsequent daily care. The hyperalimentation fluid should if possible be provided in its container ready for administration but if additions are required, these should be added in a laminar flow cabinet in the pharmacy. The fluid should be preferably used immediately, but if not should be kept at 4° C. The giving set should be changed at least every 24 hours and the fluid more frequently. If any signs of infection appear, the catheter should be removed and cultures taken as described above. Bacteraemia or fungaemia may resolve on removal of the catheter, but treatment should not be delayed if signs of infection persist. Filters are often used to reduce risks of infection from intrinsically contaminated solutions and appear to be microbiologically effective, but their value in the prevention of clinical infection remains uncertain.

Collection of clinical specimens for laboratory examination

Hazards of infection, both to patients and to staff, occur during collection of specimens, during transport to the laboratory and during examinations in the laboratory. The last of these hazards is discussed in Chapter 16 (p. 278). The following notes are not a guide to techniques for collecting laboratory specimens, but consider infection hazards in the collection and delivery of specimens and how they may be prevented.

Faulty technique during collection may result in inadequate, misleading or delayed laboratory reports which may affect a patient's treatment, including management of infection. During collection, especially of urine specimens, the patient may become infected. The nurse may be infected by contamination of the hands or clothing or by inhalation of infected aerosol material during transfer to the containers. During transit the person transmitting the specimen may be infected by contaminants on the outside of the container, or through leakage or breakage of the container. In addition the environment may become contaminated during these procedures and lead to an indirect spread of infection. Laboratory staff receiving unlabelled, potentially hazardous material (e.g. sputum from a patient with suspected pulmonary tuberculosis, or blood from one with suspected hepatitis) are also at risk. To ensure correct investigation, specimens should be correctly labelled and accompanying request forms should contain appropriate and adequate clinical details. Specimens should not be collected by inexperienced or untrained staff, unless under close supervision.

Swabs

Swabs collected from infected sites such as the throat, infected surgical wounds or vagina should be transferred carefully to the swab container and inserted slowly to avoid contamination of the rim of the container with infected material. The container should be held as near to the infected site as possible to avoid shaking infected material in the air. If a spatula has been used, this should be discarded unbroken into the waste container; the jerking movements involved in breaking a spatula may cause infected material to be released into the air. The swab should be sent to the laboratory as soon as possible. Where there is a heavy discharge of pus from an infected wound or abscess, it is preferable to send a sample of pus in a sterile universal container, rather than a swab.

Faecal specimens

These should be collected from a bedpan with a small wooden applicator, and sent as soon as possible to the laboratory. For bacteriological examination only, a small amount of faeces, approximately the size of a pea, is all that is necessary. There is no need to fill a container. A water-proofed container with a wide mouth and a tight fitting screw cap is essential, so that the specimen can be easily placed in the container and leakage does not occur. Samples of faeces collected on bacteriological swabs (especially rectal swabs) are usually unsuitable, although a sample of liquid faeces may be collected in hospital by this method. If a rectal swab is taken, ensure that faeces are actually sampled; most anal specimens are useless.

Urine specimens

The organisms which are found in urinary tract infections, apart from renal tuberculosis and typhoid fever, are not usually infective for the person collecting the specimen; faulty collection technique, however, may lead to contamination of the specimen and an erroneous diagnosis of urinary infection when this does not exist. Specimens should be collected with care, following the prescribed technique exactly and sent as soon as possible to the laboratory. Examination of the urine is necessary before contaminating bacteria begin to multiply in it.

Infection can be introduced into a patient while a specimen is collected from an indwelling catheter, and care must be taken to avoid this (see Chapter 16).

Urine is a good culture medium for bacteria; specimens collected for ward testing should not be allowed to 'go stale' but should be tested promptly or sent to the laboratory within 2 or 3 hours.

Aspirated fluids (including CSF)

Equipment used to aspirate fluids from thoracic cavity, joints, cerebrospinal space, facial sinuses etc., must be supplied sterile from CSSD. An effective skin disinfectant, such as 70% ethyl alcohol is used to prepare the site. Antibacterial agents with a strong residual effect (e.g. chlorhexidine) should preferably not be used if bacteriological examination of the aspirate is required. When cerebro-spinal fluid (CSF) is aspirated from patients with certain infectious diseases (e.g. poliomyelitis or meningococcal meningitis) a protective mask (see Chapter 9) should be worn; the organisms may be highly infectious, and some degree of aerosol production is almost unavoidable when screw caps and syringes are handled. It may also be advisable on rare occasions to wear a protective mask when aspirating purulent fluids from other sites, though in general a mask is not essential for these procedures. Wearing of gloves is not essential, but great care must be taken to avoid contamination of the skin with pus. Having collected the fluid, the operator should disconnect the needle (if any) and expel the material gently into the container, avoiding spraying of droplets or release of aerosols.

Sputum specimens

It is often difficult to obtain a specimen of sputum without contamination of the rim and outside wall of the vessel, and contamination will occur even when wide mouthed glass bottles are used. Some protection to porters and laboratory staff can be given if, after collection of the specimen, the rim and outside of the vessel are wiped with a paper tissue to remove any major contamination before putting on the lid of the container. The tissue should be discarded into a 'soiled dressing' or similar disposal bag. Should the patient be suspected of having tuberculosis, gloves should be used for handling the container, which should be placed in a small plastic bag and sealed before transport to the laboratory.

Blood specimens

In addition to hepatitis (see Chapters 5, 18 and 19) several other infection, including typhoid fever, can be acquired from blood specimens. Blood specimens should, therefore, be regarded as potentially infected and care should be taken to avoid the dispersal of droplets which occurs when the blood is squirted vigorously into the container. Before discharging blood into a container, the needle should be separated from the syringe, using forceps (DHSS, 1978). In cases of known hepatitis, some prefer to leave the needle attached; after carefully

116

discharging the contents, the syringe and needle are discarded together into a suitable container. Nozzles of syringes should not be broken before discarding, since the hazard of acquisition of the syringe by a drug addict is much less than the danger of an infected aerosol. The hands should be thoroughly washed after taking a blood sample.

For protection of the patient during collection of blood specimens, only autoclaved or presterilized disposable equipment should be used. When finger prick specimens are taken an individual needle is essential; this should preferably be disposable. The Hagedorn needle in spirit should no longer be considered acceptable as an instrument for collection of capillary blood specimens.

Bone marrow biopsy

Many laboratories still maintain and sterilize their own bone marrow biopsy equipment. While there are advantages in having the equipment readily available, it is preferable for it to be supplied by the CSSD, since the sterilizing facilities are more suitable and better needle-sharpening facilities are usually available in the CSSD. The biopsy procedure can often be carried out in an open ward without special risk of infection, but the patient (e.g. with leukaemia or aplastic anaemia) is often particularly susceptible to infection, in which case a side room should be used for the procedure (if the patient is not already under protective isolation in single-bed room). Adequate skin preparation with 0.5% alcoholic chlorhexidine or alcoholic solutions of iodine or iodophor is essential; prophylactic antibiotic cover is not necessary. A dry dressing should be placed over the puncture wound and left in place for 3–4 days.

Infective agents, including tubercle bacilli and brucella, may be present in the bone marrow; care must therefore be taken to avoid aerosols during preparation of microscope films and on expulsion of the contents of the syringe. Films should be allowed to dry naturally and not waved in the air.

Renal biopsy; liver biopsy

These procedures are rarely followed by infection if the equipment is properly sterilized and the skin adequately disinfected. In many hospitals they are performed on open wards without hazard. Masks are unnecessary; gloves are not essential but they are desirable. However, care is necessary when taking tissue for biopsies from a jaundiced patient (see above on blood specimens). Tests for hepatitis B antigen (HB_sAg) in blood should be made before liver biopsy is undertaken.

Miscellaneous procedures

Ward equipment

Cleaning and disinfection of many items of equipment, including nail-brushes, soap dishes, shaving equipment, thermometers, bedpans, urinals, suction, gastric aspiration and rectal equipment, beds, bedding and curtains are considered in Chapter 7.

117

Washing and bathing

Patients should use wash-basins in the washing areas whenever possible and their own soap, hand and bath towels and other toilet requisites. Communal towels should not be available. Bathing or showering in the bathroom is preferred to bed-baths, but if bed-baths are necessary, patients should have their own individual wash-bowls. If not possible, bowls should be disinfected between use by different patients (see Chapter 7). Water from the wash-bowls should be emptied into a sink and not into a bucket on the bathing trolley. Bathroom furniture should be simple, easily cleaned and reduced to a minimum and the bathroom should not be used as a store room.

Communal bath mats should not be used; patients should use a towel, unless disposable mats can be supplied. A routine of cleaning baths after each use should be instituted, and the nurse or orderly responsible for bathing patients should be responsible for cleaning. Instructions as to the correct method of cleaning the bath or wash-basins should be given to staff and also to patients if they are expected to clean their own bath. Cleaning is particularly important before and after a bath if the patient has an open wound; such patients should preferably not use a bath used by pre-operative patients. Showers would overcome this problem to some extent. Salt is still commonly added to the bath-water, but the practice has little if any value as an antimicrobial measure. If disinfection of the bath-water is required, add a sachet of povidone-iodine ('Steribath'); if activity is required against *Staph. aureus* only and not against Gram-negative bacilli, hexachlorophane or 'Savlon' is effective. Disinfection of the bath-water is necessary only during outbreaks in a ward or as part of the treatment for infected patients or carriers. Disinfection of the bath before and after use is still necessary even if a disinfectant is added to the bath-water.

Pre-operative preparation (see also Chapter 7, p. 73 and Chapter 10)

Patients should be admitted preferably on the day before operation and should have a shower rather than a bath. If a bath is required, this should be disinfected as recommended above. Pre-operative shaving should be carried out on the day of operation to reduce risks of infection from small cuts or abrasions. It may be possible to avoid shaving altogether by the use of clippers, a chemical depilatory cream, or possibly an electric razor. The head of the electric razor or clippers (not the motor) should be disinfected by immersion in 70% alcohol for 5 min before use. Shaving-brushes should not be used and only staff who are skilled should shave patients, so that local trauma can be reduced to a minimum. Preliminary disinfection of the operation sites in the ward is not usually necessary, but may be desirable for some orthopaedic or other special operations. A greater reduction in organisms on the skin can be obtained by repeated treatment.

Treatment of pressure areas

Staff carrying out these treatments should wash their hands between patients. Patients with bedsores should be treated as infected and nursed in isolation, if this is indicated from clinical and bacteriological examination (e.g. if profuse discharge is present; also if multiresistant organisms are isolated). All open areas should be treated as wounds. If these patients are bed-bathed, the water should be disposed of carefully without splashing since it may be heavily contaminated. Nurses carrying out these procedures should wear disposable plastic aprons. *Staphylococcus aureus* are often dispersed in large numbers from healed as well as open pressure sores.

Mouth-cleaning and dentures

The mouth and throat of ill persons, particularly on antibiotic treatment, are often colonized by Gram-negative bacilli or by *Candida*. Equipment used for mouth cleaning should be disposable whenever possible, or should be disinfected by heat (autoclaved); mouth packs can often be supplied by the CSSD. If glycerine and thymol is used, it should be supplied in small containers and discarded daily. Dentures may be stored in the patient's own preparation (e.g. 'Steradent'), but if this is not available a weak hypochlorite solution may be used (e.g. 'Milton' 1/80). Solutions should be changed daily. Paper-bags should be supplied for disposal of cottonwool, paper wipes etc.

Respiratory suction techniques

A no-touch technique with either forceps or gloves should be used for the suction procedure. In suspected cases of pulmonary or laryngeal tuberculosis, the operator should wear a mask to protect the wearer (see Chapter 9).

Disposal of sputum

Containers should be disposable and large enough to contain paper handkerchiefs discarded by the patients after wiping the mouth. Containers should be regularly discarded and the responsibility for this task should be clearly defined. Used containers should be placed in a plastic bag and well sealed to await collection (see also the section on secretion and exudate precautions in Chapter 9).

Eyes

Hands should be thoroughly washed before carrying out any procedures, and a no-touch technique should be used. Cottonwool, fluids or ointments should be sterilized (see Chapter 15).

Dead bodies

Most bodies are not infective and no special care is necessary; washing the body with soap and water is adequate. Bedding can be disposed of in the usual way, and mattresses, pillows, bed-frames may be cleaned by the recommended routine. Sterilization (or even disinfection) of these or other items associated with the patient is not necessary, unless death was due to a communicable disease. For details on disposal of infected dead bodies see Chapter 9.

A note on carpets (or soft flooring materials) in hospital wards

There is no evidence that carpets are an infection hazard in hospitals. If installed in surgical wards or similar patient areas, the carpets should have a waterproof backing and joints should be sealed. Pile fibres should be water-repellent and non-absorbent. Ease of cleaning and rate of drying are improved by having a pile

119

of short upright fibres. The carpet should be washable and not damaged by application of commonly used disinfectants. Carpet should be vacuum cleaned daily and periodically wet cleaned with specially designed equipment, e.g. steam cleaners or machines with a vacuum pick-up. Most carpets in heavily contaminated areas, e.g. units for the mentally subnormal, are inadequately maintained; carpets are not recommended in these areas unless frequent cleaning with special equipment is possible.

Appendix 8.1 Use of packs in surgical procedures

Preparation of trolley and patient. General principles

The patient is screened and the procedure is explained. The nurse washes her hands or applies 70% or 95% alcohol, and prepares the trolley. At the beginning of each dressing-round, the trolley may be either washed or wiped with 70% alcohol (or a phenolic disinfectant) and allowed to dry.

The requisite pack, supplementary packs, lotions and non-sterile items such as bandages, adhesive plaster and dressing scissors are placed on the lower shelf of the trolley. Lotions should be kept in small containers and preferably replaced daily.

The trolley is taken to the bed-side and the patient prepared. Bed-clothes and clothing are gently removed to expose the appropriate site and the patient is placed in a suitable position.

The dressing pack is opened and the inner pack is placed in the centre of the trolley top. A bag of adequate size is fixed to the side of the trolley nearest to the patient for soiled dressings, and another bag is fixed to the opposite side for soiled and unused instruments. On completion of the procedure, instruments are placed in one bag (or directly into the used instrument container) and the unused dressings and disposables are rolled up in the paper towel covering the trolley top and placed in the soiled dressings bag. In the preparation room, the instruments are discarded into a detergent disinfectant solution which is replaced daily and supplied by the CSSD. The used dressing bag is discarded into a large plastic or paper sack. Hands are washed on completion of the procedure.

Routine dressing technique

The trolley and patient are prepared as already described. The inner wrap is opened, handling corners only, and forms the sterile field. Supplementary packs are opened and the contents are gently slid onto the sterile field.

The pack contents are arranged using handling forceps and handles of instruments are placed in a small defined handling area near the edge of the trolley. The lotion, if required, is poured into the gallipot.

The adhesive plaster is loosened and the dressing is removed with handling forceps (or gloves) and discarded into the soiled dressing bag. The forceps (if not disposable) are placed in the other bag. If gloves are used to remove the old dressing, they should be removed and replaced with sterile gloves before picking up the clean dressing. Clips or sutures are removed if necessary and the dressing

120

completed using two pairs of sterile forceps. After securing the dressing, instruments and unused or soiled materials are placed in bags as described. If two nurses are available, the assistant prepares the patient, opens the outer bag of the pack and supplementary packs and pours the lotions. The dresser prepares the trolley and the sterile field and carries out the dressing technique.

Catheterization

The patient, trolley and sterile field are prepared as already described. In male patients the penis is held with sterile gauze, the foreskin is retracted if necessary and glans and external meatus are thoroughly cleaned with sterile saline. The local anaesthetic is inserted into the urethra. The nurse opens the catheter packet and the catheter is slid into a sterile receiver. A surgical drape is placed over the patient's thigh and the receiver with the catheter is placed between the patient's thighs. The penis is held with sterile gauze and the catheter is passed into the bladder. Catheters should be handled only with sterile gloves or forceps and should not be touched unless sterile gloves are worn. The catheter on removal is discarded into the soiled dressing bag.

If two nurses are available the assistant prepares the patient, opens the outer bag and supplementary packs and pours the lotion. The assistant also opens the catheter pack and slides it carefully into the sterile receiver.

Similar procedures are used for female catheterization. The vulva and urethral orifice are cleaned thoroughly with sterile saline. The labia are held apart with a gloved hand or with sterile gauze after cleaning and during the insertion of the catheter.

Lumbar puncture

The nurse, after preparation of patient and trolley, opens the inner wrap by handling the corners only. She then slides the contents of the supplementary packs onto the sterile field.

The doctor washes and dries his hands and arranges the pack contents on the sterile field with handling forceps. Sterile gloves may be worn if preferred. The nurse pours the lotion into the gallipot. The doctor arranges the surgical drapes in position, swabs the lumbar region with a 1% alcoholic solution of iodine or 0.5% solution of chlorhexidine in 70% ethyl alcohol and injects local anaesthetic. The manometer is prepared and the lumbar puncture needle inserted. Specimens are collected as required. The nurse applies a dressing after the needle has been removed.

Similar procedures are used for chest and other aspirations.

References and Further Reading

Ayliffe, G. A. J., Brightwell, K. M., Collins, B. J. and Lowbury, E. J. L. (1969), Varieties of aseptic practice in hospital wards. *Lancet*, ii, 1117.
Department of Health and Social Security (1978), *Code of Practice for the*

Prevention of Infection in Clinical Laboratories and Post-mortem Rooms, HMSO, London.

Phillips, I., Meers, P. and D'Arcy, P. F. (1976), *Microbiological Hazards in Infusion Therapy.* M.T.P. Press Ltd., Lancaster.

Taylor, L. J. (1978), Evaluation of hand washing techniques, Parts 1 and 2, *Nursing Times,* 74, 54 and 108.

CHAPTER NINE

Prevention of Infection in Wards (2) Isolation of Patients

Introduction

The spread of infection to patients in hospital can be controlled by physical protection (isolation); the extent of this control varies with the methods used. Isolation for control of infection is applied in two ways: (1) *source (or 'containment') isolation* — the isolation of infected patients to prevent the transfer of their infection to others; and (2) *protective (or 'reverse') isolation*, to prevent the transfer of infective micro-organisms to patients at special risk from infection (those with diminished resistance because of their illness or treatment — e.g. the use of immunosuppressive drugs). In some patients, e.g. those with extensive burns, combined source and protective isolation is desirable to protect patients already infected with one pathogen against infection with other pathogens.

Methods of physical protection

The methods of physical protection are:

(a) *Barrier nursing* — special nursing procedures which reduce the risks of transferring infective organisms from person to person, especially by direct contact or by way of fomites.
(b) *Segregation* in single rooms, cubicles or plastic isolators which reduces airborne spread to and from patients, and facilitates nursing techniques.
(c) *Mechanical ventilation*, which reduces the risks of airborne spread by removing bacteria from the patient's room and, in protective isolation, by excluding from the room bacteria present in the outside air.

The transfer of infection by the airborne route, e.g. respiratory infections, can be controlled only by confining the patient in a single room, whether for source or protective isolation. On the other hand, the control of diseases spread by contact, such as enteric fever, depends primarily on barrier nursing.

The term *isolation* is commonly used in the sense of segregation of the patient in a single room; it is used here to include all methods by which the patient may be physically protected, including barrier nursing in an open ward. *Barrier nursing*, like single room accommodation and mechanical ventilation, is one of the basic components of patient isolation and can be used on its own or together with the other components.

123

Modes of spread of infection in wards (Table 9.1)

Direct contact spread means transfer of infection to the patient by direct contact with an infected person or with a healthy carrier of a virulent organism. *Indirect contact spread* means transfer of such organisms on needles, instruments, bedding and other 'fomites', in food, or on the hands of staff. This includes the transfer of dysentery and other intestinal infections through faecal contamination — the 'faecal-oral' route. *Airborne spread* refers to spread of infection through the air in small droplets from the mouth, or on skin scales, or in dust particles. Some infections are transmitted by more than one route, e.g. staphylococcal infections, which can be spread by direct and indirect contact and also by airborne transfer; and poliomyelitis, which may be acquired either by inhalation or ingestion.

Infections unlikely to spread in hospital

Actinomycosis, amoebiasis, aspergillosis, brucellosis, cat scratch fever, cryptococcosis, histoplasmosis, infectious mononucleosis (glandular fever), leptospirosis, pneumonia (pneumococcal), rabies, rheumatic fever, tetanus, toxocara infections, toxoplasmosis and worm infestations are unlikely to be transmitted in hospital. *Some special precautions* are necessary for some of these diseases (see p. 136, and Chapter 13).

Varieties of accommodation for isolating patients

There are various types of isolation offering different degrees of protection:

(1) Smallpox hospitals

These provide maximum security, are reserved entirely for smallpox, and are normally independent of other hospitals.

(2) High security isolation units

These are usually part of an infectious diseases hospital, and have facilities for treating patients with highly communicable viral infections, having a high mortality rate and no definitive treatment, e.g. Lassa, Marburg and Ebola fevers. Total environmental control is usually achieved by the use of negative pressure plastic isolators. At the time of writing, there are five such units in the United Kingdom.

(3) Infectious diseases hospitals

At the present time these units are usually separate from other hospital buildings but may be situated in the grounds of a general hospital. If so, separate ventilation and nursing staff should be provided. Facilities are available for the treatment of all infections, excluding smallpox and the African vital haemorrhagic fevers. Patients are admitted both from the community and from other hospitals.

(4) General hospital isolation units

These provide source isolation facilities for hospital-acquired infections; they also provide facilities for protective isolation and for the screening of patients with suspected infections before admission to a general ward or transfer to a communicable diseases unit (1, 2 or 3 above).

(5) Single rooms of a general ward (ward side rooms)

These provide less secure *source isolation* than (3) because of close proximity to other patients and sharing of nursing and domestic staff with a general ward. Their value in *protective isolation* depends on the types of patient in the general ward, on the thoroughness of barrier nursing, on whether the room is self-contained (with w.c. and ablutions) and on the type of ventilation used.

(6) Barrier nursing in open ward

Can be effective in controlling infections transferred by contact but not by air; room isolation is preferable.

(7) Isolators in open wards

Plastic enclosures ('Isolators') for individual patients have been shown to be of value as a form of protective isolation for high risk patients and of source isolation for infected patients.

(8) Ultra-clean wards

Experimental units have been set up in special centres for organ transplantation, treatment of leukaemia, chorion-carcinoma and other diseases associated with extreme susceptibility to infection.

At present very few general hospitals have satisfactory isolation units or even a sufficient number of single rooms for the treatment of patients suffering from, or particularly susceptible to, infection. The size of a general hospital isolation unit would depend on a number of factors, including availability of single room accommodation in the general wards (which should have not less than two), proximity of a major communicable diseases unit and the size of the hospital. The number of rooms in such a unit might vary from six to twenty, depending on the above factors. A proportion of these rooms (about one third) should have an appropriate form of mechanical ventilation for the treatment of 'high-risk' patients — those with increased susceptibility to infection, e.g. patients on immunosuppressive therapy or with extensive burns, and those suffering from severe infections which are likely to spread by air. Since these wards are likely to contain ill patients from all areas of the hospital and since they are in individual rooms, a much higher nurse/patient ratio (e.g. two nurses to one patient over the 24-hour period) is required than in general wards. A specially trained team of domestic workers should be available for cleaning isolation rooms or units.

125

Table 9.1 Mode of spread of transmissible diseases in hospital

Diseases	*Routes and possible routes of transfer*		
	Airborne	*Contact*	
		Faecal–oral route	*Personal and/or fomites*
Anthrax	X		X
Campylobacter enteritis		X	X
Candidiasis			X
Chickenpox	X		X
Cholera		X	X
Diphtheria	X		X
Eczema vaccinatum	X		X
Fungal infections (skin)			X
Gastro-enteritis in babies		X	X
Gonococcal ophthalmia necnatorum			X
Hepatitis (infectious and serum)		X	X
Herpes zoster	X		X
Influenza	X		X
Legionnaire's disease	X		X
Measles	X		X
Meningitis			
(a) meningococcal	X		X
(b) viral	X	X	X
Mumps	X		X
Plague	X		X
Pneumonia (viral)	X		X
Poliomyelitis	X	X	X
Psittacosis	X		X
Q Fever	X	X	X
Rubella	X		X
Salmonella and shigella infections		X	X
Scabies			X
Smallpox	X		X
Staphylococcal disease	X		X
Streptococcal disease	X		X
Syphilis (mucocutaneous)			X
Tuberculosis (open)	X		X
Typhoid and paratyphoid		X	X
Vaccinia (see Eczema vaccinatum)	X		X
Viral haemorrhagic fevers	X	X	X
Whooping cough	X		X
Wound infection	X		X

Categories of isolation

Some infections are more likely to spread than others and a higher degree of strictness is required in the source isolation of such diseases. The term *strict isolation* is used to describe the isolation procedure for highly transmissible and for dangerous infections. The term *standard isolation* is used to describe methods used for other transmissible infections; some variation in nursing procedure is required, depending on the nature of the infection. The term *protective isolation* is used to describe methods of isolation for highly susceptible patients.

Details of these three categories of isolation* are presented below:

Standard isolation

Although it is recognized that special precautions may sometimes be necessary for certain categories of infection, e.g. respiratory or enteric, we propose a standard technique for all patients requiring isolation in a general hospital. This also includes most patients requiring protective as well as source isolation. All staff should wear a gown or apron when attending to a patient or when in close contact with the patient's immediate surroundings and should wash their hands on leaving the cubicle (also on entering if the patient requires protection). Masks are usually unnecessary and caps and overshoes are not required. Additional requirements in the ward are a bedpan washer/disinfector and a washing-up machine which reaches a suitable temperature for disinfection. Discipline of the staff is of major importance, especially in hand-washing, keeping door closed, disinfection of baths, toilets and bedpans, care in taking blood samples and disposal of materials from virus hepatitis carriers. It is easier to maintain rigid and minimal practices than to observe a long list of rules without defining priorities. However, modifications can be made if necessary, e.g. gowns or aprons are unnecessary for the common childhood infectious diseases and for most respiratory infections. A ventilation system (consisting at least of an extractor fan) is also advantageous for patients with communicable respiratory infections, especially chickenpox, and probably also for heavy staphylococcal dispersers. Enteric precautions are always necessary for diarrhoeal diseases and enteric fever. It is also necessary to ensure staff are protected against tuberculosis, poliomyelitis and rubella. Evidence of an infection with mumps, measles and chickenpox should be recorded and immunization against measles should be considered in the non-immune staff of paediatric or isolation wards.

(1) Room

If a single room is necessary, the door should be kept closed at all times, except for necessary entrances and exits. An extraction fan may be fitted. Any unnecessary furniture should be removed before admitting the patient. The room may then be equipped with special items needed to nurse the patient, e.g. pedal bins, plastic bags, thermometer, coat hangers for gowns, etc. All equipment should be kept inside the room, and the room should be kept tidy to facilitate nursing and cleaning procedures.

*Modified from US Dept. Health, Education and Welfare (1970).

(2) Gowns or aprons

Disposable plastic aprons are recommended and may under most circumstances be used in an isolation room for one day. Cotton gowns provide limited protection, but are acceptable in most circumstances. Gowns made of water-repellent materials (e.g. ventile or suitable non-woven materials) which have low permeability to bacteria give better protection. Some gowns (e.g. ventile) may be uncomfortable to wear, and disposable gowns are likely to be expensive. The gown or apron should be left hanging in the room and changed daily, or earlier when obviously soiled. Although disposable aprons are preferred, non-disposable plastic aprons may be used and should be disinfected by heat, if possible. The front of plastic aprons may be disinfected by spraying and wiping with 70% alcohol after contact with the patient. Disposable, water-repellent gowns with low permeability to bacteria are preferred to aprons for strict isolation techniques.

(3) Gloves

Conventional, disposable plastic gloves are adequate for handling infected sites or contaminated materials. Long sleeved disposable gloves may be used when protection of the arms is necessary.

(4) Masks

These are rarely necessary; if used they should be of the filter type (see Chapter 8).

(5) Hands

Hand-washing before and after contact with the patient is perhaps the most important measure in preventing the spread of infection. Either a non-medicated soap or a detergent antiseptic preparation should be adequate for routine purposes, but 70% alcohol is more effective in removing transient as well as resident flora and should be used in high risk situations, as described elsewhere (see Chapters 7 and 8).

(6) Equipment

Disposable or autoclavable equipment should be used whenever possible. Items such as the sphygmomanometer and stethoscope should be left in the room and terminally disinfected when the patient is discharged. Hard surfaces may be disinfected by wiping with a clear soluble phenolic disinfectant or a hypochlorite solution. Other equipment may be disinfected by wiping with 70% alcohol. Sphygmomanometer cuffs may be disinfected, if necessary (e.g. on discharge of the patient or when contaminated with known pathogens) by low temperature steam.

(7) Needles and syringes

These should be disposable. Both the needle and the syringe should be placed in a separate container such as a cardboard box which should be sealed before sending for disposal.

(8) Dressings

For notes on dressing techniques see Chapter 8 and Appendix 8.1; also notes on secretion and exudate precautions below.

(9) Thermometers

The thermometer should be kept in the isolation room until the patient is discharged (for treatment see Chapter 7).

(10) Linen

Avoid vigorous bed-making. Linen from infected patients should be placed in a colour-coded linen bag for transfer to the laundry. Linen which may present a hazard to laundry staff, e.g. from patients with open pulmonary tuberculosis, hepatitis or enteric fever, should first be sealed in a hot water-soluble or alginate-stitched bag. The outer bag should be labelled to indicate that the contents should not be handled. Wet linen may be placed in a clear plastic bag which is then placed in the infected linen bag (see Chapter 11).

(11) Plastic mattress covers and plastic pillow covers

See Chapter 7, p. 81.

(12) Crockery and cutlery

Disposable items may be used when a dishwasher heating the water to over 80° C is not available. Food should be placed in polythene bags and discarded with ward waste.

(13) Laboratory specimens

Some warning should be given to laboratory staff when sending blood samples from patients with infectious or serum hepatitis, faeces from patients requiring enteric precautions, suspected tuberculous material etc. Containers should be placed in a plastic bag and labelled 'Biohazard' (see Chapter 16).

(14) Charts

Patients' charts should be kept outside the contaminated areas, if only to discourage frequent visits to the room. The infective hazard of contamination from charts, however, is very small.

(15) Transporting patients

Patients should be sent to other departments only if it is essential to do so. The department in question should be notified in advance, so that they may make arrangements to prevent possible spread of infection. It may be advisable for the order in which patients visit other departments to be arranged in advance.

(16) Secretion, excretion and exudate precautions

(Precautions against infected oral or other secretions, or against pus and other infected exudates).

(a) **Oral.** Patients should be encouraged to cough or spit into paper tissue and then discard this into a plastic bag.

(b) **Exudate.** A 'non-touch' technique using forceps or disposable gloves should be used and contaminated material should be placed in sealed paper or plastic bags. Bags containing contaminated materials should be placed in a pedal-bin lined with a plastic bag.

(c) **Excretion.** For patients with enteric fever, dysentery, cholera and other infections spread by urine or faeces, disposable gloves should be worn to take the bedpan from the patient to the disposal area; it is necessary for the nurse to put on a plastic gown to prevent contamination of the uniform. The pan should be covered with a disposable paper bag before transport. Gloves should be placed in a plastic bag after use. Disposable gloves and a plastic apron or gown should be worn to handle contaminated equipment or linen, and when cleaning the perineal area (see Chapter 7 for disinfection of bedpans, etc.).

(17) Disposal of personal clothing

Clean clothing requires no special treatment (apart from clothing from patients with anthrax, typhoid and smallpox). Contaminated or fouled clothing should be transferred to the hospital laundry in a sealed hot water-soluble or alginate-stitched bag and treated by the routine method used for this category of linen (see Chapter 11). Rarely other methods of disinfection (chemical or low temperature steam) or incineration may be necessary for heat-sensitive materials. Articles from patients with anthrax should be autoclaved. Infected clothing from typhoid patients may be treated in the hospital laundry if enclosed in sealed hot water-soluble or alginate-stitched bags and not handled in the laundry prior to disinfection. Clothing from smallpox and viral haemorrhagic fever patients requires special arrangements (see Chapter 17).

(18) Disposal of the dead

When death of a person suffering from a Notifiable Disease takes place in a hospital, provision is made under Public Health Act (1936.S 163 164) to prohibit the removal of the body from the hospital, except for the purpose of being taken direct to a mortuary or being forthwith buried or cremated. Under the Act, every person having charge or control of premises where such a body may be lying must take such steps as may be practicable to prevent persons coming unnecessarily into contact with or proximity to it. Wakes over such bodies are prohibited. Furthermore a Justice of the Peace has the power to order the removal or burial of such a body subject to a medical certificate issued by the Medical Officer for Environmental Health (or other registered practitioner on his staff) that the body constitutes a risk of spread of infection. In practice the above powers are not today generally enforced except for smallpox (see Chapter 17). Cremation is perhaps the safest method of disposal of the infected dead; relatives should be encouraged to agree to this method, but it cannot be legally enforced.

Death may occur from infectious diseases which are not notifiable and the corpse may remain infectious to those who handle it. The precautions already described for handling infected patients do not become unnecessary with the patient's death. The isolation category should be stated on a card attached to the body. Porters, mortuary attendants, pathologists and funeral undertakers must be informed of the possible danger in order that appropriate precautions may be taken.

(19) Terminal disinfection of isolation rooms

All surfaces, including beds, other furniture, wash-basins etc., and the floor should be washed with a clear soluble phenolic (e.g. 1% Stericol or equivalent) (see Chapters 6 and 7, pp. 69, 75); it is unnecessary to wash walls and ceilings unless visibly contaminated. The room may be occupied when dry but should preferably be left for 24 hours.

Strict isolation techniques (in addition to the standard)

(1) Masks

Masks protective to the wearer (of a recommended filter-type) should be stored outside the room, put on before entering the room and discarded into a pedal bin before leaving.

(2) Gloves

Gloves should be used for procedures which include handling the patient or his bedding and the gloves discarded after each use. Long, disposable gloves should be used for lifting patients and for other procedures likely to contaminate forearms.

(3) Protective clothing

Water-impermeable gowns, with low permeability to bacteria, are preferred to aprons. A supply of gowns should be available outside the room, and a clean gown should be used whenever the room is entered. Sterile gowns may be advisable for maximum protective isolation. Patients with suspected/confirmed smallpox or viral haemorrhagic fevers must be transferred between hospitals only in specially equipped ambulances with crews wearing protective clothing.

(4) Double-bag technique

Contaminated articles should be removed from the room in a plastic bag (or coloured laundry bag for linen), which must be sealed before leaving the infected area. Outside the area this bag is placed in a second clean bag which may be held by a second person, or a stand may be provided for this purpose. However, this technique is rarely necessary, if care is taken not to contaminate the outside of the bag.

Protective isolation

This is used for diseases or lesions in which there is increased susceptibility to infection and in which patients need special protection from the hospital environment. The amount of protection required varies with the type of patient; maximum protection, including sterile linen, food and other supplies, may be required for immunosuppressed patients, but is not necessary for patients with eczema or burns. Protective measures available and possible indications for their use are summarized in Table 9.2.

Table 9.2 Protective Isolation: Indications and Categories (see Spiers, Gaya and Goldman, 1978)

Category	Neutrophil count per µl blood	Type of isolation	Notes
1	> 1000	Single room	May use ward bathroom
2	< 1000 > 200	Single room with bathroom and toilet	Patient should not leave the room unless special precautions are taken
3	≤ 200	Maximum isolation precautions in plenum ventilated room (8–10 air changes/hour), with bathroom and toilet *or* Positive pressure isolator	Mouth and other orifices, gut and skin decontamination may be advised. Sterile food, bedding, books, etc. Staff wear sterile protective clothing.

NB Transient or chronic neutropenia are not necessarily indications for strict protective isolation.

(1) Gowns

Long sleeved gowns or suits of small-pore, water-impermeable materials, e.g. ventile or certain non-woven fabrics, should be worn by attendants to protect the high risk patient against contact contamination. Sterile gowns may be advisable for patients in category 3 (see Table 9.2); for categories 1 and 2 plastic aprons may be worn instead of gowns.

(2) Gloves

When handling patients requiring maximum protection (category 3), gloves should be worn by all attendants who handle the patient and objects that come in contact with the patient. Gloves are not necessary for handling patients in categories 1 and 2, provided the hands are thoroughly washed or disinfected.

(3) Hands

Hands must be washed or disinfected before entering the room; as it is uncertain whether the patient has already acquired infection, hand-washing on leaving the room is also necessary.

(4) Equipment

Items such as sphygmomanometer, stethoscope, thermometer, wash-bowl, bedpan and urinal should be reserved for the patient and left in his room.

(5) Crockery and cutlery

These items should either be disposable or disinfected by heat before taking them into the room.

(6) Dressings

Normal non-touch sterile technique should be used (see Chapter 8).

(7) Secretion, excretion and enteric precautions

No special precautions are necessary unless infection has already been acquired.

(8) Linen

Clean linen from the laundry will usually be satisfactory, but in some circumstances should be sterile (e.g. in category 3).

(9) Laboratory specimens

No precautions needed, unless hepatitis B infection or carriage of HB_sAg has developed.

(10) Masks

Masks may be worn for patients requiring maximum (category 3) protection, or those with burns treated by the exposure method or exposed at change of dressings (see Chapter 8).

(11) Charts

Charts should remain outside the room.

(12) Visitors

If visitors are admitted to the isolation room, they should be given detailed instructions and should take similar precautions to staff. If suffering from any infection, they should be excluded.

(13) Staff

Staff including medical and auxiliary staff should be excluded if they have any infection. In some instances screening for staphylococcal carriage may

133

be advisable. In a mixed source and protective isolation ward, staff nursing source-isolated patients should preferably not nurse patients in protective isolation in the same span of duty.

(14) Transporting patients

The patient should not be transported to any other department in the hospital unless unavoidable.

Suggested labels for categories of isolation

Adhesive labels are recommended to be used for patients in isolation. These should be attached to the door of the isolation room. This will help to inform members of staff going into the room of the measure to be taken. The labels, which are held by the Ward Sister, are colour-coded as follows:

(1) Red — strict isolation
(2) White — protective isolation
(3) Blue — standard isolation

If excretion or secretion precautions are needed a *brown card* marked *secretion* or *excretion precautions* is attached. The 'comments' line is left blank so that the Ward Sister may enter details pertaining to the individual patient. In a general hospital isolation unit, coloured cards without instructions are useful for the staff, particularly for domestic staff when cleaning cubicles in an agreed order; protective isolation cubicles should be cleaned before source isolation cubicles.

The *visitors* line only should be translated into other languages as required.

Strict source isolation

VISITORS:	PLEASE REPORT TO SISTER'S OFFICE BEFORE ENTERING ROOM
SINGLE ROOM: Necessary	*Door must be kept closed* *Patient must not leave the room*
GOWNS (IMPERVIOUS):	Must be worn.
MASKS:	Must be worn (filter type).
HANDS:	Must be washed on leaving.
GLOVES:	Must be worn.
ARTICLES:	Normal supplies. Disposed in waterproof containers.
COMMENTS:	RED LABEL

Standard source isolation

VISITORS: PLEASE REPORT TO SISTER'S OFFICE
BEFORE ENTERING ROOM

SINGLE ROOM: Necessary; for all infections transferred by air, and preferred, when available, for all infections, including those not transferred by air. Door must be kept closed.

GOWNS OR
PLASTIC APRONS: Must be worn when attending to patients

MASKS: Not necessary, except for persons susceptible to the disease (filter type).

HANDS: Must be washed on leaving.

GLOVES: Not necessary (except for contact with infected area, or when excretion or secretion precautions necessary).

ARTICLES: Normal supplies. Disposed in waterproof containers.

COMMENTS: | BLUE LABEL |

Protective isolation*

VISITORS: PLEASE REPORT TO SISTER'S OFFICE
BEFORE ENTERING ROOM

SINGLE ROOM: Door must be kept closed; patient must not leave the room.

GOWNS (IMPERVIOUS):   Must be worn on entry.

MASKS: Must be worn.

HANDS: Must be washed *before* handling the patient and his surroundings.

GLOVES: Must be worn by those handling the patient or with objects coming in contact with patient.

ARTICLES: For immunosuppressed patient all items, including food, should be sterile. No special precautions when removing from room.

COMMENTS: | WHITE LABEL |

*See summary of protective isolation (p. 132). Masks, gloves and sterile food and clothing are probably not essential in categories 1 and 2.

Isolation methods for individual diseases

Isolation for infections

This section lists diseases in alphabetical order, the category of isolation and special nursing procedure, if any required. Abbreviations used:

HIU — Hospital Isolation Unit
HSIU — High Security Isolation Unit
IDH — Infectious Diseases Hospital
SR — Single-bedded Side-room

Actinomycosis　　　　　Isolation unnecessary
　　　　　　　　　　　　Exudate precautions

Amoebiasis　　　　　　Isolation unnecessary
　　　　　　　　　　　　Excretion precautions

Anthrax

Category of isolation:	Strict (pulmonary or systemic); standard (cutaneous).
Period of isolation:	Length of illness (e.g. until completion of successful chemotherapy).
Place of isolation:	HIU, IDH, or SR, for cutaneous infection.
Comments:	Laboratory must be warned of any specimens sent for examination. Notify Medical Officer for Environmental Health.

Aspergillosis　　　　　See Fungal infection.

Brucellosis　　　　　　Exudate precautions only if a draining lesion.

Campylobacter enteritis

Category of isolation:	Standard.
Period of isolation:	Until diarrhoea stops.
Place of isolation:	SR, HIU, or IDH.
Comments:	Excretion precautions.

Candidiasis　　　　　　See Fungal infection.
(moniliasis, thrush)

Cat scratch fever　　　No special precautions required.

Chickenpox

Category of isolation:	Standard (in room with extractor fan).
Period of isolation:	Seven days from start of eruption.
Place of isolation:	HIU or IDH.
Comments:	Take precautions with secretions. Staff who have not had the disease must be excluded. Visitors who have not had the disease must be warned of the risks.

Cholera

Category of isolation:	Standard.
Period of isolation:	Length of illness.
Place of isolation:	IDH.
Comments:	Notify Medical Officer for Environmental Health. Excretion precautions.

Common cold

See Influenza.

Conjunctivitis (gonococcal)

See Ophthalmia neonatorum and Venereal Diseases.

Diarrhoeal disease of unknown origin

Category of isolation:	Standard.
Period of isolation:	Duration of illness.
Place of isolation:	SR or HIU.
Comments:	Excretion precautions.

Diphtheria

Category of isolation:	Strict.
Period of isolation:	Until bacteriologically negative.
Place of isolation:	IDH.
Comments:	See section on Contacts. Notify Medical Officer for Environmental Health.

Dysentery, bacillary (shigellosis)

Category of isolation:	Standard.
Period of isolation:	Until three consecutive negative stools after acute phase, whenever possible.
Place of isolation:	HIU or IDH.
Comments:	Notify Medical Officer for Environmental Health. Excretion precautions for stools.

Dysentery (Amoebic)

Isolation unnecessary.
Excretion precautions for stools.

Comment:	Notify Medical Officer for Environmental Health.

Ebola virus disease

See Viral haemorrhagic fevers.

Eczema vaccinatum and generalized vaccinia

Category of isolation:	Strict.
Period of isolation:	Length of illness, until crusts separate.
Place of isolation:	HIU or IDH.
Comments:	Children with eczema should be prophylactically treated with human specific immunoglobulin if exposed to vaccinia infection.

137

Food poisoning

Staphylococcal and clostridial	No special precautions. Notify Medical Officer for Environmental Health
Salmonella	See p. 142.

Fungal infections

Aspergillosis, crypto-coccosis, histoplas-mosis	No special precautions.
Ring-worm	Precautions against contact transfer. Isolation in a cubicle may be advisable especially in children's wards.
Candidiasis	Standard isolation for candidiasis in neonatal wards.

Gastro-enteritis in babies

Category of isolation:	Standard.
Period of isolation:	Length of illness or until stools are negative.
Place of isolation:	HIU, or IDH, or SR.
Comments:	Excretion precautions are important. Nappies must be sealed in plastic bags. Notify Medical Officer for Environmental Health in Northern Ireland only.

Gas gangrene

No special precautions. See p. 153.

Gonorrhoea

See Venereal diseases.

Herpes simplex

Category of isolation:	Standard (children's wards only).
Period of isolation:	Length of illness.
Place of isolation:	SR or HIU.
Comments:	Staff with infection should be excluded from neonatal, maternity or children's wards and should cover cuts or abrasions on fingers if in contact with infected child.

Herpes zoster

Category of isolation:	Standard.
Period of isolation:	Length of illness (when lesions stop discharging).
Place of isolation:	SR or HIU.
Comments:	Staff who have not had chicken-pox must be excluded. Visitors who have not had the infection should be warned of the risk.

Infectious hepatitis

Category of isolation:	Standard
Period of isolation:	Isolation probably not required once jaundice has

	developed. However, patients are infectious in early febrile phase of illness.
Place of isolation:	SR or HIU.
Comments:	Excretion precautions. See also section on Serum hepatitis (p. 296). Notify Medical Officer for Environmental Health.

Infectious mononucleosis

Oral secretion precautions only.

Influenza

Category of isolation:	Standard (if admitted with disease).
Period of isolation:	Length of illness.
Comments:	Isolation not necessary if acquired in hospital or if other patients with the disease are in the ward.

Lassa fever

See Viral haemorrhagic fevers.

Legionnaire's disease

Category of isolation:	Standard.
Period of isolation:	While in hospital.
Place of isolation:	HIU, IDH or SR.
Comment:	Diagnosis usually retrospective except in outbreak. Person-to-person transfer is unlikely.

Leprosy

Category of isolation:	Standard.
Period of isolation:	Length of hospital stay.
Place of isolation:	HIU or IDH.
Comments:	Not infectious following adequate treatment. Exudate secretion precautions. Notify Medical Officer for Environmental Health.

Leptospirosis

Isolation unnecessary.
Notify Medical Officer for Environmental Health.
Excretion precautions (urine).

Listeriosis

Not known to spread in hospitals: isolation unnecessary.
No special precautions.

Malaria

Isolation unnecessary.
Notify Medical Officer for Environmental Health.

Marburg disease

See Viral haemorrhagic fevers.

Measles

Category of isolation:	Standard.
Period of isolation:	Five days from onset of rash.
Place of isolation:	SR, HIU, or IDH.
Comments:	Secretion precautions.
	Notify Medical Officer for Environmental Health.
	If outbreak in paediatric ward, do not admit children who are not immune until 14 days after the last contact has gone home (see section on Contacts).

Meningitis (meningococcal)

Category of isolation:	Standard (with masks).
Period of isolation:	48 hours after onset of treatment (if sensitive strains).
Place of isolation:	HIU or IDH.
Comments:	Secretion precautions. See section on Contacts.
	Notify Medical Officer for Environmental Health.

Meningitis (tuberculous)

See Tuberculosis, p. 144.

Meningitis (viral) and meningo-encephalitis

Category of isolation:	Standard.
Period of isolation:	Length of acute illness.
Place of isolation:	HIU or IDH.
Comments:	Excretion precautions.
	Notify Medical Officer for Environmental Health.

Meningitis (pneumococcal, haemophilus, coliform and other causes)

No isolation required.
Notify Medical Officer for Environmental Health.

Mumps

Category of isolation:	Standard.
Period of isolation:	Nine days after onset of parotid swelling.
Place of isolation:	SR,HIU, or IDH.
Comments:	Secretion precautions.
	Exclude staff who are not immune.
	Warn visitors who are not immune, and provide masks if necessary.

Nocardiosis

No isolation required unless immunosuppressed patients are in the ward.
Exudate and secretion precautions.

Ophthalmia neonatorum (see also Venereal diseases)

Category of isolation:	Standard.
Period of isolation:	Length of illness (24 hours after start of chemo-therapy).
Place of isolation:	SR.
Comments:	Secretion precautions.
	Notify Medical Officer for Environmental Health.

Orf No isolation required.
Exudate precautions.

Paratyphoid fever See Typhoid and paratyphoid.

Plague

Category of isolation:	Strict.
Period of isolation:	Until bacteriologically negative.
Place of isolation:	IDH.
Comments:	Secretion and exudate precautions.
	No visitors if pneumonic.
	Notify Medical Officer for Environmental Health.

Pneumonia No isolation or special precautions required for lobar (unless due to antibiotic-resistant strains of *Strep. pneumoniae*) or primary atypical (mycoplasma) pneumonia. For other causes see staphylococcal infection, plague and psittacosis, Legionnaire's disease.

Poliomyelitis

Category of isolation:	Standard (with masks in early stages).
Period of isolation:	Until stools negative for poliovirus (or seven days from onset).
Place of isolation:	IDH.
Comments:	Excretion precautions. Visitors wear masks in early stages and avoid contact.
	Notify Medical Officer for Environmental Health.

Psittacosis

Category of isolation:	Standard (with masks).
Period of isolation:	For seven days after onset.
Place of isolation:	SR, HIU, or IDH.
Comments:	Secretion precautions.
	Notify Medical Officer for Environmental Health.

Puerperal sepsis

Category of isolation:	Standard.
Period of isolation:	Until bacteriologically negative (48 hours or longer).
Place of isolation:	SR.

141

Comments: Exudate precautions.
                              Notify Medical Officer for Environmental Health.

Q fever   As for Psittacosis.

Rabies
Category of isolation: Strict (though person-to-person transfer is unlikely)
                              (see Chapter 17).
Period of isolation: Length of illness.
Place of isolation: IDH or SR in Intensive Care Unit.
Comments: Secretion precautions.
                              Notify Medical Officer for Environmental Health.

Rheumatic fever   No isolation or special precautions required.

Ringworm   See Fungal infections.

Rubella
Category of isolation: Standard.
Period of isolation: Five days from onset of rash.
Place of isolation: SR or HIU.
Comments: Secretion precautions.
                              Exclude young women staff or visitors who may be
                              pregnant unless they are immune. The congenital
                              rubella syndrome is highly infectious. See section on
                              Contacts.

Salmonella infections (food poisoning)
Category of isolation: Standard.
Period of isolation: Until three stools negative, whenever possible.
Place of isolation: SR, HIU, or IDH.
Comments: Excretion precautions.
                              Visitors avoid contact with patients.
                              Notify Medical Officer for Environmental Health.
                              Carriers: send home and inform Medical Officer for
                              Environmental Health.

Scabies
Category of isolation: Standard until successfully treated (p. 147).
Comments: See sections on Contacts, and on Insect and Mite
                              Infestation (pp. 146, 156).

Scarlet fever   See Streptococcal infections.

Schistosomiasis   No isolation or special precautions.

Shigellosis   See Dysentery.

142

Smallpox (or suspected smallpox)

Category of isolation:	Strict.
Period of isolation:	Length of illness.
Place of isolation:	Smallpox Hospital.
Comments:	See Chapter 17 (notes on Smallpox) and section on Contacts.
	Notify Medical Officer for Environmental Health *by phone.*

Staphylococcal infection (epidemic or highly resistant strains) including pneumonia

Category of isolation:	Standard.
Period of isolation:	Until the organism is no longer isolated from the lesion.
Place of isolation:	SR or HIU.
Comments:	Exudate and secretion precautions (and see section on Prevention of Spread of Hospital Sepsis, p. 148).

Staphylococcal infection (sensitive, or resistant only to penicillin)	Barrier nursing; exudate and secretion precautions. No isolation room needed, unless in maternity and neonatal wards.

Streptococcal infection (including scarlet fever and erysipelas)

Category of isolation:	Standard.
Period of isolation:	Until organism no longer isolated, following chemotherapy (or not less than three days).
Place of isolation:	SR or HIU.
Comments:	Exudate and secretion precautions (and see section on Prevention of Spread of Hospital Sepsis, p. 148). Scarlet fever and in Scotland, erysipelas: Notify Medical Officer for Environmental Health.

Syphilis	See Venereal diseases.
Tapeworm	No isolation needed. Excretion precautions.
Tetanus	No special source isolation precautions, but patient should be in SR, for medical reasons. Notify Medical Officer for Environmental Health.
Threadworms	No isolation needed. Excretion precautions.
Tonsillitis	See Streptococcal infection.

Toxocara	No isolation needed. Excretion precautions.
Toxoplasmosis	No isolation or special precautions.
Trichomoniasis	No isolation needed. Excretion and exudate precautions.

Tuberculosis (open, including pulmonary, urinary or draining lesions)

Category of isolation:	Standard (with masks for bedmaking and other nursing procedures involving close contact with patient).
Period of isolation:	Until *M. tuberculosis* no longer found in direct films of sputum, urine or exudate or three weeks after treatment has commenced.
Place of isolation:	ID (or special) H, or HIU.
Comments:	Secretion, excretion and exudate precautions. Staff and visitors who are not immune should be warned of risk and given suitable protection. See section on Contacts. Notify Medical Officer for Environmental Health.

Tuberculosis (closed)	Isolation and special precautions not needed. Notify Medical Officer for Environmental Health.

Typhoid and paratyphoid (and carriers)

Category of isolation:	Standard.
Period of isolation:	Until six negative stools, and urines if applicable, are taken with 24 hours between specimens whenever possible.
Place of isolation:	IDH.
Comments:	Excretion precautions. Notify Medical Officer for Environmental Health. It is not necessary to keep the patient in hospital until he is no longer excreting typhoid bacilli.

Vaccinia	See Eczema vaccinatum.

Venereal diseases (syphilis (mucocutaneous) and gonorrhoea)

Category of isolation:	Standard.
Period of isolation:	Until bacteriologically negative; this will occur after 48 hours in syphilis, and after 24 hours in gonorrhoea unless the strain is resistant to the antibiotic.
Place of isolation:	Ward SR or HIU.
Comments:	Use of gloves for handling secretions or infected sites.

Varicose ulcers (with sepsis)   See wounds.

Viral haemorrhagic fevers

Category of isolation:	Strict.
Period of isolation:	Until virus no longer isolated.
Place of isolation:	HSIU.
Comments:	See p. 293.
	Notify Medical Officer for Environmental Health.

Whooping cough

Category of isolation:	Standard.
Period of isolation:	Three weeks after onset of paroxysmal cough, or seven days after appropriate chemotherapy (e.g. erythromycin or amoxycillin).
Comments:	Secretion precautions.
	Notify Medical Officer for Environmental Health.

Wounds   See section on Prevention of Spread of Hospital Sepsis (p. 148).

(i) Extensive wounds (with sepsis caused by epidemic or highly antibiotic-resistant *Staph. aureus* or Gram-negative bacilli):

Category of isolation:	Standard.
Period of isolation:	Until wound is healed or sepsis resolved.
Place of isolation:	SR or HIU.
Comments:	Exudate precautions.

(ii) Minor wounds:

Category of isolation:	Standard.
Period of isolation:	Until wound is healed.
Place of isolation:	Ward.
Comments:	Exudate precautions.

Worm infestations (see also tapeworm, threadworm and toxocara)   Isolation not necessary
Excretion precautions only.

Isolation for susceptible patients

Neutropenic, leukaemic and immunosuppressed patients

Category of isolation:	Protective.
Period of isolation:	Duration of illness or period of immunosuppression.
Place of isolation:	SR, ultra-clean unit or isolator.
Comments:	Protective technique as listed (see summary, p. 132).

Burns   See p. 153.

Generalized eczema

Category of isolation:	Combined protective and standard source isolation.
Period of isolation:	Duration of hospital stay or until remission.
Place of isolation:	SR or HIU.

Management of contacts of infected patients in hospital

Chickenpox

If indicated, an injection of human specific immunoglobulin may be given to patients suffering from, or contacts of, chicken-pox who are on steroid therapy or receiving cytotoxic or immunosuppressive drugs (e.g., patients with leukaemia).

Cytomegalovirus infection

Pregnant staff should be kept away from patients (usually children or the immunosuppressed, especially following renal transplantation) with CMV infection. Screening for antibodies determines the non-immune.

Diphtheria

Throat and nasal swabs should be taken from all close contacts of patients who develop diphtheria while in hospital; they should be given prophylactic erythromycin. Active immunization of contacts if not known to be immune should be started (see also Chapter 13). All contacts should be kept under surveillance, and if any develop sore throat or nasal discharge, antitoxin should be given.

Infantile (Escherichia coli) gastro-enteritis

If an outbreak of gastro-enteritis due to enteropathogenic *E. coli* occurs, stools should be cultured from all contacts, and admissions to the ward must be suspended. Children who are well enough to go home should be discharged as soon as possible. The isolation of a gastro-enteritis serotype of *E. coli* in the laboratory from a child without symptoms should not cause alarm, but is an indication that this child should be kept away from any susceptible children (under two years old) in the ward. Nurses working in a ward where cases of gastro-enteritis are present should not be transferred to other wards.

Intestinal infections (including typhoid fever, other salmonellosis, cholera and bacillary dysentery)

Other patients and staff in the ward should be kept under surveillance and stool samples should be obtained from those developing signs of the disease. Under certain circumstances it may be necessary to close a ward or unit. When typhoid contacts, in whom the incubation period may be prolonged to three weeks, are discharged from hospital, the general practitioner should be made aware of the contact so that cases are not missed. The Occupational Health Department should be informed of contacts among members of staff.

Legionnaire's disease (see p. 153)

A potentially severe respiratory infection usually acquired from an inanimate source, e.g. air conditioning systems. Person-to-person spread appears to be unusual, but isolation is advisable because of the severity of the disease, and close contacts should be kept under surveillance.

Measles

Contacts under two years of age and other children in whom measles might be particularly dangerous (e.g. those suffering from chronic or debilitating diseases, leukaemia or receiving corticosteroid drugs) should be given an injection of human normal immunoglobulin as soon as possible after contact. It may be necessary to close a children's surgical ward because operations on children with measles can be dangerous. Admissions should be limited to children who have had a definite attack of measles.

Meningococcaemia

Close contacts should be kept under surveillance and throat swabs should be taken; a prophylactic course of minocycline or rifampicin should be given. Only use sulphonamide if the organism is known to be sensitive.

Poliomyelitis

All contacts, staff and patients, should be offered oral poliomyelitis vaccine.

Rubella

Rubella is generally a benign disease, but infection during the first four months of pregnancy is associated with a significant incidence of abnormal foetuses. In such persons, estimation of the antibody titres in the blood can be helpful and should be done without delay. Immunoglobulin is not recommended.

Scabies

When scabies is diagnosed in a patient admitted to hospital, arrangements must be made for all home contacts to be treated.

Smallpox

As soon as smallpox is suspected, the appropriate Medical Officer for Environmental Health must be notified immediately. He will arrange for the patient to be seen by a member of a Panel of Smallpox Consultants and advise on vaccination and surveillance of contacts. Under no circumstances must the patient be moved without permission of the Medical Officer for Environmental Health (see Chapter 17).

Tuberculosis (open pulmonary)

The names of all patient contacts of a case of sputum-positive tuberculosis should be notified to the appropriate Medical Officer for Environmental Health. Staff contacts are reported to the hospital control of infection or occupational health departments.

147

Viral hepatitis

Human normal immunoglobulin gives protection against infectious (Virus A) hepatitis but not against serum (Virus B) hepatitis: 500 mg should be given to debilitated contacts and pregnant women. Human specific immunoglobulin, conferring protection against Virus B hepatitis, is available for those at risk by reason of accidental exposure to infection (see Chapter 18, p. 304).

Visiting of patients in isolation hospitals

Infected patients

In general, patients in hospital suffering from infection should be allowed visitors in the normal way, and daily visiting of small children by their parents is encouraged. However, under certain circumstances, some restrictions may have to be imposed for the protection of visitors or to prevent the spread of disease. It is sometimes necessary for the visitor to wear a gown or plastic apron, e.g. if handling a child with an intestinal infection, and instruction must be given on hand-washing. Language and cultural difficulties may have to be considered in some cases. Visitors must not visit patients other than those whom they have come to see. It is unwise to allow children to visit patients in isolation or communicable diseases units, and adults who are not considered to be immune to a particular condition should be excluded from contact with that disease. Pregnant women should not visit patients suffering from rubella. Visitors are not allowed in a smallpox hospital.

Patients in protective isolation

Parents may visit children, but contact should be restricted, especially in visits to immunosuppressed patients. Plastic isolators may be helpful in allowing parents to touch their children without breaking isolation. If the intending visitor has infection of the respiratory or intestinal tract, boils or other septic lesions, the visit should be postponed.

Prevention of spread of hospital sepsis

Infection due to Staphylococcus aureus in general hospital wards

Except in special units, where staphylococcal infection is still common, *Staph. aureus* is today less often transmitted in hospital. Certain strains of *Staph. aureus* have a propensity for spreading and causing sepsis in a ward and are known as 'epidemic strains'. These are usually resistant to two or more antibiotics; not all multiple-resistant strains, however, spread readily to other patients. Antibiotic-sensitive strains (or strains resistant to penicillin only) rarely spread in wards (apart from neonatal units), but may be responsible for infection in the operating theatre or for self-infection of the patient. People are the most important source of infection; staphylococci multiply in noses, on the skin (e.g. perineum) and in lesions, but not in the inanimate environment. Nevertheless, staphylococci, which can survive for some time outside the body, especially in dry conditions,

148

may spread from the inanimate environment; e.g. bedding and baths are sometimes important reservoirs. Some infected patients and occasionally healthy people, who may be carriers, are responsible for heavy environmental contamination; they are known as 'dispersers' and are a special hazard in a ward or operating theatre. Staphylococci may be transferred by direct (i.e. personal) or indirect (i.e. fomite-borne) contact, or through the air. Transfer of organisms from an infected patient on the hands or clothing of members of staff is an important mode of transmission. Strains carried in the noses of staff are rarely responsible for wound infection acquired in the ward, but people with concealed lesions, such as a boil in the axilla or on the buttock, may be an important source of infection.

Control of infection

Control of infection is based on a good reporting system, high standards of aseptic technique and immediate isolation or removal from the open ward of any patient with hospital-acquired sepsis.

Isolation

All patients with an infection due to a multiple-resistant strain, especially if resistant to fusidic acid, gentamicin or methicillin, should, if possible, be transferred to the Hospital Isolation Unit, or to a single-room (preferably equipped with appropriate mechanical ventilation) or, if clinically feasible, sent home. The doors of cubicles or side-wards should be kept closed. Isolation should include precautions against contact transfer as well as against airborne transfer.

Priority of isolation

Since isolation facilities are limited in most hospitals, priorities or alternative methods of controlling infections must be considered, as follows:

(1) Major open staphylococcal sepsis (e.g. generalized eczema, chest infection, urinary tract infection, profusely discharging wounds, generalized furunculosis or skin sepsis, burns, enterocolitis, bed-stores) due to multiple-resistant (especially epidemic) strains; in particular, strains resistant to methicillin, clindamycin, fusidic acid or gentamicin.
(2) Sepsis due to multiple-resistant epidemic strains or strains resistant to penicillin only.
(3) Sepsis due to strains sensitive to antibiotics or penicillin-resistant only.

Since some strains of *Staph. aureus* may be resistant to five or more antibiotics, often including methicillin or cloxacillin, it is worthwhile isolating patients treated with certain antibiotics (e.g. fucidin or clindamycin) to which resistance has not yet emerged in the hospital, so that, if resistance emerges, the resistant organisms will not be spread to other patients.

Isolation facilities are usually limited, but even when single-rooms are available, priority is often not given to infected patients; too frequently they are used for difficult patients, for private patients, or for social or ill-defined medical reasons, whilst infected patients are nursed in open wards. Patients with major open sepsis caused by a multiple-resistant strain should be isolated in single-rooms,

149

since barrier nursing measures in an open ward are of limited value in reducing the spread of infection (especially staphylococcal infection) from such patients.

Other measures if no isolation facilities are available

If no isolation facilities are available or single-bed wards are already occupied with high priority patients, some measures may help to limit the spread of infection. Topical chemoprophylaxis of burns with an effective agent contributes much more to the exclusion of hospital infection in a burns unit than isolation methods (see Chapter 15). In the absence of an outbreak (i.e. more than two or three infections due to the same phage type), a good aseptic technique and adequate covering of a wound may be sufficient for preventing spread of infection from patients with minor sepsis. However, infection can be spread from a patient with a small septic lesion (e.g. bedsores); since even a healed lesion, or a 'healthy' nasal or skin carrier of a multiple-resistant strain, can sometimes disperse large numbers of staphylococci, 'source isolation' cannot be used for all potential sources of infection.

Additional measures which can be used for treating patients with sepsis or dispersing epidemic strains in the open wards are as follows:

(1) **Treatment of nasal carriers.** Apply a cream containing neomycin and chlorhexidine ('Naseptin' or one of equal effectiveness) to the anterior nares four times a day for two weeks or until the staphylococcus is removed. If neomycin-resistant staphylococci are present in the hospital, 1% chlorhexidine or hexachlorophane cream or ointment may be used.

(2) **Skin treatment.** An effective antiseptic detergent preparation, e.g. 4% chlorhexidine detergent solution ('Hibiscrub'), should be used for bathing and washing. 1 oz of 10% hexachlorophane solution or an iodophor ('Steribath') added to bath water reduces the hazard of transfer of infection through contamination of the bath. Patients who are perineal carriers should wash the perineum and 'bathing-trunk area' daily with an effective detergent antiseptic preparation, e.g. 'Hibiscrub' (see Chapter 7).

(3) **Open wounds and lesions (excluding burns).** Open and drained wounds, ulcers of the skin, pressure sores (however small) should be liberally dusted with 'Hibitane' powder (1% chlorhexidine in sterile calcium phosphate); or dressings soaked with 0.1% solution of chlorhexidine in water or impregnated with chlorhexidine ('Bactigras') may be applied. These may be effective against *Staph. aureus* but not against many Gram-negative rods. (Note: hexachlorophane and chlorhexidine ('Hibitane') are different compounds: hexachlorophane has toxic properties and must *not* be applied to open wounds.) An iodophor spray may also be used. Sprays or powders containing neomycin and bacitracin may be used in an emergency, but for short periods and only if neomycin-resistant strains of staphylococci are not present in a hospital. Open or drained wounds and lesions should be covered with bacteria-proof dressings.

(4) **General measures.** Careful handling and disposal of bedding and dressings is important, i.e.

    (a) Bedding and clothing should be changed daily if possible, or every two days. Bedding should be carefully removed and transferred at the bed-side to a container or bag which is immediately closed and sealed.

(b) Contaminated dressings must not be handled with fingers but should be placed with forceps immediately into a bag and sealed. Large dressings are best handled with disposable gloves. Contaminated instruments should be placed into a disinfectant solution immediately after use.

(c) Urine bottles used by patients with staphylococcal urinary infection should be handled carefully with gloves and the bottles should be disinfected after use, preferably by heat.

(d) Wash-bowls, bedpans, baths and the barber's razor should be disinfected after use by an infected patient (see Chapter 7). The infected patient should preferably retain his own equipment which is terminally disinfected on discharge from hospital.

(5) Special prophylactic measures

(a) *Patients:* In the presence of a severe outbreak of staphylococcal infection it may be advisable to treat prophylactically the noses of all patients in the ward twice daily with the special antibiotic cream or ointment (see above); all patients should also use antiseptic soap and take antiseptic baths (see Chapter 7). Hexachlorophane or chlorhexidine powder should be applied daily to the groins, trunk, buttocks and upper thighs of bed-ridden or long-stay patients; *hexachlorophane must not be applied to open lesions.* Lesions and open wounds, whether infected or not, should be treated as described in the previous section. Treatment of uninfected, dry, undrained operation wounds is not necessary, since these are unlikely to acquire infection in the ward.

(b) *Staff hand-washing:* All staff working in the ward (including physiotherapists, radiographers and laboratory technicians) should wash their hands with povidone-iodine 'surgical scrub', or with a chlorhexidine detergent solution, or disinfect with a solution of 70% alcohol rubbed on until hands are dry, before and after handling any patient or his immediate environment (see Chapter 7).

Sepsis and nasal carriers in hospital staff

Members of staff carrying an epidemic strain of *Staph. aureus* in the nose or on the skin, especially if dispersers or with a septic lesion caused by any strain of *Staph. aureus*, require treatment. This should be controlled by the Staff Medical Officer and the Microbiologist. It is not necessary to treat a nasal carrier of a strain which has not caused an infection. A member of the staff with a septic lesion should be excluded from the wards until this is healed. Minor cuts and abrasions should be covered with a waterproof dressing. Prophylactic nasal treatment of staff is rarely required. Nasal carriers requiring treatment should be treated with nasal cream and antiseptic soap (see section on Treatment of nasal carriers). If there is evidence of skin carriage of an epidemic strain or repeated septic lesions, daily baths with chlorhexidine detergent solution or another recommended antiseptic detergent preparation should be taken for one week, and the hair should be washed twice weekly with chlorhexidine detergent or povidone-iodine or cetrimide shampoo in addition to the routine treatment.

If the staphylococci are not removed after two weeks, a further course of nasal treatment should be given and chlorhexidine detergent solution should be continued. If eradication proves difficult it may be necessary to continue treatment for long periods.

Closure of wards

If there are many infections and carriers of an epidemic strain in a ward, and if measures have failed to control an epidemic, it may be necessary to close a ward. The ward should be cleaned, and when it is re-opened patients should be screened for the presence of the epidemic strain before they are admitted to the clean ward. Screening is particularly important if patients are transferred to the clean ward from another hospital or from another ward in the same hospital. Unless required for aesthetic reasons, cleaning of walls and ceilings is unnecessary.

Neonatal units

Staphylococci are particularly apt to be transferred on the hands of staff. A baby with any infection, however small, irrespective of the antibiotic sensitivity pattern, should be isolated in a single-room with full precautions against airborne and contact spread. If an outbreak occurs, all babies should be treated with hexachlorophane powder (e.g. 'Ster-Zac') or chlorhexidine powder at each napkin change or twice daily (if this is not already routine procedure). The buttocks, groins, lower abdomen, umbilicus and axilla should be powdered. Povidone-iodine or a 4% chlorhexidine detergent solution or 70% alcohol solution rubbed to dryness should be used for all handwashing by the staff. Hexachlorophane detergent or liquid soap may still be used for staff hand-washing, but not for bathing babies. If a nursery has an outbreak involving more than two or three babies, no new babies should be admitted until all occupants are discharged and the room and equipment have been cleaned. Routine screening of staff for *Staph. aureus* is not worthwhile, but in an outbreak carriers of the epidemic strains should be treated (see Chapters 2 and 15).

Infections due to Gram-negative bacilli (other than intestinal pathogens)

Gram-negative infection is often due to self-infection from the patient's own bowel flora but cross-infection is also common (including infections first acquired by the patient's intestinal flora from food). Gram-negative bacilli are usually transferred by contact; airborne spread is rare. Transfer on the hands of staff is probably the main route of spread, although contaminated solutions or equipment are sometimes responsible for infection. Precautions against contact transfer should be taken for all infections, but for patients infected with Gram-negative bacilli (with some exception for *Pseudomonas aeruginosa* and highly resistant *Klebsiella* spp.) isolation in a single-room should be given a lower priority than in patients with staphylococcal infection; combined infection of wounds with staphylococci and Gram-negative bacilli are common. Although airborne spread of *Ps. aeruginosa* is uncommon, *Pseudomonas*-infected patients in special units, e.g. neonatal, intensive care (especially in the presence of patients with tracheostomy), ophthalmic, neurosurgical, or where patients are treated with immunosuppressive drugs, should be isolated in single-rooms because of the difficulty of preventing infection and the high susceptibility of the patients. If infection occurs in a ward where patients are particularly susceptible, staff should use povidone-iodine, a chlorhexidine detergent, or 70% alcohol preparation for hand-washing, and if it is necessary to bathe patients with discharging wounds, an iodophor (e.g. 'Steribath') should be added to the bath water (see also Chapter 16, section on Urological units).

Infections due to Group A β-haemolytic streptococci (*Streptococcus pyogenes*)

Haemolytic streptococci can spread both by contact and through the air. All patients with streptococcal infections in maternity units should be isolated in a Hospital Isolation Unit or in single-rooms and treated with an appropriate antibiotic. If an infection occurs, staff and patients should be screened (nose and throat swabs) and carriers should be excluded from the ward and treated with an appropriate antibiotic (see Chapter 12). Patients in other wards, particularly surgical, with profusely discharging wounds or extensive skin sepsis due to this organism should be given a high priority for isolation.

Infections due to *Clostridium welchii* and other gas gangrene bacilli

Hospital-acquired infection with *Cl. welchii* is almost always postoperative and derived from the patient's own bowel flora. Gas gangrene is rare, but it occasionally follows orthopaedic operations on the leg (especially above the knee) when the arterial blood supply is defective, and may occur after certain abdominal operations.

Because gas gangrene bacilli which are no different from those that cause infection are carried in abundance by most healthy people in their bowel flora and are also commonly found in the environmental air and dust, there is no reason to close a theatre after operations on patients with clostridial infection; all that is needed is a thorough routine cleaning of the theatre after the operation. Though, for the same reason, isolation to prevent cross-infection with *Cl. welchii* is unnecessary, a patient with gas gangrene should be nursed in an isolation room because he is dangerously ill, and requires special nursing care.

Isolation of patients with burns

Patients with burns are commonly thought to require protective isolation before the burns become infected, and to require source isolation if they do become infected. In practice, the burns are infected for at least 24 hours before this state can be recognized by bacterial cultures. Moreover, a patient may be infected with one pathogen (e.g. *Staph. aureus*) but for the moment free from other pathogens (e.g. *Ps. aeruginosa*) from which he should be protected. For these reasons it is logical to use combined source and protective isolation for extensive burns.

Many burns, especially those of small or moderate extent, can be kept free from bacterial colonization for long periods by topical chemoprophylaxis (e.g.

153

with 0.5% silver nitrate solution or silver sulphadiazine cream). Segregation in cubicles, even with mechanical ventilation, has been shown to have little protective value for burned patients in a burns unit. Good barrier nursing techniques (especially the use of gloves for handling the patient) and topical chemoprophylaxis are of particular importance for such patients. Strict isolation in single-bed rooms facilitates the aseptic handling of extensively burned patients and should be adopted. Such single-bed rooms should, ideally, have plenum ventilation and an exhaust ventilated air-lock; if no air-lock is provided, the extracted air should not be discharged into the ward. For smaller burns, given effective local chemoprophylaxis, barrier nursing in an open ward with exudate precautions is acceptable, provided the dressings can be changed in a mechanically ventilated dressing room.

If a patient with burns, whether small or extensive, is in a general surgical ward, it is of the greatest importance that he should be source-isolated in a single-bed room. If a patient is nursed in such a room, it should be remembered that while staphylococci are commonly transferred by air, most Gram-negative burn infections, when not acquired from the patient's faecal flora, are acquired by contact. Barrier nursing techniques are more effective in preventing cross-infection of the patient than physical segregation by the walls that surround him, though this will facilitate barrier nursing and reduce the risk of cross-infection by discouraging unnecessary visits.

Legionnaire's disease

This is a potentially severe respiratory infection which has recently been described and is caused by a Gram-negative bacillus *Legionella pneumophila* (Balows and Frazer, 1979). The organism is widely distributed in nature and is commonly found in soil and surface waters. Colonization of static water is likely, and the organism may be found in hospital water tanks without any evidence of infection in patients or staff. Outbreaks are usually associated with air-conditioning systems, particularly with cooling-towers, and sometimes with showers. Outbreaks are usually reported in hotels or hospitals, and in the UK usually in new hospitals. Sporadic cases also occur with no recognized source. Although the epidemiology of the disease remains to some extent uncertain, there is no evidence of person-to-person spread, and infection is not acquired by ingestion. Infection is usually acquired by inhalation of contaminated aerosols and tends to occur in particularly susceptible patients, e.g. immunosuppressed or with chronic respiratory disease. In the event of an outbreak, antibody levels should be measured in patients and staff likely to have been exposed to the source of infection. Depending on the probable source, cooling-towers, humidifiers, and showers should be cleaned and disinfected with hypochlorites (a final concentration of five parts per million should be adequate). Hot water storage tanks should be maintained above 55° C. Isolation of the infected patient is unnecessary, but source isolation may be indicated in hospital because of the severity of the disease and the publicity associated with it. The organism has probably been a cause of pneumonia in susceptible patients for many years. The risks of acquisition in hospital have been considerably exaggerated.

154

Ambulance services: general procedures for control of infection

Many diseases are infectious before symptoms appear and contact with a sick person before a final diagnosis is made will always carry some risk of infection. Most infections, e.g. bronchitis, pneumonia, abscesses, and urinary tract infection, will not be transferred to normal healthy staff and the risk of acquiring infection is minimized by immunization and basic hygienic techniques. The inanimate environment within the ambulance is unlikely to be an infection hazard and the risk of transfer of infection from one occupant to the next is remote. The minimal measures required are:

(1) Immunization of ambulance staff (if not already immune) against polio-myelitis, tuberculosis and tetanus.
(2) Hand-washing after a patient and his belongings have been removed from the ambulance.

Bedding (blankets, sheets and bed-covers) should be sealed in a plastic bag and laundered after use by a patient with a notifiable disease, or if soiled with blood, secretions or excreta (whether the patient has a known infection or not). Spillage should be removed with disposable wipes, which should be sealed in plastic bags for incineration.

Disposable plastic aprons and gloves should be available for handling contaminated patients (e.g. with diarrhoea and vomiting) or cleaning up contaminated surfaces. A phenolic disinfectant may be used for cleaning contaminated surfaces.

Additional procedures for special infections

A few infections are potentially dangerous to staff as well as to patients and require special care. These include typhoid, dysentery, serum hepatitis, diphtheria and open tuberculosis. For highly dangerous infections, e.g. Lassa, other haemorrhagic fevers and smallpox, see Chapter 18.

Suggested procedures

(a) Typhoid, dysentery and other gastro-intestinal infections
Bedpans, urinals, vomit bowls, etc., should be either washed in a bedpan washer with a steam disinfection cycle or washed in a phenolic disinfectant. Disposable cups should be used. If surfaces are extensively contaminated the ambulance should be taken out of service and all surfaces cleaned with a phenolic disinfectant. Surfaces should be dry before the ambulance is re-used. Fumigation with formaldehyde is unnecessary.

(b) Infectious or serum hepatitis
As above, but disinfect with 1% hypochlorite (containing 0.1% available chlorine).

(c) Tuberculosis
As above. Sputum containers and wipes used for removing secretions

155

from patient should be sealed in a plastic bag and incinerated.

(d) Diphtheria

As above. Prophylactic antibiotics may be recommended by the Medical Officer for Environmental Health.

If an ambulance is specially designated for transport of infected patients it is advisable:

(1) to remove any equipment not considered necessary, e.g. spare stretcher;
(2) to seal equipment locker with adhesive tape (terminal cleaning of inside will not then be necessary);
(3) to seal clean blankets and bedding in a plastic bag and carry in bag and to seal box containing resuscitation equipment, so that only the outside of the box will require cleaning or disinfection.

Respiratory resuscitation equipment should be returned to a hospital CSSD or equipment cleaning and disinfection department for processing.

Infestation by insects and mites

Although insects and mites are unlikely to transfer infection in hospital in the United Kingdom, the problem of infestation is often referred to infection control staff.

Insecticides used for environmental treatment or application to the skin are potentially toxic and only those approved by the Pesticides Safety Precautions Scheme should be used and directions should be carefully followed.

Fleas

Infestation is usually with the cat flea, which will bite humans in the absence of the primary host. The human flea is more likely to be introduced from outside the hospital, but it is now uncommon. Fleas are able to survive for some weeks in the environment without feeding.

Control measures

Patient admitted with fleas

(a) Remove all clothing and bedding and seal in a bag. Whenever possible, process linen in the laundry in a washing machine using conventional heat treatment. A hot water-soluble plastic bag will allow transfer to the machine without handling. Clothing not suitable for washing may be sealed in a laundry bag and treated with low temperature steam. Autoclaving at higher temperatures is satisfactory but is likely to damage some materials. This is the process commonly used by environmental health authorities.
(b) Use aerosol dispensers containing insecticide to kill visible fleas and for spraying surfaces in the environment concerned.

156

Infestation in a hospital ward

(a) Identify flea if possible, and if it is a cat flea take steps to find and remove stray cats from the environment.

(b) Treat clothing and bedding as described above.

(c) Vacuum clean floors, carpets, upholstery, fabrics etc. and treat with a residual insecticide.

(d) Treat inaccessible areas such as ducting, hard surfaces and under fixtures with a residual insecticide.

Lice

These may be head, pubic (crab) or body lice. Head and pubic lice are usually found in specific areas, e.g. scalp and pubic hair, but can occur in the axillae, beard, and eye-brows; the eggs are firmly attached to hair and not easily removed. Body lice are found mainly in clothing, but also on the body surface especially in axillae and around the waist. Secondary superficial infection due to scratching is common.

Control measures

(1) Carefully remove all clothing of patients with body or pubic lice. Disposable gloves and a plastic apron should be worn.

(2) Treat clothing and bedding as described for fleas or fumigate with ethyl formate.

(3) In infestation with head or crab lice, treat the specific areas of the host with an appropriate insecticide such as carbaryl or 0.5% malathion, and repeat within seven to ten days. Patients with body lice do not require specific treatment but should be bathed.

(4) No special treatment of the environment is required as spread is mainly by direct contact, e.g. on combs or shared linen or clothing. If unfed, lice usually die in the environment at room temperature within a few days.

Mites (scabies)

Scabies is caused by a small mite (0.3–0.4 mm) which burrows into the skin. Burrows may occur anywhere, but are mainly on the hands and arms, particularly finger webs. An associated hypersensitivity rash may also occur, mainly in the groins, inside thighs and around the wrists and waist. Transmission is by person-to-person contact and is usually assumed to require fairly prolonged and intimate contact. Spread from bedding, clothing or fomites is unlikely. However, spread of 'Norwegian' scabies to staff and patients in hospital wards, particularly geriatric wards, has occasionally been reported. This is believed to be due to large numbers of immature parasites on the skin.

Control measures

(1) Apply 1% gamma benzene hexachloride, or benzyl benzoate 25% cream to all areas of the skin below the chin immediately after a hot bath. Do not wash off for 24 hours. If benzyl benzoate is used repeat the treatment after

157

seven days. Benzyl benzoate may also cause skin irritation, and toxic effects have been reported with gamma benzene hexachloride, particularly if used excessively.

(2) Treat bedding and clothing as described for fleas. Mattresses should be enclosed in impermeable covers which can be washed, or if not enclosed should be left for 10 days before further use.

(3) No special environmental control measures are necessary.

(4) Inform the Medical Officer for Environmental Health so that members of the family can be treated.

References and Further Reading

Bagshawe, K. D., Blowers, R. and Lidwell, O.M. (1978), Isolating patients in hospital to control infection. *Brit. med. J.*, ii, 609, 684, 744, 808, 879.

Balows, A. and Fraser, D. W. (eds) (1979), *International Symposium on Legionnaire's Disease*, Atlanta, Georgia (November), *Annals of Internal Medicine*, 90, 487-707.

Public Health Act (1936. S 163 164).

Spiers, A. S. D., Gaya, H. and Goldman, J.M. (1978), *Clinical Leukaemia Practice*. ICI, Macclesfield.

Tyrrell, D. A. J., Phillips, I., Goodwin, C. S. and Blowers, R. (1979), *Microbial Disease: the Use of the Laboratory in Diagnosis, Therapy and Control*. Edward Arnold, London. pp. 289-304.

US Department of Health, Education and Welfare (1970), *Isolation Techniques for Use in Hospitals*, PHS Publication No. 2054, Washington DC.

CHAPTER TEN

Asepsis in Operating Theatres

Clinical wound infection (sepsis) occurs in a small proportion of patients (often 1-5%; see Cruse and Foord, 1973; Ayliffe *et al.*, 1977) having operations on 'clean' areas (e.g. soft tissues, muscle, bone). Such infections are often *exogenous*, i.e. acquired from extraneous sources by cross-infection or, more rarely, due to contamination with bacteria from the inanimate environment; many are caused by *Staphylococcus aureus* and related bacteria, though other organisms, including Gram-negative bacilli, may be involved, sometimes in mixed infection with staphylococci. Operations on hollow viscera, especially the colon and rectum which contain enormous numbers of bacteria, have a higher incidence (commonly 10-20%) of postoperative infection; most infections following such operations are *endogenous* and caused by the patient's intestinal flora, the predominant species present being the anaerobic non-sporing bacillus, *Bacteroides fragilis*; *Escherichia coli* and other aerobic Gram-negative bacilli are also abundant. If operation is delayed, some of the intestinal organisms are likely to be strains acquired in hospital and commonly resistant to antibiotics which are usually active against similar organisms found in the intestines of persons outside hospital.

Special forms of postoperative infection are pseudomembranous enterocolitis, gas gangrene and tetanus. Pseudomembranous enterocolitis has recently been found to be caused by the toxins of *Clostridium difficile*, an organism sometimes present in normal faeces (George *et al.*, 1978); its proliferation in the gut is apparently promoted by oral administration of certain antibiotics, especially clindamycin and ampicillin. Postoperative gas gangrene is a special hazard after orthopaedic operations or amputations on ischaemic lower limbs; infection is usually endogenous, arising from contamination of the skin with faecal *Cl. welchii* (perfringens) which is resistant to standard skin antisepsis and readily transferred to the wound at operation. Postoperative tetanus, by contrast, is more often exogenous, a rare and sometimes epidemic consequence of heavy air-borne contamination (e.g. during building works) or of the use of contaminated materials; in former times catgut was a well-recognized source. Early post-operative infection, occurring in wounds that are closed without drainage before the patient returns to the ward, can be regarded as having been acquired in the operating theatre.

In addition to these *endemic* infections, which are caused by a variety of organisms, outbreaks of *epidemic* infection occur from time to time due to the presence of a particular strain of a virulent organism carried by some member of the staff or present in materials (e.g. eye-drops) that should be sterile. Established aseptic methods have been shown to reduce these hazards, but the common development of sepsis after clean operations shows the limitations of aseptic methods and the need for meticulous standards. An 'epidemic' increase in the incidence of postoperative wound sepsis may also be caused by some failure in aseptic technique or sterilization; such outbreaks are associated with an increased incidence of sepsis caused by different types of bacteria, not by one epidemic strain.

The protection of patients in the operating theatre against hazards of exogenous infection involves the application of a large number of methods to prevent the contamination of wounds (*asepsis*) and to enhance the patient's resistance. Some of the methods are described in the chapters on sterilization and disinfection in this handbook (see Section B). Protection of patients against endogenous infection with bacteria normally resident in the hollow viscera and in the upper respiratory tract, when indicated (e.g. in resections of colon or rectum), requires the administration, for short periods, of antibiotics or other antimicrobial chemotherapeutic agents by the systemic route, or by mouth, or by both routes, the antimicrobials being selected for their activity against the organisms likely to infect. Infection of operation wounds with bacteria that happen to be present on the skin of the operation or infusion site can also be regarded as endogenous; protection against this hazard involves effective pre-operative skin disinfection, and asepsis of the infusion site.

Methods of preventing infection in the operating suite can be considered under the following sub-headings (Medical Research Council, 1968):

(a) the operating suite and equipment;
(b) preparation of the surgical team; and
(c) preparation and protection of the patient.

The operating suite and equipment

Design

A report to the Medical Research Council (1962) recommended six basic requirements for control of infection in operating suites: (i) separation from the general traffic and air movement of the hospital; (ii) a sequence of increasingly clean zones from the entrance to the operating and sterilizing areas; (iii) easy movement of staff from one clean area to another without passing through 'dirty' areas; (iv) removal of dirty materials from the suite without passing through clean areas; (v) air flow from clean to less clean areas; and (vi) heating and ventilation to ensure safe and comfortable conditions for patients and staff.

These conditions are best achieved by having the theatres in an operating suite, with a number of operating rooms sufficient to allow adequate time for cleaning (e.g. one theatre for 25–30 surgical beds), and with protective, clean, aseptic and disposal zones. Some of these recommendations are more important than others, and the need for the recommendations is diminished if dirty items are removed from the suite in sealed impervious bags.

Ventilation

Ventilation should remove airborne bacteria released in the theatre suite and prevent the entry of bacteria, especially from the corridors and other indoor areas, but also from outside the hospital. It should provide comfortable conditions, and control the humidity to reduce the risk of electrostatic sparks. Recommended ventilation systems for standard operating theatres are plenum ventilation at 1000–1500 ft^3/min in the aseptic area and sterile supply room (or 20 air changes per hour) with lower input into anaesthetic and scrub up rooms, and no input (or low input) in the entrance lobby, changing rooms and recovery rooms. The efficiency of the ventilation system should, when possible, be monitored daily by use of an airflow switch, which indicates on the theatre panel that the correct volume of air is being supplied by the plant. When this equipment is not present, measurement of air flow at grilles (by an anemometer) and of room pressure at test points is desirable, and should be recorded in a log book. Measurements of ventilation rate should be made periodically by an engineer; a reduced pressure and air turnover indicate probable blockage of the filters, which require immediate replacement if blocked. A hygrometer in the theatre should be read daily to ensure that the relative humidity does not fall to levels of electrostatic spark hazard (below 55%). Discomfort should be recorded.

For operations which present a special hazard of infection (e.g. hip replacement with a prosthesis), special operating enclosures ventilated with unidirectional (laminar) flow at a high turnover (300 air changes per hour), sometimes used with body exhaust clothing, have been recommended by some surgeons. Operating isolators in which the surgeon stands outside the plastic enclosure and uses glove ports have also been used for operating on 'high risk' patients. In a multi-hospital trial still in progress, of ultra-clean air systems in theatres for total hip replacement operations, the incidence of wound and joint infection has in most centres been very low in both ultra-clean air and control series. The results of this trial, which require follow-up for late infection, will not be available until 1981. Meanwhile the value of ultra-clean air systems, including the Charnley-Howorth and laminar flow systems which have been installed in many hospitals, cannot be regarded as adequately established; further evidence from experimental study is needed before they can be recommended for routine use for total hip replacement.

Storage of equipment

The amount of equipment should be kept to a minimum, including operating table, lights, conduits for anaesthetic gases, diathermy and suction; an instrument table and trolley are included if there is no setting-up room. Articles needed for servicing a list of operations are kept in the anaesthetic room, the scrub-up annexe and setting-up room. Stored items are arranged to require a minimum of movement by staff.

Maintenance of sterility of sterile supplies depends on adequate wrapping of packs and on the minimum exposure. Double wrapping prevents contamination during opening of packs, which must also be protected against moisture; if not used promptly, packs should be kept in a cabinet or box with a well-fitting lid. Instruments should not be kept in disinfectant solutions. Items of equipment

161

(X-ray, diathermy, etc.) must be stored under clean conditions and be cleaned or disinfected regularly.

Laying-up of trolleys in advance of the operation involves some risk of contamination. When instruments are arranged for individual operations on preset trays, wrapping can be removed in the operating room immediately before use.

Sterilization of instruments

The methods of sterilizing instruments are described in Chapters 4 and 5. In many theatre suites instruments and bowls are rapidly sterilized unwrapped in downward displacement pressure steam sterilizers, which should conform to BS 3970, Part 3. Boiling 'sterilizers' should not be used. For sterilization and disinfection of cystoscopes and other endoscopes see Chapter 7.

Cleaning of the operating suite

The principles of cleaning and disinfection are given in Section B. Surfaces should be kept free from visible dirt, and special attention should be given to areas which are likely to become heavily contaminated (i.e. upward facing surfaces). In practice, it is advisable to clean the floor of theatres after each operating session. A disinfectant should be used after known contamination of floors with material from infected patients, but for routine cleaning, mopping with water and a detergent is satisfactory. Floors should be rinsed occasionally with clean water after washing or disinfection, otherwise deposit may build up and reduce antistatic properties. A suitable floor-scrubbing machine may be used at the end of the day (see Chapter 7). For other surfaces, normal housekeeping methods are adequate — e.g. daily damp cleaning of ledges and shelves. Walls with intact surfaces acquire very few bacteria even if left unwashed for long periods; they must not, however, be allowed to grow visibly dirty, and washing at least every three months should be adequate for this purpose. If areas of paint peel off, the wall must be repainted or covered with a new wall finish. The operating lamp should be cleaned daily; oiling is unnecessary.

Disinfection of anaesthetic apparatus and mechanical ventilators

Items which enter or come near to the patient's respiratory tract (e.g. endotracheal tubes, airways, rebreathing bags and face pieces) should be disinfected after every use. These items should be disinfected in the Hospital Sterilizing and Disinfecting Unit, or in a special department with technical staff appointed for this work under the supervision of the Superintendent of the HSDU. Care must be taken to avoid contaminating the anaesthetic trolley, which should have a discard receptacle.

For details of disinfection of anaesthetic and respiratory ventilating equipment and of methods for preventing contamination of respiratory ventilators, see Chapter 7 and Appendices 7.1 and 7.4.

Operating rooms for 'clean' and 'septic' cases: order of operation

When there is no proper ventilation system in the theatre suite, operations on septic cases should preferably be performed in a separate operating theatre, though the risk of transfer from one patient to the next in a general surgical list is small. In theatre suites with plenum ventilation at 1000–1500 ft³/min an interval of five minutes, during which the room is thoroughly cleaned, should make it safe for the next patient; no special 'septic' theatre is required. No special cleaning precautions are required after operations on patients with gas gangrene, since these do not contaminate the theatre any more than operations in which the intestine is opened.

Septic patients should, when possible, be placed at the end of an operating list.

Suction apparatus (see also Chapter 7)

In free-standing units, a filter (BS 4199, Part 1, 1967) for electrically driven apparatus should be fitted between the collection bottle and the pump; this will prevent froth and spray contaminated by infective aspirates from being dispersed into the theatre; the filter should not be in the outlet to the atmosphere, because the pump may become clogged with coagulated protein if not protected by a filter.

If piped suction is installed, a filter at each peripheral suction point is required to prevent contamination of the pipeline and the exhaust discharge. Venturi suction units powered by piped oxygen also need protection by a filter between the collection jar and the suction pump. Steam-powered Venturi pumps are probably self-disinfecting and safe to use without filtration, provided the tubes leading to them are removed and sterilized after each operating session.

Contamination of fluids

To prevent contamination of fluids with *Pseudomonas aeruginosa*, *Serratia* or other Gram-negative bacilli, aqueous solutions of cetrimide and chlorhexidine should be stocked in the Pharmacy in concentrated solutions and diluted for issue with fresh distilled or sterilized water, with the addition of 7% isopropyl alcohol as a preservative. If the solutions will withstand heat, the provision of sterilized antiseptic solutions is desirable. Stock and issue bottles should be covered with a screw cap without cork liners; corks must never be used. Once open, a bottle should be in use for no longer than one day. All bottles should be sterilized or adequately disinfected before being refilled (unless disposable containers are used). Fluids used in ophthalmic surgery should be supplied, when possible, autoclaved in their final containers and in small volumes, so that none are stored in bottles that have been opened for use. Heat labile solutions should be sterilized by filtration.

Sterile water for topical use should be supplied autoclaved in bottles. Tank water sterilizers and piped systems are liable to contamination and should generally be avoided.

Infection transmitted by blood

See notes on serum hepatitis in Chapters 5, 18 and 19.

Preparation of the surgical team

Definition of team movements

All persons — surgeons, anaesthetists, operating room nurses and others — who
enter the aseptic zone of the theatre during an operation are described as members of the team. They are divided into 'scrubbed' and 'unscrubbed' members.

To reduce the hazard of contamination from dispersers of virulent staphylococci the team should be kept as small as possible; no one whose presence is not
essential should be admitted to the operating room.

Movements in the theatre should be reduced to a minimum; in particular, it
should be unnecessary to fetch materials from outside the theatre or to remove
instruments for resterilization before the end of an operation. Doors should be
kept closed during the operation.

Fitness of the members of the team for duty

No one with a boil or septic lesion of the skin or eczema colonized with *Staph.
aureus* should remain at work in an operating theatre. Protection cannot be
achieved by covering the lesion with an adhesive dressing. When the lesion is
cured, it is desirable to use an antiseptic detergent preparation or soap for all
ablutions, so that the staphylococci which caused the lesion can be removed
from the skin.

When there has been an outbreak of infection with a particular phage-type of
Staph. aureus and there is evidence to suggest that the infection was probably
acquired in the theatre, nasal or lesion carriers should be sought and treated,
nasal carriers with nasal antibacterial creams (containing neomycin or other
agent or combination of agents shown to be effective; see Chapter 9).

Respiratory infections in the team may cause respiratory infection in the
patient at a time when he is particularly susceptible, and it is preferable for persons with such infection to be excluded from the team; the hazard from respiratory infection applies especially to anaesthetists. A surgeon infected with *Strepto coccus pyogenes* (e.g. streptococcal tonsillitis) must not operate.

Bathing and showers

It has been shown that showers tend to increase rather than reduce the number
of bacteria-carrying particles dispersed from the skin. Staff should, therefore,
not take showers immediately before operations.

Removal of everyday clothes

It is rational to remove the outer clothes before putting on operating room
clothes. There is no evidence, however, that the removal of underclothes reduces
the amount of contamination from the body, and this may be left to the discretion of the individual.

Operating room clothes

Operating suits and gowns (Hambraeus and Laurell, 1980). Conventional operating clothes give some protection against contact contamination (if dry), but do
not reduce the amount of airborne contamination with bacteria from the wearer's

164

skin. Bacteria escape through pores in the fabric and (if trousers are worn) at the ankles; few escape from the openings at the neck, waist and sleeves. The use of an operating suit made of a woven fabric with pore size of 7–10 μm (e.g. Ventile) and the securing of trousers around the ankles greatly reduces the dispersal of bacteria. Gowns made of Ventile or similar closely woven fabric are available. In addition to preventing the transfer of bacteria, this type of fabric resists wetting. To retain non-wetting properties the fabric must be reproofed after about thirty launderings. Wearers have found these fabrics uncomfortable. A more comfortable disposable type of operating clothes has been developed from unwoven cellulose fibre. With the Charnley-Howorth ultra-clean air enclosure, a body exhaust ventilated operating suit made of a small-pore woven fabric has been used by the operating team and found comfortable. When ordinary cotton gowns are used, they must be changed if they become soaked with blood or other liquids.

The reduction of airborne bacterial contamination is greater when both scrubbed and unscrubbed staff wear special operating clothes which reduce the dispersal of bacteria than when these are worn only by the operating team. However, the necessity for such special operating clothing in routine general surgery is uncertain.

Footwear. Linen overshoes prevent contamination only if the theatre floor is dry. Footwear with impervious soles (e.g. rubber or plastic boots, or overshoes made of waterproof material) should therefore be worn in the aseptic zone; the shoes should fit, so that bellows action may be avoided.

Mats with tacky or disinfectant surfaces at the entrance to theatres are not recommended, as they have been found to offer little protection against bacterial contamination of operating room floors. If not regularly changed they may increase the numbers of organisms transferred into the theatre.

Headgear. The hair should be completely covered by a close-fitting cap (preferably made of an impervious plastic, paper or Ventile).

Masks. To prevent the impaction of large numbers of droplets from the mouth into the operation field, it is the usual practice to wear a mask; formerly it was recommended that an impervious 'deflector' type of mask should be worn, but current practice is to use a disposable mask that acts as a filter and, to some extent, as a deflector. Some disposable paper masks offer poor protection. A fresh mask should be worn for each operation, and masks that become damp should be replaced. Special masks with an aspirator to draw off expired air are appropriate for use in operations on high risk patients. Special operating clothes, footwear etc., must be discarded on leaving the theatre suite (see Chapter 8).

Hands and gloves. Details on pre-operative cleaning and disinfection of the hands are given in Chapter 7. An antiseptic soap or detergent preparation — e.g. 4% chlorhexidine detergent solution ('Hibiscrub') or povidone-iodine 'surgical scrub' (e.g. 'Betadine', 'Disadine') — should be used. An alternative method, which is more effective and less expensive, is to rub 10 ml (in two applications of 5 ml) of

165

0.5% chlorhexidine in 95% ethyl alcohol with 1% glycerol into the skin of hands and forearms until evaporated to dryness. A two minutes' scrub with a detergent antiseptic preparation such as 'Hibiscrub' and a sterile brush, is recommended for the first operation on the list, and detergents must be used to remove visible dirt or blood. The disinfection must be systematic and cover all areas of hands and forearms.

A metal scraper may be used to remove dirt from under finger nails. Care must be taken to avoid contaminating the contents of soap or detergent dispensers (e.g. by the use of a foot-operated dispenser).

The scrubbed team should wear new gloves which have been sterilized once only. On the appearance of a visible tear they must be removed and replaced with new gloves after washing the hands with an antiseptic detergent preparation; a fresh gown must also be put on, because the sleeves become contaminated on changing the gloves. If it is necessary for gloves to be resterilized and used again they must first be tested for invisible holes by inflation with a foot-pump and immersion under water, or by inflation with water. It is desirable to remove rings before putting on surgical gloves.

Preparation of the patient and performance of the operation

Fitness of the patient for operation: susceptibility to infection

Risks of infection vary with the operation and with certain general factors; e.g. there is a greater risk in the obese, cachectic, or elderly, in those who spend a long time in hospital before operation, in patients with uncontrolled diabetes (especially in operating on limbs, because of impaired circulation), and in those treated with corticosteroids or immunosuppressive drugs; the chances of contamination are greater in patients with existing infection. For such 'high risk' patients additional aseptic precautions are advisable, such as segregation and treatment for staphylococcal carriage before operation, perhaps the use of specially ventilated operating enclosures and, in some circumstances, chemoprophylaxis (see below, p. 169).

Protection against 'self-infection'

An operation wound may become infected with bacteria carried by the patient in his nose, gut or skin; e.g. gas gangrene in patients having amputation of a leg with poor arterial blood supply is usually caused by faecal organisms present on the skin. Urinary infections and wound infections in bowel surgery are often due to coliform bacilli from the gut (see below, under Chemoprophylaxis, p. 169).

There is a particular hazard if the patient has an active staphylococcal infection, especially if it is near the operation site. In these circumstances the patient's operation should, if possible, be delayed till the infection is over, or if this cannot be done an appropriate antibiotic should be used for prophylaxis (see below). Other measures, such as covering the lesions with a bacteria-impermeable dressing and disinfecting the surrounding skin, may also be helpful. Protection against staphylococci carried by patients who have no infection is unnecessary except during an outbreak of staphylococcal sepsis caused by an epidemic strain, when a nasal antibacterial cream and a disinfectant soap should be used for a few days before operation (see below).

Protection of the operation site

Methods of cleansing and disinfection of the skin are described in Chapter 7. The agents recommended for routine use on skin are 0.5% chlorhexidine or 1% iodine in 70% alcohol or alcoholic povidone-iodine applied with friction for at least two minutes; where there is a special hazard from clostridia, a compress of 10% aqueous povidone-iodine should be applied for 30 minutes. The skin should be washed with soap and water and dried before disinfection, after removing hair with a razor. Soap for shaving should be applied with a sterile gauze swab, not with a shaving brush. Because of the risk of causing small abrasions which may become heavily colonized by bacteria, it is advisable to defer shaving until the day of the operation. There is some evidence that there is less wound infection if the skin is not shaved at all (Cruse and Foord, 1973).

For disinfection of mucous membranes an aqueous solution of iodine (e.g. Lugol's or povidone-iodine) or aqueous chlorhexidine is generally recommended; alcohol appears to have little or no action against bacteria on the oral mucous membranes, probably because of dilution by saliva.

For disinfection of the urethra, 1 ml of 1% chlorhexidine obstetric cream should be instilled immediately before the patient is taken to the theatre for cystoscopy or before catheterization; the instillation of a diluted solution (1/5000) of chlorhexidine for disinfection of the bladder after gynaecological operations is also useful. A pad of plastic foam kept moist with chlorhexidine jelly may be attached to indwelling catheters at the urethral meatus in female patients.

Transport of the patient to the operating suite

The patient should be provided with freshly laundered theatre clothes and disinfected blankets immediately before he is taken to the operating suite. The porters should hand over the patient on his trolley to theatre staff in the interchange area; there is no evidence that the transfer of the patient to a clean trolley reduces the chances of contamination of the theatre, so this procedure (and the availability of a trolley transfer area in the theatre suite) can be omitted. (See Ayliffe *et al.*, 1969; Hambraeus and Laurell, 1980).

Towelling techniques

Sterile drapes provide sterile cover for areas away from the immediate site of the operation and for instrument trays and other equipment. To prevent the loss of protectiveness on wetting, a layer of sterilized waterproof material under the drape or the use of waterproof towels is advantageous. There is evidence that adhesive plastic drapes do not protect the wound against contamination from the adjacent skin or reduce the incidence of sepsis (Wheeler, 1979); their use for the prevention of infection can therefore not be recommended.

Operations on contaminated organs

The incidence and mortality from sepsis is higher after operations on the bowel

167

than after operations on other sites. It is therefore rational to remove colonic bacteria when this can be done without risk. Colonic washouts have been widely used, but are unlikely to reduce the density of colonic bacteria or the incidence of sepsis. Non-absorbed aminoglycoside antibiotics (neomycin, framycetin) given by mouth can greatly reduce the aerobic flora, but they are ineffective against anaerobes; metronidazole has been shown to reduce the incidence of anaerobic postoperative sepsis, and a short course in combination with an aminoglycoside is an effective prophylactic (see below, and Chapter 12).

In operations involving section of the alimentary tract or other heavily colonized viscera, gross soiling of tissue should be avoided by careful technique and by the use of packs (perhaps containing a layer of impervious material) and swabs. Instruments used on the opened viscus must be regarded as contaminated and should be kept separate from the rest of the instruments in the tray; they should be discarded after completion of anastomosis or excision.

Tissue handling techniques

Tissues must be handled gently, and no more foreign material must be left in a wound than is essential for the success of the operation. Careful haemostasis is important; dead tissue and haematoma must be removed, and their formation must be prevented.

The practice of picking up with artery forceps only the bleeding vessel with little or no surrounding tissue, and the use of diathermy to coagulate the smaller bleeding points reduces the amount of dead or foreign material in the wound. The thinnest ligature which has the required strength should be chosen.

Whenever primary suture is intended care must be taken to avoid contamination from the skin.

Wound drainage

A wound that is drained is more likely to become infected than a closed wound; drainage should therefore be used only when there is a definite indication for it — e.g. to prevent accumulation of fluid such as when a serous cavity has been opened, when infection is present, when there is a fistula, or when there is much oozing of blood, lymph or serum into the wound.

The risk of infection may be reduced by the use of a closed system of drainage. The drain should be removed as soon as possible; e.g. oozing of blood will stop after a few hours, and a drain inserted to meet this hazard can normally be removed after 24 hours or less. It is better for drainage tubes to be too large than too small (small tubes without suction and corrugated drains are inadequate except for very superficial wounds). For deeper wounds the drain should be long, extending to a bottle below the level of the bed; an underwater seal should be used for chest drains. Suction drainage provides a closed system which should help to prevent ascending infection.

Disposal of used material

Contaminated swabs and other articles should be placed in impermeable bags,

168

which are sealed to prevent liberation of bacteria during handling and removal for cleaning and sterilization.

Chemoprophylaxis (see also Chapter 12)

When the antibiotics were new they were often used uncritically and needlessly for prophylaxis in surgery. This indiscriminate use encouraged the emergence of a predominantly resistant hospital flora. There was evidence, too, that patients were obtaining no clinical benefit from such prophylaxis, and when sepsis appeared it was likely to be caused by organisms resistant to the available antibiotics. The outcome was a general and somewhat uncritical condemnation of chemoprophylaxis in surgery.

A number of controlled trials and microbiological studies in recent years have led to a reappraisal of the situation. While routine systemic chemoprophylaxis is still seen as likely to do more harm than good, the use in selected patients of antibiotics which are likely to cover the range of probable invaders can undoubtedly give valuable protection; selective prophylaxis against known organisms of usually predictable sensitivity, used as an adjunct of careful asepsis, is appropriate when the consequence of infection would probably be serious. The drug should be given in standard or large doses, starting not long before the operation and continuing for, at most, a few days afterwards; such a short period of treatment is unlikely to encourage the emergence of resistant variants, but it protects the patient during his most vulnerable period of exposure.

Since the first edition of this Handbook there have been many publications which show the great importance of non-sporing anaerobic bacilli as a cause of postoperative sepsis after operations on the gastro-intestinal tract; such organisms greatly outnumber the aerobic organisms, including *Escherichia coli*, in the faeces, and they are resistant to the aminoglycoside antibiotics, such as neomycin, which have been in common use for pre-operative disinfection of the gut. Willis (1979) quotes researches which show that, in patients having major colonic surgery, prophylactic metronidazole may confidently be expected to eliminate anaerobic sepsis after operations in which the anaerobic sepsis rates are usually about 50%; similar prophylactic results were obtained in patients having appendicectomies and hysterectomies. Others (e.g. Keighly and Burdon, 1979) have found that short systemic courses of metronidazole or lincomycin combined with an aminoglycoside (neomycin, tobramycin) gave good protection in colorectal surgery. Oral administration of these antimicrobial drugs can cause a large reduction in the bacterial flora of the faeces, but postoperative sepsis and pseudomembranous enterocolitis are reported to occur more often in patients given oral prophylaxis than in those protected by systemic antibiotics.

Chemoprophylaxis is indicated in patients having colorectal operations because they are exposed to massive contamination. Detailed recommendations for chemoprophylaxis in abdominal surgery are presented in Chapter 12 (p. 195). In operations on ischaemic lower limbs (e.g. amputation for diabetic gangrene) a short course (five days) of prophylaxis with a narrow-range antibiotic active against *Clostridium welchii* and other gas gangrene clostridia (usually a penicillin) is indicated because of the known risks of gas gangrene through contamination of ischaemic muscle with *Cl. welchii* (faecal contaminants) on the skin of

169

the buttocks and thighs. Other operations in which chemoprophylaxis is recommended include dental operations in patients with endocardial disease, to prevent infective endocarditis (penicillin or, in penicillin-sensitive patients, erythromycin or cephalosporin, are appropriate agents). Patients with infected urine should have prophylaxis with an antibiotic selected on the basis of sensitivity tests before operation. In patients undergoing operations for insertion of heart valve prosthesis, prophylactic treatment is indicated, e.g. with a penicillinase-tolerant penicillin, continuing the treatment for as long as three months (until the valve cuff becomes epithelialized).

The use of volatile sprays containing neomycin, bacitracin and polymyxin has been found to reduce the incidence of sepsis in general surgery and in neurosurgery. It has also led to the emergence, through selection, of staphylococci resistant to neomycin and bacitracin. This method should therefore be used only in 'high-risk' patients; its use should be controlled by the microbiologist and the antibiotics chosen should be active against all the staphylococci and most of the Gram-negative bacilli isolated in the hospital. The use of povidone-iodine spray is an appropriate alternative to topical antibiotics which appears to have some value. Instillation into the wound before closure of 1 g cephaloridine in 2 ml water has been reported to reduce the incidence of sepsis. Resistant bacteria are likely to emerge if this method is used, so it should be reserved for patients in whom there is a high risk of infection (see Chapter 12). Oral premedication with antibiotics before colonic operations is discussed above (operations on contaminated organs); superinfection with resistant organisms not only reduces the value of this method but may be a dangerous complication. Nasal chemoprophylaxis with neomycin-containing creams has been found effective when combined with other methods, but should be reserved for 'high-risk' or epidemic situations. Disinfection of the urethra before instrumentation may prevent postoperative infection of the urinary tract and bacteraemia.

After total hip and knee replacement operations deep infection may develop as much as two or three years later. Short courses of systemic chemoprophylaxis by cloxacillin or by a combination of antibiotics have been reported to reduce this hazard. Another method which has been associated with exceptionally low sepsis rates is the use of acrylic cement containing gentamicin, which is released very slowly and does not lead to any detectable concentration of the antibiotic in the blood after the first few days. The prophylactic value of antibiotic-loaded cement and the freedom from hazards of patient-sensitization and microbial resistance still need to be assessed.

References and Further Reading

Altemeier, W. A. (1963), Prevention of post-operative infections: operating theatre practice. In: *Infection in Hospitals* (eds R. E. O. Williams and R. A. Shooter), p. 207. Blackwell, Oxford.

Altemeier, W. A., Burke, J. F., Pruitt, B. A. and Sandusky, W. R. (1976), *Manual on Control of Infection in Surgical Patients*. Lipincott, Philadelphia.

Ayliffe, G. A. J., Babb, J. R., Collins, B. J. and Lowbury, E. J. L. (1969), Transfer areas and clean zones in operating suites. *J. Hygiene*, 67, 417.

Ayliffe, G. A. J., Brightwell, K. M., Collins, B. J., Lowbury, E. J. L., Goonati-lake, P. C. L. and Etheridge, R. A. (1977), Surveys of hospital infection in the Birmingham Region: effect of age, sex, length of stay and antibiotic use on normal carriage of tetracycline-resistant *Staphylococcus aureus* and on post-operative wound infection. *J. Hyg. Camb.*, 79, 299.

British Standards, BS 3970 Part 3, BSI (in draft).

British Standards (1967), *Electrically operated surgical suction apparatus of high vacuum and high air displacement type.* BS 4199 Part 1, BSI.

Cruse, J. P. E. and Foord, R. (1973), A five-year study of 23,649 surgical wounds. *Archs. Surg.*, 107, 206.

George, R. H., Symonds, J. M., Dimock, F., Brown, J. D., Arabi, Y., Shinagawa, N., Keighley, M. R. B., Alexander-Williams, J., and Burdon, D. W. (1978), Identification of *Clostridium difficile* as a cause of pseudomembranous colitis. *Br. med. J.* i, 695.

Hambraeus, A. and Laurell, G. (1980), Protection of the patient in the operating suite. *J. hosp. Infect.* 1, 15.

Keighley, M. R. B. and Burdon, D. W. (1979), *Antimicrobial Prophylaxis in Surgery*, Pitman Medical, London.

Medical Research Council (1962), Design and ventilation of operating suites. *Lancet*, ii, 943.

Medical Research Council (1968), Aseptic methods in the operating suite. *Lancet*, i, 705, 763, 831.

Walter, C. W. (1958), *The Aseptic Treatment of Wounds*, MacMillan, New York.

Wheeler, M. H. (1979), Abdominal wound protection by means of plastic drapes. In: *Surgical Sepsis* (eds C. J. L. Strachan and R. Wise), Academic Press, New York.

Willis, A. T. (1979), Infections with obligate anaerobes. In: *Recent Advances in Infection*, 1 (eds D. Reeves and A. Geddes), Churchill Livingstone, Edinburgh, London and New York, pp. 205-21.

CHAPTER ELEVEN

Laundry, Kitchen Hygiene and Refuse Disposal

Laundry hygiene and handling of contaminated linen (see DHSS, 1971)

Contaminated laundry may be an infection hazard to patients and staff in the ward, to the portering staff during transport, and to laundry staff during sorting and washing. Inadequately disinfected or recontaminated clean laundry may be responsible for transferring infection from the laundry to the patient.

Many organisms, mostly non-pathogenic, can be isolated from soiled linen and clothing. *Staphylococcus aureus* is the commonest and one of the most important of the potential pathogens there, since it survives much better in the environment in dry conditions than Gram-negative bacilli and most viruses. Healthy staphylococcal carriers or dispersers are not commonly recognized, so that care must be taken in the handling of all soiled linen. Linen from patients infected with other pathogens, e.g. *Salmonella* sp., *Shigella* sp., and myco-bacteria is likely to be a greater hazard, especially if visibly soiled with excretions or discharges, but the infections are usually recognized and treated with due care. The DHSS report suggests that laundry should be divided into two categories (1) *foul or infected* and (2) *soiled*. However, all hospital linen should be disinfected by heat in the washing process or, if this is not possible, by some other method; hypochlorite or another disinfectant may be added to the rinse water.

To reduce the risk of cross-infection in the ward, bedding should be carefully removed and placed in a suitable sack at the bed-side. Foul or infected linen should be sealed in a waterproof bag of a distinctive colour, e.g. red; alternatively the waterproof bag should be placed in an outer coloured laundry bag.

Since linen may look clean and yet be heavily contaminated with pathogenic organisms, all laundry should be completely sealed in a bag which is not permeable to micro-organisms. Sealed impermeable bags may be carried through open wards or public corridors and transferred to the laundry with very little risk of infection. If intermediate storage areas are required between the clinical area and the laundry, these should be built for the purpose, providing protection from the weather, and should have facilities for cleaning (see p. 180, Disposal of refuse). If possible, dirty and clean laundry should be transported in different vehicles. This is less important if both dirty and clean linen are transported in impermeable bags or containers, but cleaning of the interior of the vehicles is

172

required if clean linen is transported after dirty.

The ward staff are responsible for placing laundry in the correct bag and adequately closing it. This should reduce sorting of infected linen in the laundry to a minimum and reduce the risk of infection to the laundry staff. Although handling of foul or infected linen should not be necessary, it is apparently unavoidable owing to the presence of miscellaneous items, e.g. forceps, which would damage the machines; gloves should always be worn by handlers. The ward staff must be trained to remove any such items and to realize the harmful effect it might have on the health of the laundry staff if further sorting is required. This applies particularly to certain categories of infected linen which should be placed in clearly identified bags and *never* handled by the laundry staff. This includes linen from all patients in strict isolation (see Chapter 9), with enteric diseases, dysentery, infectious or serum hepatitis and open tuberculosis. Linen in this category should be placed in alginate stitched or hot water-soluble plastic bags and transferred unopened into the foul sluicing machine. Infested linen (e.g. with lice or fleas) should be similarly handled. Linen from patients with hepatitis or with hepatitis antigen-positive blood should be clearly labelled. Linen from patients with anthrax should be autoclaved before washing. Linen from patients with dangerous infections, such as Lassa fever, also requires special treatment (see Chapter 17). A member of the infection control team should contact the laundry manager and wards if any such patients are present in the hospital or if there is any doubt as to precautions required.

If sorting of foul linen in the laundry is unavoidable, it may not be worthwhile separating foul from soiled in the ward, although the infected linen as described above must never be sorted by laundry staff. The development of a suitable metal detector could reduce the need for sorting. However, there is no evidence of an increased risk of infection in laundry workers who sort foul linen.

Sluicing of infected linen should take place in a separate area and in special machines. Water from foul or infected sluicing machines should be discharged directly into a drain so that splashes or aerosols do not contaminate the laundry environment. If linen is sent to a commercial laundry or a laundry in another hospital, it is important to ensure that safe foul washing machines are available. If not, linen should be disinfected by sluicing and heat before it is sent out.

All linen should be disinfected during the washing process. Thermometers on machines should be correctly sited, and times and temperatures of the disinfection process checked with every cycle. Thermometers with pen recorders should be placed on machines used for infected laundry.

During the disinfecting stage of the cycle, the temperature of the items in the machine should be maintained at at least 65° C (150° F) for 10 min or 71° C (160° F) for 3 min. Linen from patients with serum hepatitis should be heated to at least 93° C (200° F) for 10 min. Mixing times of 4 to 8 min should be included, depending on the size of the machine. Since the recorded temperature does not necessarily correspond to the temperature of the load, it is important that the efficiency of the disinfection process should be checked bacteriologically in new machines and at intervals afterwards (e.g. twice yearly). Small numbers of organisms surviving the washing process may be killed at a later stage by the heat-drying and finishing process.

173

Chemical methods of disinfection are less reliable than heat, but may occasionally be necessary for heat-labile materials. Hypochlorites and quaternary ammonium compounds are readily inactivated by organic materials during the washing process, but may be effective if added during the rinse process (e.g. if hypochlorites are added to a final concentration of 250 ppm in the second rinse). Chemical methods of disinfection are not generally accepted alternatives to heat, and the use of heat-labile clothing should be discouraged. If staining is reported when chlorhexidine-contaminated linen is bleached, sodium perborate should be used instead of hypochlorite as a bleaching agent.

It is also important that clean linen should not be recontaminated on storage or during transport to the ward. Although physical barriers between soiled and clean areas are not indicated, the air-flow should be adjusted by extractor fans so that the flow is from clean to contaminated areas. The routes for soiled and clean laundry should be separate so that transmission of contamination by contact is not possible.

The risk of infection to the laundry staff is not great, provided the required precautions are undertaken, and it is probably no greater than to the nursing staff. Staff should wear aprons, gloves and overalls for sorting and should be provided with adequate personal washing facilities. Training in personal and hospital hygiene is important. Staff should be offered BCG if Mantoux or Heaf tests are negative, and immunization against poliomyelitis. Staff with superficial sepsis should not handle clean laundry.

Kitchen hygiene (see DHSS, 1974)

All patients usually receive food from one kitchen, and poor hygiene in food preparation may be followed by an outbreak of infection involving the whole hospital. Infection from contaminated food is particularly hazardous in debilitated or aged people and can cause severe illness or even death. It is also important to prevent food-borne infection among the staff, since subsequent transfer to patients would have similar unfortunate results. Every effort should be made to prevent the serving of contaminated food to patients or staff. Bacterial food poisoning is usually caused by *Salmonella* sp., or the toxins of certain strains of *Staph. aureus* and *Cl. welchii.* These organisms, especially *Salmonella* sp., may be transferred to the patient directly from contaminated raw foods (e.g. meat and poultry if inadequately cooked) or indirectly to initially uncontaminated food on the hands of staff or from inadequately cleaned surfaces or equipment. Staphylococcal and salmonella carriers on the staff may also contaminate food if their personal hygiene is poor. Inadequately cooked food which is left without refrigeration for several hours, and particularly if subsequently warmed, is an important source of infection; any food capable of supporting bacterial growth should be stored either below $6°$ C ($43°$ F) or above $65°$ C ($149°$ F).

Good personal hygiene of kitchen staff and effective methods of cleaning food preparation areas and equipment is of major importance in preventing the spread of infection. The general kitchen structure, e.g. walls, floors and ceilings, though of little direct relevance in the spread of infection, should be kept clean and in good condition.

174

Medical staff examination

The prospective employee should be questioned for a past history of typhoid or paratyphoid fever, dysentery, persistent diarrhoea or attacks of diarrhoea and vomiting lasting for more than two days within the past two years, tuberculosis, boils, skin rashes, discharges from eye, ear, nose or other site, also the place and date of visits abroad. A questionnaire on the above illnesses and other relevant information is filled in by the Catering Manager or a member of the occupational health department and signed by the proposed employee (see Appendix 11.1). If otherwise suitable, the Catering Manager may provisionally accept him pending a satisfactory assessment by a medical officer, who may require a more extensive medical examination. A tuberculin skin test is advisable and, if negative, BCG should be offered. Examination of blood, faeces, other laboratory tests or a chest X-ray need not be carried out unless indicated by past history. The microbiologist or control of infection officer should be consulted if laboratory tests are considered necessary. If an examination of faeces is required, at least three samples on successive days should be examined.

Sickness

A member of the staff suffering from diarrhoea and/or vomiting during working hours should immediately report to the Catering Manager, who will refer him to the staff medical officer. If the employee prefers to see his own general practitioner, he should still report to the Catering Manager, staff medical officer or a member of the infection control team (or when these are not available, the senior member of the nursing staff on duty) before leaving the hospital so that arrangements can be made for collecting a sample of faeces if necessary. Staff suffering from a skin rash, boils, any other skin lesion, or discharge from any site, should likewise cease work and be referred by the Catering Manager to a medical officer as soon as possible. Employees referred because of infection or suspected infection should only return when a certificate of clearance signed by a medical officer is produced. Details of the infection need not be disclosed to the Catering Manager or other lay staff if this is preferred by the employee.

Employees should also report to the Catering Manager (1) on returning to duty after an illness involving diarrhoea and/or vomiting, or any of the conditions mentioned above; (2) after returning from holiday which included an attack of diarrhoea and/or vomiting lasting for more than one day; and (3) if any member of his household is suffering from diarrhoea and/or vomiting.

If in any doubt about these circumstances or any other disease, e.g. infectious hepatitis or poliomyelitis, the Catering Manager should refer the employee to a medical officer, who then must certify him as free from infection before he returns to work. If a diagnosis of *Shigella* or *Salmonella* infection has been made or suspected, at least three consecutive negative faeces samples should be obtained before allowing the member of the staff to return to duty. More tests will be required following typhoid fever. The employee should also sign a form agreeing to report any of the relevant infections or conditions (see Appendix 11.2). The success of the arrangements depends on the ready availability of a medical opinion. Hospitals should make arrangements for a staff medical officer or a member of the infection control staff to be accessible for this purpose. To encourage employees to report illnesses rapidly at any time of the day or night, they should not receive their pay until seen by a staff medical officer or their own general practitioner, and certified as fit or not for return to work.

Training

All food handlers should be given training in personal and kitchen hygiene on employment and at intervals afterwards. A booklet containing rules of hygiene should be provided for each member. Posters demonstrating different aspects of hygiene should be prominently displayed in catering food storage areas and changed at frequent intervals (see Appendix 11.3).

Personal hygiene

The main route of transfer of infection to food is on the hands of staff. Hands should be washed frequently, especially after using the toilet and before handling food. In addition to the hands and particularly nails, the face and other parts of the body likely to come into contact with food should be kept clean, e.g. the hair and scalp, and the forearms when short sleeves are worn. The nose, lips and hair should not be touched while handling food. Nails should be kept short. Hands are not necessarily completely free from pathogenic organisms after washing, and food should be handled as little as possible. Hands should be washed in hot water using the recommended soap or detergent and must then be well rinsed and thoroughly dried on a fresh paper towel. Nail brushes should only be used if hands are heavily soiled, and, if used, brushes should be nylon (not bristle) and stored in a dry state (and preferably autoclaved daily). Their use should be avoided if possible, because they tend to damage the skin. Washbasins must be provided in each food preparation area and plain bar or liquid soap or detergent provided. If liquid soap dispensers are used they must be thoroughly cleaned at regular intervals and must not be refilled without prior cleaning and disinfection. The liquid soap should contain a preservative. Antibacterial soaps (e.g. chlorhexidine detergent preparations, iodophors, hexachlorophane or Irgasan DP300 for staphylococcal infections) may be required during an outbreak of infection, but should be used only on advice from a microbiologist. The catering staff should be provided with good changing and sanitary accommodation. Food handlers should keep their personal clothing and overalls clean and should change their protective clothing daily or more frequently if necessary. The protective clothing should only be worn for catering duties and should not be worn in other departments. Laundering should be arranged by the hospital authorities. Uniforms and other protective clothing should not be taken home for laundering or any other purpose. Staff should not smoke while handling food or while in a room where there is 'open' food. All cuts and grazes must be completely covered with a waterproof dressing.

Cleaning and maintenance

Detailed schedules should be produced defining methods and responsibility. Floors should be constructed to facilitate cleaning and should be well maintained. Walls and ceilings should have smooth impermeable surfaces and cooking equipment should be so sited that areas below and around can be easily cleaned.

All cleaning should be carried out with a freshly prepared and accurately diluted detergent solution. Cleaning equipment, e.g. scrubbing machines and mops, should remain in the kitchen area (for methods of disinfection see Chapter 7) and should be examined at defined intervals. If worn or damaged, equipment should be repaired or replaced. Special attention should be paid to the cleaning of food preparation surfaces and meat slicers. Preparation surfaces should be impervious to water and should be maintained in a good condition. Stainless steel surfaces are advised, although composition chopping boards and blocks are suitable. Wherever possible, preparation surfaces should be used for one purpose only. Food requiring no further cooking, e.g. sandwiches, cooked meat etc., should not be prepared on surfaces which have previously been used for the preparation of raw meat, fish, poultry or vegetables. In small units with limited working areas, it may be necessary to use surfaces for more than one purpose; thorough cleaning and drying between different uses is required in such cases. Preparation surfaces should always be cleaned with a recently prepared hot cleaning solution and an unused disposable or freshly laundered cloth. There is little point in providing separate surfaces for different preparations if all surfaces are cleaned with the same cleaning solution and cloths; contamination will be transferred from one surface to another. Each individual surface should be dried with a disposable or freshly laundered dry cloth; most Gram-negative bacilli die on drying, if the surface is initially clean.

Disinfectants are usually unnecessary, but may be recommended by the Control of Infection Officer or microbiologist during outbreaks of infection (hypochlorite solutions containing at least 250 ppm available chlorine are often used.)

Transfer of contamination from one product to another is particularly likely with meat mincers and slicers. Cooked and uncooked meats must never be processed on the same machine without thorough cleaning between operations.

Crockery and cutlery; pots and pans

Crockery and cutlery should be machine-washed at a minimum temperature of $60°$ C ($140°$ F) and a final rinse of at least $82°$ C ($180°$ F). A central washing-up machine is preferred and washing up by hand on the ward should be avoided whenever possible. A washing-up machine on the ward is, however, a satisfactory alternative.

Until machine washing is available, crockery and cutlery can be washed by hand, but twin sinks should be used to ensure efficient rinsing. Detergent solutions and rinsing water should be changed frequently and should be as hot as possible. The use of washing-up cloths should be discontinued, and replaced by disposable cloths. Nylon brushes, washed and thoroughly dried after each use, are preferable to cloths, but should not be used in preference to disposable materials.

It is important that all crockery, cutlery, pots and pans and kitchen equipment should be thoroughly dried after cleaning. The use of linen drying cloths (tea towels) should be discontinued whenever possible and replaced by a system of heat drying or air drying in racks. When drying by hand is necessary, a disposable towel is preferred.

177

Crockery, cutlery, pots and pans should be examined regularly. Worn, chipped, stained or broken items should be replaced. When not in use, clean crockery, cutlery, pots and pans should be stored so that recontamination is limited as much as possible.

Storage of food and transportation

Certain food, such as raw meat, fish and poultry, may be contaminated with harmful bacteria and should be properly prepared and cooked before serving; periodic checking of temperatures with a probe thermometer in the coldest part of the food is recommended. Poultry may be contaminated with *Salmonella* sp., and inadequate thawing of frozen poultry before cooking may enable those organisms to survive the cooking process. The multiplication of bacteria should be prevented by careful storage of food at the correct temperature before and after cooking, e.g. *Clostridium welchii* is a common cause of food poisoning and its spores may survive the cooking process. These bacteria may multiply if cooked food is left without refrigeration for longer than two hours. Subsequent reheating may further increase the numbers of bacteria, and when large numbers are eaten, toxins (poisons) may be released into the intestine and cause food poisoning.

Food must be stored so that raw meat, fish and uncooked vegetables (whether prepared or unprepared) do not come in contact with food which is to be served without further heat treatment. These foods must be separated by storing in separate refrigerators or in closed compartments within the same refrigerator or cold room. Food must not be stored on the floor of cold rooms or below foods which may be spilt or leak.

Food requiring cooling must not be left in the kitchen area but should be transferred to a cooling area and cooled rapidly to at least 8° C (46° F). The food should also be protected from recontamination. Food which is transported within the hospital, e.g. from stores to kitchen, or from kitchen to ward, should be transported under clean conditions and properly covered to prevent contamination. Vehicles used for this purpose should be properly designed, kept clean and in a good state of repair. Contaminated materials, such as refuse or soiled linen, must not be carried in these vehicles. Food should be carried in a clean closed container, especially if the vehicle is used for other purposes.

Refuse and food waste (swill) must not be allowed to accumulate in the kitchen, and should be removed at frequent intervals (see below under Disposal of refuse and food-waste).

The amount of time during which food is allowed to stand on hot plates and trolleys must be kept to a minimum. Trolleys, hot cupboards and containers must be maintained at the correct temperature, and checked at regular intervals, e.g. monthly.

Food should be served by staff trained in food hygiene. Clean overalls should be worn and adequate serving equipment should be provided to prevent unnecessary handling. Patients should not take part in food preparation or washing-up procedures. This applies particularly to psychiatric hospitals where it is difficult to instruct patients in good food hygiene. Left over food in ward refrigerators should be discarded daily and swill must not be retained or stored on the ward.

Centralized frozen or chilled meal services

Centralization of any catering service increases the number of meals produced in one area and subsequently the risk of a major outbreak of infection. When the food has been cooked, it must be artificially cooled as rapidly as possible. Portioning should be carried out under strictly controlled hygienic conditions and as quickly as possible.

The time interval from removing the food from the oven and chilling and freezing should not exceed two hours. Detailed schedules of time of cooking, preparation and cooling should be produced for each batch as well as appropriate temperatures. A probe thermometer should be used to confirm that the necessary temperatures are reached in each stage of the process. The temperature of the warmest part of the chilled pack should not rise above $10°$ C ($50°$ F) during transport and insulated containers or refrigeration may be necessary. If refrigeration is not available maximum transport times should be agreed and checked at each delivery. After delivery, the food should be heated to defrost it adequately and the temperature should be raised to a safe level. The time required for each pack should be calculated from temperature measurements and rigid control must be maintained. If rules are rigorously enforced a service of this type can provide food which may be safer than that produced by conventional methods.

Responsibility

The Catering Manager is responsible for hygiene and cleaning in his department. The responsibility for maintenance of structure and equipment should be clearly defined. At least one annual inspection should be made by the Catering Manager, the Infection Control Officer or another competent person and a member of the engineering or building staff to examine aspects of hygiene in the catering area. Occasional inspections should also be made by an environmental health officer, who may be invited to visit the hospital catering department at any suitable time. However, the Infection Control Officer and Committee are responsible for advising the administration on all hygienic matters including catering, and reports should be referred to them before action is taken.

Infestation: eradication and control

The infestation of hospital premises (kitchens, canteens, laundries, nurses' homes, etc.) with pests, particularly cockroaches, Pharaoh's ants and mice, is common. Although it is extremely difficult to keep premises free of pests, every effort should be made to control them. The role of pests in the transmission of hospital acquired infection is uncertain, but reports indicating the carriage of specific pathogens, including *Salmonella* spp. are numerous. Apart from the possibility of disease transmission, food may be tainted and spoiled, and fabrics and building structure damaged. Pharaoh's ants have been responsible for the penetration of sterile packs and the invasion of patients' dressings including those *in situ*.

Treatment with insecticides and rodenticides alone is insufficient, and attention must also be paid to good hygiene and structural maintenance. Pests require food, warmth, moisture, harbourage, and a means of entry; hospital staff should be encouraged to enclose food, remove spillage and waste, and to avoid

179

accumulations of static water. Buildings should be of sound structure and well maintained, drains should be covered, leaking pipework repaired, and damaged surfaces made good. Cracks in plaster and woodwork, unsealed areas around pipework, damaged tiles, badly fitting equipment and kitchen units, are all likely to provide excellent harbourage. Close-fitting windows and doors, the provision of fly screens and bird netting etc., all help to exclude pests from hospital buildings.

Many pests are nocturnal, e.g. cockroaches and mice, and infestation surveys are often best carried out at night. In addition to seeing the pests themselves, droppings, nests, runs, smears, insect fragments, structural and fabric damage all indicate signs of infestation. The use of pyrethrum aerosols is useful for flushing cockroaches and other insects from their harbourage, and liver baiting is useful for assessing infestation with Pharaoh's ants. In most hospitals the task of pest control is given to a commercial company specializing in this work. Nevertheless, the hospital should appoint an officer to investigate and record complaints and sightings, carry out preliminary and routine assessments of control measures, and negotiate and comply with the recommendations of the servicing company regarding maintenance and hygiene.

It is usual and desirable for contracts with servicing companies to contain details of methods of eradication or control of specified 'nuisance' pests over an agreed period. The contract should follow a preliminary survey of the extent of infestation; the contract should state the frequency of subsequent surveys and visits for the application of control treatments. The use of specific insecticides and rodenticides should be stated, and these should satisfy the requirements of the Pesticides Safety Precautions Scheme (Ministry of Agriculture, Fisheries and Food). Arrangements should also be made for emergency visits and the provision of detailed reports submitted to the authorized hospital officer. A hospital authority may prefer to carry out its own pest control techniques and advice should be obtained from an official body (MAFF and the DHSS in the United Kingdom). This applies particularly to the types of insecticide or rodenticide used.

Disposal of refuse and food-waste

The risk of infection in hospital from refuse and swill (food waste) is not great but it should be properly enclosed and safely transferred from wards and departments to the main disposal area as quickly as possible. Waste-bags must be protected from the weather and from damage by vermin when stored before and after transfer to the central disposal area.

A clearly defined policy for the collection and disposal of refuse and swill should be produced for each hospital or group and one person should be responsible for implementation of the policy.

Refuse (household and clinical)

Dressings and clinical refuse should be sealed in plastic bags. Household rubbish should be placed in paper sacks made of good quality bitumen impregnated or other paper of good wet strength, or plastic bags. These bags should be mounted on stands with lids. The sealed plastic bags containing contaminated dressings etc., can be placed in paper sacks for removal from the ward area. The risk of infection from the contents of a sealed plastic bag is slight. Needles require special treatment (see Chapter 8). Paper sacks should not be overfilled and the ward staff should be responsible for adequately closing the bags with staples. Bags should be removed from wards and clinical areas at least twice daily and preferably transported directly to the central incineration or compactor site.

If intermediate storage sites are necessary, these should be purpose built, roofed and provided with a washable floor, adequate drainage and a water supply. The areas must be kept clean at all times and care must be taken that spilt rubbish is immediately cleared up.

Food refuse (swill)

This should be sealed in plastic bags and returned to a central area for disposal. A waste disposal unit associated with a central washing-up machine is recommended. If no central disposal unit is available the plastic bags should be taken to the main disposal area for incineration, or small waste disposal units might be provided in wards of small units. Ideally swill should not be sold to contractors, but if sold it should be disposed of only to contractors licensed in accordance with the requirements of The Diseases of Animal (Waste Food) Order, 1973.

If intermediate storage sites (e.g. outside kitchens) are necessary, these should be purpose built as described above for general refuse.

Appendix 11.1 Questionnaire for catering staff

Have you ever had any of the following:					
(1) Typhoid fever? Paratyphoid fever? Dysentery? Persistent diarrhoea? Tuberculosis?	Yes	No	When (year)	How long off work	If yes Name of doctor or hospital
(2) Have you suffered from any of the following within the past two years: Diarrhoea and/or vomiting for more than 2 days?					

Continued overleaf

181

Skin rash?					
Boils?					
Discharge from eye?					
ear?					
nose?					
Other infections?					

(3) Have you ever been abroad?   Yes   No

    If yes: Where   When

I declare that all the foregoing statements are true and complete to the best of my knowledge and belief.

                . . . .

---

(4) *Investigations:*

    Chest X-ray

    Faeces

    Blood

    Other

    Comments

Appendix 11.2 Catering staff agreement to report infection

I agree to report to the Catering Officer or his deputy

(1) If suffering from an illness involving:
Vomiting
Diarrhoea
Skin rash
Septic skin lesions (boils, infected cuts etc., however small)
Discharge from ear, eye or nose
(2) After returning and before commencing work following an illness involving vomiting and/or diarrhoea, or any of the above conditions.
(3) After returning from a holiday during which an attack of vomiting and/or diarrhoea lasted for more than two days.
(4) If another member of my household is suffering from diarrhoea and/or vomiting.

I have read (or had explained to me) and understood the accompanying rules on personal hygiene.

Signed   Date

Appendix 11.3 Kitchen and food-handling staff: rules of personal hygiene

Patients in hospital may develop severe infection with germs which are not harmful to healthy people.
The following rules must be observed to prevent germs from entering food:

(1) *WASH THE HANDS FREQUENTLY*, ESPECIALLY AFTER USING THE TOILET AND BEFORE HANDLING FOOD. THIS IS THE MOST IMPORTANT METHOD PREVENTING THE SPREAD OF INFECTION. In addition to hands and particularly nails, the face and other parts of the body likely to come into contact with food should be kept clean, e.g. the hair and scalp, and the forearms when short sleeves are worn. Avoid touching the nose, lips and hair while handling food.
(2) Personal clothing and overalls must be kept clean. Protective clothing provided by the Hospital must be worn.
(3) All open cuts and grazes must be completely covered with a waterproof dressing.
(4) You must not smoke while handling 'open' food or while in a room where there is such food.
(5) Other hygienic rules as indicated by the Catering Manager.

References and Further Reading

Department of Health and Social Security (1971), *Report on Hospital Laundry Arrangements*, (HM(71)49).

Department of Health and Social Security (1974), *Health Service Catering Manual*, Vol. 2, *Hygiene*.

Hobbs, B. C. (1974), *Food Poisoning and Food Hygiene*, 3rd edn, Edward Arnold, London.

Chemotherapy, Chemoprophylaxis and Immunization

CHAPTER TWELVE

Use of Antibiotics and Chemotherapeutic Agents

In this chapter the word antibiotic refers to both synthetic compounds (anti-microbial chemotherapeutic agents) and naturally produced agents (antibiotics). These substances have *selective toxicity* against many living agents pathogenic to man. Selective toxicity means that the drugs are less poisonous to the tissues of the body than they are to micro-organisms. Some substances (e.g. the penicillins) are almost without toxicity to man (except for those rare persons who are hypersensitive to them) but will kill many pathogenic bacteria. Certain antibiotics (e.g. bacitracin, neomycin) are so toxic that they cannot be safely given parenterally and are general reserved for topical treatment of superficial infections when the infected area is not extensive, or for oral administration to remove intestinal bacteria, provided that the antibiotic is not absorbed from the intestine.

If a patient is known or suspected to be suffering from an infection the clinician must decide which organism is known or likely to be responsible and to which antibiotic it will probably be sensitive. Other factors which must be considered include the expected value of treatment and the possible side-effects of the antibiotic.

The aim of chemotherapy is principally to aid the natural defences of the body to eliminate the microbes from tissues by preventing their multiplication. The blood and infected tissues must contain a concentration of the antibiotic higher than the *minimal inhibitory* (i.e. *bacteristatic*) *concentration* (MIC) of the antibiotic for the infecting organism. In septicaemia, endocarditis, osteomyelitis, pyelonephritis, and infections in patients with poor natural defences or in those receiving immunosuppressive drugs or steroids, chemotherapy must aim to *kill* the infecting organisms, i.e. tissue fluids must contain more than the *minimal bactericidal* (i.e. *killing*) *concentration* (MBC) of the antibiotic. To achieve this the drug must be given by the proper route; (e.g. drugs not absorbed from the intestine must not be given by mouth except for their local action in the bowel). If the drug does not reach the tissues (e.g. the meninges) in sufficiently high concentration, local (e.g. intrathecal) administration may occasionally be required in addition to systemic therapy. If high blood levels are important, as in severe infections, injection rather than oral administration is preferable, and for the initial treatment of life-threatening infections the route should be intravenous.

Antibiotic-resistant strains of certain organisms are common in hospital. *Staphylococcus aureus* and certain Gram-negative bacilli causing hospital

187

infection have become increasingly resistant to the commonly used antibiotics during the past twenty years. These resistant organisms may have appeared either as the result of the selection of intrinsically resistant strains by extensive and often indiscriminate use of antibiotics, or by mutation of previously sensitive bacteria, and selection following exposure to the antibiotics. Some organisms, especially Gram-negative bacilli, can transfer antibiotic resistance to other bacteria. Streptomycin is particularly likely to cause the emergence, by selection, of resistant strains of bacteria. Whereas the majority of hospital staphylococci and also many strains in the community are now resistant to penicillin, all haemolytic streptococci of *group A (Streptococcus pyogenes)*, clostridia and the treponema of syphillis remain sensitive to this antibiotic — an example of the extreme variability of bacterial resistance.

In view of the large number of available antibiotics, there is need for guidance on their use. This chapter provides concise information about antibiotics and recommendations for their safe and effective administration in treatment and (where indicated) in prophylaxis. Methods of delaying the emergence of resistance (especially by avoidance of unnecessary or inefficient use) are stressed. (For detailed information on antibiotics see Garrod, Lambert and O'Grady, 1981 and Kucers and Bennett, 1979.)

Classification of antibiotics

Antibiotics can be classified as *'broad spectrum'* or *'narrow range'* agents. The former act against a wide range of Gram-positive and Gram-negative bacteria and include the tetracyclines, the aminoglycosides and ampicillin, while the latter include agents primarily active against Gram-positive organisms (penicillin G and erythromycin), certain Gram-negative bacilli (the polymyxins), and specific groups of organisms, such as fungi (amphotericin B, nystatin), *Mycobacterium tuberculosis* (isoniazid, ethambutol) and anaerobes (metronidazol).

Antibiotics can also be classified as *bactericidal* (killing bacteria) or as *predominantly bacteristatic* (preventing their growth). The latter are satisfactory for most purposes, but the former are required for the successful treatment of severe infections or in patients with poor natural resistance. Some bactericidal agents (penicillins) may be antagonized by bacteristatic agents and are best not used in combination with them.

Use of individual antibiotics

For guidance on complex treatment and its control, the clinician should consult the bacteriologist or a physician experienced in chemotherapy. The British National Formulary should be available in all wards and departments as it contains up-to-date information on all available antibiotics.

Application of antibiotics to tissues

Most infections with sensitive organisms respond to systemic antibiotic therapy. However, there are times when local application of chemotherapeutic agents

188

may be indicated. Bladder infections can often be contained or prevented in patients with indwelling catheters by the twice daily instillation of framycetin in a dose of 500 mg diluted in 100 ml of sterile water. Chloramphenicol or neomycin drops are used for the treatment of purulent conjunctivitis. Suppurative external ear conditions are treated with antibiotic ear drops. 0.5% silver nitrate solution is an effective chemoprophylactic agent for severe burns; silver sulphadiazine cream is a more convenient and very effective application for this purpose, though sulphonamide-resistant bacteria may be selected through its use in a burns unit. Topical polymyxin has prophylactic value against *Ps. aeruginosa*, and though it is an antibiotic its use does not lead to the emergence of resistant variants. Its cost prohibits use on extensive burns. Gentamicin should not be used topically for routine prophylaxis because of the risk of promoting resistance. Streptococcal infections of burns should be treated with a systemic antibiotic and not topical therapy; in general it is best to avoid applications of penicillins or neomycin to the skin as sensitization may result. Intrathecal administration of antibiotics is occasionally valuable in treating pneumococcal or tuberculous meningitis, but is not necessary in other forms of pyogenic meningitis. Antibiotics may be instilled into the pleural cavity in addition to parenteral therapy in the treatment of purulent effusions.

Antibiotic combinations

Most infections respond satisfactorily to treatment with a single antibiotic. There are, however, occasions when combined therapy may be valuable:

(1) Prevention of development of bacterial resistance

Tuberculosis is an example.

(2) Infections caused by more than one organism (mixed infections)

Intra-abdominal sepsis is usually caused by both aerobic and anaerobic bacteria, and for this reason a combination of gentamicin and metronidazole is commonly used; cefoxitin has a similar spectrum.

(3) Septicaemia and endocarditis

Combinations of antibiotics are sometimes required for treatment of septicaemia and certain forms of endocarditis. A combination of penicillin and gentamicin may be used to treat endocarditis caused by *Streptococcus viridans*, and penicillin or ampicillin and gentamicin for *Strep. faecalis* endocarditis. Ticarcillin and gentamicin may be combined (but must be separately injected) for the treatment of pseudomonas septicaemia, and combined regimes (e.g. penicillin G and fusidic acid) can be employed for staphylococcal septicaemia. Severely ill neonates are frequently treated with both gentamicin and ampicillin (or cloxacillin). However, most infections mentioned under this heading *can* be treated successfully with a single antibiotic.

(4) When a combination is superior to a single agent

Trimethoprim and sulphamethoxazole (co-trimoxazole) is such a combination. Laboratory tests are available for synergy testing of chemotherapeutic agents.

(5) When the organism is unknown and the patient is seriously ill

The development of a febrile episode in a neutropenic patient is a possible indication for combination therapy.

Selection of an antibiotic

The selection of an antibiotic should never be a haphazard choice but must be based on careful consideration of the following factors:

(1) The sensitivity (or probable sensitivity) of the infecting organism

Severe infections such as endocarditis require detailed sensitivity testing, including the determination of the MIC and MBC of the organism. Before the organism and its sensitivity are known it may be possible to predict its probable identity and antibiotic sensitivity by consideration of the clinical picture; e.g. in subacute bacterial endocarditis, where the commonest infecting organism is *Strep. viridans*, or in purulent meningitis, in which the organisms are usually meningococci, pneumococci or *Haemophilus influenzae*.

(2) The clinical pharmacology of the various antibiotics

Particularly important factors are their absorption, excretion and distribution. Certain antibiotics, e.g. ampicillin, are excreted in bile and urine while some, e.g. chloramphenicol and the penicillins, penetrate the inflamed 'blood–brain barrier' and pass into the cerebrospinal fluid (CSF). Antibiotics which are poorly absorbed from the gut are sometimes used for treating intestinal infections and for bowel preparation prior to colonic surgery.

(3) Route of administration

Oral therapy is satisfactory for the treatment of many infections. Severe infections, however, require intramuscular or intravenous injections. To achieve adequate blood levels antibiotics given intravenously should be administered by 'bolus' and not added to the drip bottle. Topical application of antibiotics may be sufficient for certain eye, superficial skin and external ear infections.

(4) Toxicity of antibiotics

All antibiotics have side-effects and toxic drugs should not be used when safer agents are available. Chloramphenicol, for example, can cause fatal aplastic anaemia and should normally be reserved for the treatment of typhoid fever and *H. influenzae* meningitis. Aminoglycoside antibiotics cause eighth nerve damage if blood levels are allowed to exceed accepted safe levels; in the presence of renal failure longer intervals between doses are

190

required to prevent toxic blood levels. Tetracyclines should not be given to be given to children under the age of 12 or to pregnant women because of their ability to stain and possibly cause hypoplasia of growing teeth.

(5) There are relatively few well-defined indications for prophylactic antibiotics (see p. 194)

Antibiotic prophylaxis should not be given as a routine to unconscious patients or before 'clean' surgical operations, or to patients with bladder catheters.

(6) Cost of antibiotics

When other factors are equal the least expensive drug should be selected.

Treatment of specific infections

Urinary tract infections

Many infections acquired outside hospital are caused by *Escherichia coli* strains sensitive to sulphonamides. If the organism is sulphonamide-resistant, ampicillin or co-trimoxazole are satisfactory alternatives in domiciliary practice. Patients with chronic or recurrent infections and those with hospital-acquired infections often have organisms in their urine resistant to many antibacterial agents and the choice of antibiotic must then be made after the results of sensitivity testing are available. Acute pyelonephritis must be treated as soon as the diagnosis is suspected with a parenteral drug active against a wide range of Gram-negative bacilli, such as gentamicin or co-trimoxazole.

Alimentary tract infections

Antibiotics are *NOT* indicated for the treatment of most gastro-intestinal infections. Exceptions to this rule are: (a) severe infantile gastro-enteritis caused by enteropathogenic *E. coli* where a combination of oral and intramuscular gentamicin may be indicated, and (b) invasive salmonella infections. Typhoid fever is treated with chloramphenicol or co-trimoxazole. Co-trimoxazole and ampicillin are effective in invasive infections caused by salmonella organisms other than *Salmonella typhi* and *Salmonella paratyphi B*. (c) Staphylococcal enterocolitis is treated with flucloxacillin. (d) Co-trimoxazole is indicated for *severe* bacillary dysentery. (e) Perforation of the bowel (including the appendix) leads to peritonitis, often with a mixed flora, the principal organisms being Gram-negative bacilli and anaerobic bacteria especially *Bacteroides* spp. The treatment of choice is gentamicin plus metronidazole (or clindamycin, or cefoxitin). (f) Acute cholecystitis and cholangitis should be treated with gentamicin or a cephalosporin. (g) Campylobacter enteritis, if severe, is treated with erythromycin.

Tuberculosis

Material such as pus, sputum, or CSF from which tubercle bacilli may be cultured, should be sent to the laboratory *before* chemotherapy is commenced. A single dose of antibiotic may prevent the isolation of *Mycobacterium tuberculosis* and failure to determine the antibiotic sensitivities may prejudice the result of treatment. Tubercle bacilli readily acquire resistance to the three principal

191

drugs (isoniazid, rifampicin and streptomycin) and also to the drugs of second choice (e.g. ethambutol) which are used when the infecting strain is resistant to the standard drugs. For this reason two or three drugs must always be used in combination. Treatment should be supervised by a physician with experience in the management of tuberculosis.

Respiratory tract infections (other than tuberculosis)

Upper respiratory tract infections are frequently viral, and antibiotic therapy is only indicated when a bacterial aetiology is known or suspected. The commonest bacterial cause of acute sore throat is the haemolytic streptococcus of group A for which benzylpenicillin or phenoxymethylpenicillin are the drugs of choice. Acute sinusitis and otitis media usually respond satisfactorily to erythromycin or ampicillin. For oral candidiasis (thrush), local applications of nystatin are effective.

Acute infections of the lower respiratory tract acquired outside hospital are usually due to *Strep. pneumoniae* or *H. influenzae*. Both organisms are usually sensitive to ampicillin and co-trimoxazole. Benzylpenicillin is the drug of choice for pneumococcal infections. Many pneumococci and *H. influenzae* strains and also some haemolytic streptococci are resistant to tetracycline. In debilitated patients or those suffering from viral infection such as influenza, *Staph. aureus* may cause a fulminating pneumonia which should be treated with high doses of flucloxacillin and/or fusidic acid. Acute epiglottitis is a very serious and some-times fatal condition which is usually caused by *H. influenzae* and should be treated with parenteral chloramphenicol or high doses of ampicillin. Acute bronchitis and exacerbations of chronic bronchitis are treated with ampicillin or cotrimoxazole. Specific pneumonias are treated as follows:

Staphylococcal	flucloxacillin or fusidic acid
Pseudomonas	gentamicin, ticarcillin, amikacin, mezlocillin or azlacillin
Mycoplasma	tetracycline or erythromycin
Psittacosis	tetracycline

Wound infections

Wounds are frequently colonized by bacteria without being grossly infected, and these respond satisfactorily to local measures, such as removal of sutures, drain-age, application of antiseptics and frequent saline bathing.

Severe wound infections with spreading cellulitis and/or systemic illness are treated with an antibiotic, depending on sensitivity testing. Infected abdominal wounds in patients who have had operations of the gastro-intestinal tract (includ-ing appendix and gall-bladder) are likely to be due to the patient's bowel flora, including aerobic and anaerobic organisms. Infections of clean stitched wounds when the intestine has not been opened are usually staphylococcal and should be treated with flucloxacillin. A combination of gentamicin and metronidazole may be necessary for 'mixed' wound infections or those where the severity is such that treatment must be commenced before the results of sensitivity testing are available.

Burns must be cultured regularly and treated according to the results obtained. The isolation of *Staph. aureus, Ps. aeruginosa* or other Gram-negative bacilli is not an indication for chemotherapy except when there is evidence of clinical sepsis (severe illness, septicaemia, cellulitis). If *Strep. pyogenes* is isolated, treatment with benzylpenicillin may fail, even though the organism is sensitive, because of inactivation of the penicillin by penicillinase produced by staphylococci and other organisms present in the burn. Flucloxacillin, erythromycin or clindamycin should be used rather than penicillin G for *Strep. pyogenes* burn infections, for which chemotherapy is obligatory on all full-thickness lesions because of destruction of skin grafts by this organism.

Meningitis

Bacterial meningitis caused by identified organisms should be treated as follows:

Meningococcal. Benzylpenicillin 2 000 000 u every 4 to 6 h for 48 h by 'bolus' intravenous injection, reducing to 1 000 000 u every 6 h by i.m. injection for a further 7 days.

Pneumococcal. As for meningococcal.

Haemophilus influenzae. Almost invariably occurs in children under the age of five. Give chloramphenicol 50–100 mg/kg body weight/day (reduction in dose for neonates). Ampicillin in dose of 400 mg/kg/day is an alternative, but ampicillin-resistant strains are being isolated.

Other forms of meningitis treated according to predicted or known sensitivity of the organism. If organism unknown, give chloramphenicol or ampicillin to children and benzylpenicillin or chloramphenicol to adults.

Infections in neonates

Most superficial infections such as septic spots, 'sticky' eyes and umbilical sepsis respond to local treatment. Systemic infections are frequently caused by Gram-negative bacilli, including *Pseudomonas* spp., and also by penicillin-resistant staphylococci. A combination of cloxacillin with gentamicin should be used to treat seriously ill neonates with an undiagnosed infection.

Puerperal sepsis (and septic abortion)

Usually due to streptococci or anaerobic organisms, but also sometimes caused by Gram-negative bacilli. Initial treatment with a combination of metronidazole and gentamicin until results of cultures available.

Eye infection

Gonococcal ophthalmia is treated with a combination of topical and parenteral penicillin. Most other forms of purulent conjunctivitis respond to topical chloramphenicol.

Ear infection

Acute bacterial otitis media is usually caused by *Strep. pyogenes*, pneumococci and *H. influenzae*. The majority of cases respond to benzylpenicillin or to

193

erythromycin; children under the age of five should be given amoxycillin as
H. influenzae is a common pathogen of that age group.

Septicaemia and endocarditis

These are serious and potentially fatal conditions which should be treated with
a parenteral bactericidal antibiotic as soon as the diagnosis is suspected on *clinical* grounds. It is often possible to predict the probable infecting organism by
consideration of the clinical features of the illness. For example, acute pyelonephritis or cholangitis may be complicated by Gram-negative septicaemia and
segmental pneumonia may be associated with pneumococcal septicaemia. Acute
osteomyelitis is frequently secondary to staphylococcal septicaemia which can
also accompany wound infection and skin sepsis. Subacute bacterial endocarditis is usually caused by *Strep. viridans*, while acute endocarditis may be due to
various organisms including staphylococci, pneumococci and *Strep. faecalis*.
Strep. faecalis may enter the patient's blood-stream during operations on the
genito-urinary tract or catheterization and may cause endocarditis in elderly
males after cystoscopy or prostatectomy, and in young women following
gynaecological procedures.

When an organism is cultured from the blood it is important to carry out
detailed sensitivity testing, including MIC and MBC determinations, with appropriate antibiotics. When possible, serum levels of the antibiotic selected should
be determined during treatment of endocarditis or septicaemia to ensure that
adequate concentrations are obtained in the blood.

Fungal infections

Most fungal infections seen in this country involve skin, nails or mucous membranes; systemic fungal infections (or mycoses) are relatively rare although they
occasionally occur in debilitated patients.

The commonest superficial fungal infection is candidiasis or thrush caused by
Candida albicans which responds satisfactorily to topical applications of nystatin
or miconazole. Systemic candida infection is treated with intravenous injections
of amphotericin B, a toxic antibiotic which may cause drug fever, nausea, vomiting and an increase in blood urea. Flucytosine is an alternative or may be used in
combination with amphotericin B.

Actinomycosis is treated with benzylpenicillin.

Griseofulvin has a specific action against dermatophytes and is used for the
treatment of fungal infections of hair and nails.

Indications for prophylaxis with antibiotics

Systemic chemoprophylaxis

(1) Absolute indications
   (a) Dental extraction or manipulation in patients with valvular heart
       diseases or prosthetic valves. Give benzylpenicillin 1 000 000 u i.m.
       1 h *before* operation and continue with amoxycillin 500 mg 6 hourly

for 24 hours. If a patient is allergic to penicillin or already receiving penicillin for rheumatic fever prophylaxis — give erythromycin or vancomycin. For gynaecological and genito-urinary procedures in patients with heart valve abnormalities, give gentamicin (dose depends on weight of patient) plus 500 mg of ampicillin 30 min before operation, and 2 doses at 8-hourly intervals if renal function is normal.

(b) Operations on ischaemic legs and in pelvic region. For prophylaxis against gas gangrene give benzylpenicillin 1 000 000 u i.m. every 6 h for 2 doses before operation and for 5 days thereafter.

(c) Wounds (including burns) contaminated with soil or road dust and patients with extensive devitalization of tissue. For prophylaxis against tetanus and gas gangrene — as in (b) (but see Chapter 13, p. 223); also to forestall probable invasive infection with *Ps. aeruginosa* or other pathogens already colonizing extensive burns in severely ill patients. The indication for chemoprophylaxis against tetanus has been reduced with the increasing availability of human ATG.

(d) For non-immune diphtheria contacts — give erythromycin 500 mg 4 times a day for 1 week.

(e) For contacts of meningococcal infection — give minocycline or rifampicin (or sulphonamide if strain is known to be sensitive).

(f) Following acute rheumatic fever, for at least 5 years or until child leaves school, give phenoxymethyl penicillin (penicillin V) in a dose of 125 or 250 mg twice a day by mouth.

(g) Before artificial rupture of the membranes in pregnancy, in certain categories of patient — give ampicillin 500 mg 6 hourly i.m. commencing 12 h *before* membranes rupture (to allow adequate concentration in liquor) and continue for further 24 h.

(h) Before colonic surgery (see below).

(i) Following splenectomy, especially in children, give long-term oral penicillin.

(2) Relative indications (used by some clinicians, or only in specific circumstances)

Arterial grafts, cardiac surgery, neurosurgical operations involving foreign materials. Wide cover is required not only against recognized pathogens but also against organisms which are not normally pathogenic. Combined therapy is therefore necessary.

(3) Chemoprophylaxis in abdominal surgery

(a) Indications (Keighley and Burdon, 1979). Prophylaxis against surgical sepsis is advisable whenever an internal organ, the contents of which contain more than 10^4 viable bacteria/ml, is opened. The type and extent of bacterial colonization within the gastro-intestinal tract is related to the site, and the nature of any underlying disease. Prophylaxis should be used for the following groups of operations:

(i) Operations on the stomach or oesophagus in patients with carcinoma or bile reflux gastritis.

    (ii) Cholecystectomy in selected patients who have infected bile. Patients at risk for sepsis can be selected on the basis of a history of jaundice, rigors, recent acute cholecystitis, age over 70, or a previous biliary operation. An alternative method of selection is by immediate Gram stain of a sample of bile aspirated from the gall-bladder early in the course of the operation.

    (iii) All intestinal resections in patients with inflammatory bowel disease.

    (iv) All colorectal operations involving resection and/or anastomosis.

    (v) Patients with a perforated or gangrenous appendix should be given a therapeutic course of antibiotic. The need for prophylaxis in non-perforated, non-gangrenous appendicitis is not yet established.

    (vi) Abdominal and vaginal hysterectomy.

(b) Timing and route of prophylaxis. Prophylaxis is effective only if high blood and tissue levels of an appropriate antibiotic are present at the time of bacterial contamination of the surgical wound, or in some cases when large amounts of antibiotic are applied locally to the wound. Prophylaxis should not continue after completion of the operation. Intramuscular drugs should be given 1 h before the start of surgery and i.v. drugs during induction of anaesthesia.

(c) Choice of chemotherapeutic agent. This should be based upon the nature of the organisms likely to contaminate the operative field. For patients in groups (i) and (ii), the organisms most likely to cause sepsis are streptococci, *Escherichia coli* and other aerobic Gram-negative bacilli. Operations in groups (iii), (iv) and (v) require antibiotics active against anaerobic bacteria, *E. coli* and other aerobic Gram-negative bacilli. Anaerobic bacteria are mainly responsible for pelvic sepsis in group (vi) patients. Suitable prophylactic regimes for the above groups are:

Group i. A single pre-operative dose of gentamicin or a cephalosporin by i.m. or i.v. injection.

Group ii. A single pre-operative injection of gentamicin or cephalosporin i.m. or i.v.

Groups iii and iv. A single pre-operative injection of gentamicin i.m. or i.v. and metronidazole i.v. is recommended. Pre-operative oral bowel preparation with antibiotics is often effective, but, with the possible exception of neomycin plus erythromycin, is not recommended because of the risk of emergence of resistant Gram-negative bacilli.

Group v. Metronidazole given as a suppository or i.v. is the most rational prophylactic for appendicectomy.

Group vi. Metronidazole is the most effective prophylaxis against pelvic sepsis.

    Chemoprophylaxis with antibiotics will almost inevitably lead to the selection of bacteria resistant to the prophylactic agent. For this reason indiscriminate prophylaxis should be avoided; narrow-range rather than broad-spectrum antibiotics should be used whenever possible (e.g. in prophylaxis against a particular pathogen, such as *Strep. pyogenes* or *Cl. welchii*); short-term or single-dose prophylaxis should be used to cover short periods of hazard, such as exposure to microbial contamination during an operation; and a careful watch must be kept for the appearance of resistant bacteria.

(4) Peritoneal dialysis

The dialysis fluid is an excellent culture medium for bacteria and may become infected from the outside (faulty technique) or the inside (preexisting peritoneal infection or transperitoneal spread). Prophylactic addition of antibiotics to dialysis fluid is *not* recommended. The effluent fluid should be sent for culture every 24 hours. In this way warning of infection is usually obtained before it is clinically evident and treatment can be given with an antibiotic appropriate to the organism cultured. The presence of bacteria in the fluid is not in itself an indication to stop dialysis; antibiotics should be put into the fluid and dialysis continued. Penicillins, particularly ampicillin, rapidly lose activity in dialysis fluid because of the pH which is approximately 5.5.

Topical chemoprophylaxis

Local treatment of severe burns with 0.5% silver nitrate compresses, one of the most effective means of preventing infection with *Ps. aeruginosa* and *Proteus* spp, is less often used today than in the late 1960s. Patients having this treatment need supplements of electrolytes by mouth and laboratory control of serum electrolyte levels. Silver sulphadiazine cream is less effective against *Ps. aeruginosa* and *Proteus* spp, but more effective against many other Gram-negative bacilli. It is a valuable alternative to silver nitrate compresses, easier to use and more appropriate for the treatment of infants, also for smaller burns. Mafenide acetate (11%) cream applied daily and left exposed is an alternative to 0.5% silver nitrate compresses which can be used if silver nitrate solution is not appropriate (e.g. if serum electrolytes cannot be kept at normal levels); it is painful on burns in which the nerve-endings are not destroyed. A cream containing 0.5% silver nitrate and 0.2% chlorhexidine gluconate is also effective and involves no hazard of emergence of resistant bacteria (Lowbury, 1976).

Formulation of antibiotic policy

There are several reasons for having in each hospital an agreed policy for prescribing antibiotics.

(1) The restrained use of antibiotics means that the appearance of resistant organisms is delayed and their incidence in hospital is kept low. Resistant staphylococci remain a problem, and strains resistant to clindamycin, fucidin, gentamicin or methicillin are found in some units. In recent years gentamicin-resistant Gram-negative bacilli, especially *Klebsiella aerogenes* and *Ps. aeruginosa*, have caused cross-infection problems in urological, intensive care and burns units. Resistance among Gram-negative bacilli is complicated by the fact that it is commonly transferred from one organism

197

to another, even when the organisms are unrelated. Transferable resistance to one antibiotic is often linked with resistance to other antibiotics, so that excessive use of one antibiotic may be the cause of a high incidence of resistance to several others in the hospital population of organisms.

(2) Up-to-date information should be provided for the prescriber, and adverse reactions should be reduced by restricting the use of certain potentially toxic agents.

(3) Prescribing costs are reduced by controlling the use of expensive agents.

The type of policy must be adapted to the needs of the staff, the type of patients treated and the prevalent organisms in the hospital or unit. It must therefore be flexible and where necessary adapted to the needs of individual units, e.g. burns and intensive care. The policy could have the following components.

Personal advice and example

By this is meant the effect which daily discussion between senior and junior doctors has on prescribing habits. Effective use of antibiotics requires experience and this is not readily obtained. Most hospitals have doctors (usually a Medical Microbiologist or Infectious Diseases Consultant) with a special interest in and knowledge of antibiotics which should be available to other members of staff. Regular review of individual patients is also necessary and is aided by indicating the antibiotics given on the temperature chart.

General advice and education

Education of antibiotic prescribers can also be helped if some *aide memoir* is available on the wards. The British National Formulary is one source of information. Some hospitals or even regions have their own booklets. It is particularly important that advice is available on the use of topical agents, on prophylaxis and on expensive preparations. Postgraduate lectures on chemotherapy are also helpful, but less important than personal advice and discussion.

Provision of survey data

The antibiotic policy depends to a considerable extent on the sensitivity pattern of currently isolated strains of bacteria. When the clinician sees that a large number of strains is resistant to a particular antibiotic, he is unlikely to prescribe it for an infection with the bacterial species in question even if he has no knowledge of the sensitivity of the individual strain causing the infection. The type of report which can be made available to clinicians is shown in Tables 12.1 and 12.2. Variations between the hospitals can be seen in both tables. It is clear from this example that the percentage of *Staph. aureus* and Gram-negative bacilli resistant to a number of antibiotics varies greatly in the two hospitals. Similar variations will occur from time to time in the same hospital. Regular (e.g. quarterly) reports can be prepared from information available in most laboratories where sensitivity

Table 12.1 Examples of survey data from two hospitals: percentage of strains of Gram-negative bacilli and of *Staphylococcus aureus* resistant to antibiotics (1971).

Antibiotic	*Escherichia coli*		*Proteus* sp.‡		*Klebsiella* sp.		*Staphylococcus aureus*	
	DRH* (853)	BAH† (218)	DRH (282)	BAH (268)	DRH (167)	BAH (215)	DRH (204)	BAH (9325)
Ampicillin	35	41	24	53	98	76		
Benzylpenicillin							85	82
Carbenicillin		42		53		83		
Cephaloridine		24		53		78		
Chloramphenicol		15		7		17		
Colistin (polymyxin)	1		98		3			
Erythromycin							22	91
Fusidic acid							2	0.3
Gentamicin		0.9		0.4		5		0.6
Kanamycin (and neomycin)	4	16	4	71	9	56	25	90
Lincomycin (and clindamycin)							22	74
Methicillin							7	3.3
Nalidixic acid	5	2	6	3	23	4		
Nitrofurantoin	6	34	64	98	19	77		
Streptomycin	31	18	36	11	38	30		
Sulphonamides	31	31	17	38	41	46		
Tetracycline	36	48	88	94	46	72	38	82
Trimethoprim		7		15		12		1.3

*Dudley Road Hospital
†Burns Unit, Birmingham Accident Hospital
‡at BAH *Proteus mirabilis* only

Table 12.2 Examples of survey data from two hospitals: percentage of strains of Gram-negative bacilli and of *Staphylococcus aureus* resistant to antibiotics (1979).

Antibiotic	*Escherichia coli*		*Proteus* sp.		*Klebsiella* sp.		*Staphylococcus aureus*	
	DRH* (328)	BAH† (89)	DRH (57)	BAH (164)	DRH (118)	BAH (105)	DRH (157)	BAH (3648)
Ampicillin	45	27	13	5	73	71	—	—
Benzylpenicillin	—	—	—	—	—	—	91	95
Carbenicillin	3	35	—	0.6	5	85	—	—
Cephalosporins	—	18	7	5	—	52	—	—
Chloramphenicol	—	15	—	1.2	—	51	—	—
Erythromycin	—	—	—	—	—	—	12	25
Fusidic acid	—	—	—	—	—	—	<1	<1
Gentamicin	—	1.1	—	0	—	11	1	<1
Kanamycin (and neomycin)	—	5.6	—	0	—	27	11	23
Lincomycin (and clindamycin)	—	—	—	—	—	—	<1	21
Methicillin	—	—	—	—	—	—	.1	22
Nalidixic acid	3	4.5	3	0	3	7	—	—
Nitrofurantoin	2	—	100	—	11	—	—	—
Sulphonamides	43	58	4	24	56	67	—	—
Tetracycline	—	30	—	93	—	65	14	26
Trimethoprim	13	2	2	5	42	36	—	<1

*Dudley Road Hospital
†Burns Unit, Birmingham Accident Hospital

tests are carried out, and knowledge of the current resistance patterns gives the clinician a valuable guide to the therapy most likely to be of use. This type of information is complementary to that provided by the individual report on a particular patient; it enables the doctor to choose an appropriate antibiotic before he knows the result of sensitivity tests, and warns him of the appearance or the increased incidence of strains resistant to currently used antibiotics.

The same type of information can be made available to general practitioners. Table 12.3 shows the resistance pattern of urinary tract organisms isolated from domiciliary urinary tract infections. Such information need only be made available once a year in general practice because of the small changes in resistance of bacteria among the general community as compared to that found in hospitals.

Table 12.3 Examples of sensitivity of organisms isolated from urine in domiciliary practice

Antibiotic	*Escherichia coli* (571 strains)	*Percentage resistant:* *Klebsiella* spp. (28 strains)	*Proteus* spp. (81 strains)
Ampicillin	22	93	3
Sulphonamides	26	39	11
Nitrofurantoin	< 1	7	95
Nalidixic acid	2	4	4
Cotrimoxazole	5	11	25
Cephalexin	2	0	1

Reservation of antibiotics

Some hospitals may find it valuable to classify antibiotics into different categories in order to hold some in reserve for particular organisms or specific types of patient. There is no doubt that such a policy of restricting the use of specific compounds can preserve the useful life of an antimicrobial agent; in large hospitals, where there is a resident population of organisms 'waiting to acquire resistance' and large amounts of antibiotics may be used, it is essential to keep some in reserve.

An example of the way in which antibiotics can be classified for this purpose is shown in Table 12.4a, which summarizes the policy adopted in a general hospital for 1971, and a similar policy for a hospital with different resistance patterns. The table was distributed widely to members of the staff. This policy was not rigidly enforced, but prescribers were quite satisfied to be guided by its recommendations.

Table 12.4b is a more recent policy from a general hospital. It was felt that category 2 in the original policy was not effective and should be strengthened. Although a restricted antibiotic (category 3) can be used by a clinician if he requires it, the Microbiologist (or Infectious Diseases Consultant) can often

Table 12.4a Example of Antibiotic Policies (1971).

Category	Availability of antibiotic	Reason for choice	Antibiotics	
			1) Dudley Road Hospital	2) Birmingham A.H. (Burns)
(1)	With no special restrictions in treatment of sensitive infections when clinically required	Long in common use, and effective; little change in resistance patterns in recent years; inexpensive; relatively non-toxic	Benzylpenicillin Tetracyclines Sulphonamides Nitrofurantoin	Benzylpenicillin Erythromycin Sulphonamides Nitrofurantoin
(2)	On general prescription, but special restraint must be exercised	Because of increasing incidence of or readily acquired resistance of *Staph. aureus* and/or Gram-negative rods and/or because of toxicity	Ampicillin Streptomycin Kanamycin Cloxacillin or flucloxacillin Erythromycin Novobiocin Cephalosporins Nalidixic acid Colistin Chloramphenicol	Streptomycin Cotrimoxazole Flucloxacillin Novobiocin Nalidixic acid Colistin (poly-myxin)

| (3) | Reserved for use only in: (a) Severe infection by sensitive bacteria when other antibiotics are inadequate or (b) As antibiotic for 'blind' use before or without sensitivity test results: on consultant's signature or recommendation only. (*Source isolation, or, if this is impossible, barrier nursing for patients on these drugs.*) | (a) To *preserve activity* when all or most strains of susceptible pathogens are sensitive (e.g. when an antibiotic is new), or | Gentamicin Ticarcillin Fucidin Rifamycins Vancomycin Lincomycins Cotrimoxazole | Gentamicin Fusidic acid Chloramphenicol Rifamycins Lincomycins Vancomycin |
| | | (b) to *restore activity* when many or most strains are resistant. | 'Ampiclox' Topical neomycin | Tetracyclines Carbenicillin Kanamycin and neomycin Ampicillin Cephalosporins |

Table 12.4b Example of Antibiotic Policy (1979)

Category	Reason for choice	Antibiotics for use
1. With no special restriction in treatment of sensitive infections when clinically required	Long in common use, inexpensive and relatively non-toxic	Benzylpenicillin Phenoxymethylpenicillin Ampicillin/amoxycillin Cloxacillin/flucloxacillin Metronidazole Topical neomycin Erythromycin Cotrimoxazole and sulphonamides Nalidixic acid Nitrofurantoin Tetracycline/oxytetracycline
2. Requires signature of senior member of staff (advice of microbiologist should be obtained whenever possible)	Because of increasing incidence of resistance, or to preserve activity when all or most strains are sensitive, or because of toxicity or cost	Aminoglycosides (apart from reserve in category 3) Fusidic acid Cephalosporins (one systemic and one oral) Chloramphenicol (systemic) Lincomycin/clindamycin Tetracyclines (other than in category 1) Mecillinam Cefoxitin Colistin
3. Restricted antibiotics; requires signature of senior member of staff; pharmacy reports to microbiologist before issuing		Amikacin (for gentamicin-resistant strains only) Ticarcillin (or other penicillins or cephalosporins with activity against *Ps. aeruginosa*) Topical fusidic acid or gentamicin Vancomycin Fixed combinations Other cephalosporins

persuade him against it if a suitable non-restricted alternative could be offered.

Purchasing policy

New agents should be carefully considered by a pharmacy committee and only purchased if superior in one or more respects to existing drugs. In particular, by this means the clinician can be guided in the use of the numerous penicillins and cephalosporins now marketed.

Changes in antibiotic policies

Action when resistance to an important antibiotic becomes common

Sometimes stopping the use of the antibiotic in question will lead to a large reduction or even elimination of the resistant organisms. This happened more often

204

in the early years of the antibiotic era, before multiple and genetically linked resistance became common in hospital bacteria. When multiple resistance is present, all of the antibiotics involved in the resistance pattern should, if possible, be withdrawn and not used again until these strains are eliminated. This manoeuvre was effective in the outbreak of transferable multiresistance at the Birmingham Accident Hospital's Burns Unit described above (Lowbury, Babb and Roe, 1972). In other outbreaks withdrawal of antibiotics has not been effective; transfer of all patients carrying or infected with strains showing the resistance pattern to one ward, which is kept closed to new admissions until all carriers of the resistant strain have been discharged, may be effective in such a situation.

The resistance pattern is constantly changing in hospital and it is necessary to change a policy with alterations in resistance. Often one unit in the hospital may require a policy different from that used by other units. For example, in a unit frequently prescribing gentamicin, resistant strains may emerge. A change could then be made to a cephalosporin or cefoxitin, with or without a penicillin active against *Ps. aeruginosa*.

Antibiotics for 'blind' treatment of severe or dangerous infections

Knowledge of the site of the infection will help the clinician when deciding on a suitable antibiotic, e.g. metronidazole would be appropriate for a pelvic abscess. The most recent quarterly resistance report should also be consulted, and until results of sensitivity tests are available, appropriate antibiotic or antibiotics most often active against the bacterium or bacteria considered or known to be causing the infection should be used, e.g. in Dudley Road Hospital in 1971 a severe wound infection with a strain of *Klebsiella* could be treated with kanamycin; in the Burns Unit of the Birmingham Accident Hospital, however, kanamycin would be an incorrect choice, but cotrimoxazole would be appropriate for use under category 2, while if the patient was dangerously ill the reserve antibiotic (category 3), gentamicin, would be an appropriate choice. Since 1971, the use of kanamycin has been generally replaced by other aminoglycosides. In 1979 (Table 12.4b) methicillin (or flucloxacillin) would not be the first choice for treating a suspected or severe staphylococcal infection in the burns unit, but would be in the general hospital. Trimethoprim resistance has increased since 1971 and trimethoprim would not be the first choice for an unknown Gram-negative infection in either hospital, particularly if it was likely to be due to *Klebsiella*. Where mixed streptococcal and staphylococcal infections are likely to occur, systemic erythromycin or flucloxacillin should be used for treatment of *Strep. pyogenes* infections; streptococcal sensitivity tests are necessary, because resistance of *Strep. pyogenes* to erythromycin very occasionally occurs.

Antibiotics and the laboratory

The hospital clinician can use antibiotics rationally only if adequate laboratory services are available. There are several ways in which the laboratory can give such assistance:

205

Accurate sensitivity reports on isolates from individual patients

Most laboratories use disc tests for assessing routine antibiotic sensitivity tests and, if controls are adequate, reliable results are obtained. Laboratory errors which can be avoided include performing sensitivity tests to inappropriate antibiotics (e.g. using nitrofurantoin sensitivity tests for respiratory pathogens), using discs containing the wrong antibiotic concentration for the site of infection (e.g. 2 μg disc of ampicillin in urinary infections), and testing with agents which are difficult to interpret (e.g. using cloxacillin in testing for methicillin-resistant staphylococci). Sensitivity tests are often performed on organisms which are non-pathogens but are either normal inhabitants of the body (e.g. *Strep. viridans* in the mouth) or are replacing the normal flora in patients receiving antibiotics (e.g. *Klebsiella* in the mouth of patients receiving ampicillin or *Proteus* sp. in the mouth of patients receiving tetracycline). Evidence, such as clinical signs of infection or of a predisposing cause, such as tracheostomy, should be sought before performing sensitivity tests. Clinicians often assume that because a test is reported the bacteriologist thinks the organism is important and should be treated. Although the interpretation of most tests is relatively straightforward, some, such as sulphonamide sensitivity and penicillinase-production, are more liable to error and need special care (see Reeves *et al.*, 1978).

Survey data on currently isolated strains

Antibiotic therapy is frequently given in hospital before laboratory reports are available. The provision of survey data on current sensitivity patterns (see section above on Antibiotic policy) enables the clinician to choose the agent most likely to be of value.

Monitoring of therapy

If facilities are available for monitoring therapy, this will enable the clinician to use a wider range of agents. Certain antibiotics are toxic if blood levels slightly exceed the therapeutic level; unless therapy is monitored, these agents are likely either to be avoided or to be used in too small a dose to ensure therapeutic levels in the body. Most large laboratories have facilities for estimating serum levels of aminoglycoside antibiotics. Some laboratories with a particular interest in chemotherapy will also carry out special tests of bactericidal activity for organisms from patients with endocarditis or other severe infections and tests of bactericidal activity of antibiotic combinations against specific pathogens. Clinicians should be encouraged to refer chemotherapy problems to the laboratory.

Appendix 12.1 Antibiotic names, prices and dosage (Feb. 1980)

Approved name	Trade name	Average daily dose (adults)	Preparation	Cost (in £) for 5 days (approx.)
Penicillins				
Amoxycillin	Amoxil	3 x 250 mg	capsules	1.87
Amoxycillin	Amoxil	3 x 250 mg	syrup	2.37
Amoxycillin	Amoxil	3 x 500 mg	injection	8.34
Ampicillin	Penbritin	4 x 250 mg	capsules	1.12
Ampicillin	Penbritin	4 x 250 mg	syrup	1.68
Ampicillin	Penbritin	4 x 250 mg	injection	5.96
Ampicillin + cloxacillin	Ampiclox	4–6 x 500 mg	injection	23.47
Ampicillin + flucloxacillin	Magnapen	4 x 500 mg	capsules	3.79
Ampicillin + flucloxacillin	Magnapen	4 x 500 mg	syrup	6.68
Ampicillin + flucloxacillin	Magnapen	4 x 500 mg	injection	17.88
Benzylpenicillin (penicillin G)	Crystapen	4 x 300 mg	injection	1.84
Carbenicillin	Pyopen	4 x 5 g	injection	147.26
Cloxacillin	Orbenin	4 x 500 mg	capsules	5.60
Cloxacillin	Orbenin	4 x 500 mg	syrup	5.00
Cloxacillin	Orbenin	4 x 250 mg i.m.	injection	15.06
Cloxacillin	Orbenin	4 x 500 mg i.v.	injection	24.54
Flucloxacillin	Floxapen	4 x 250 mg	capsules	3.49
Flucloxacillin	Floxapen	4 x 250 mg	syrup	6.20
Flucloxacillin	Floxapen	4 x 250 mg	injection	15.06
Mecillinam	Selexidin	4 x 400 mg	injection	20.40
Mezlocillin	Baypen	3–4 x 5 g	injection	201.00
Phenoxymethylpenicillin	V-Cil-K	4 x 250 mg	tablets	0.26
Phenoxymethylpenicillin	V-Cil-K	4 x 250 mg	syrup	0.67
Phenoxymethylpenicillin	V-Cil-K	4 x 250 mg	capsules	0.32

Approved name	Trade name	Average daily dose (adults)	Preparation	Cost (in £) for 5 days (approx.)
Phenoxymethylpenicillin	Crystapen V Stabillin VK Compocillin VK Icipen	4 × 250 mg		
Pivmecillinam	Selexid	4 × 200 mg	tablets	3.76
Pivmecillinam	Selexid	4 × 200 mg	suspension	6.78
Talampicillin	Talpen	3 × 250 mg	tablets	1.39
Talampicillin	Talpen	3 × 250 mg	syrup	2.61
Ticarcillin	Ticar	3–4 × 5 g	injection	205.50
Cephalosporins and Cephamycins				
Cefaclor	Distaclor	3 × 250 mg	capsules	3.49
Cefaclor	Distaclor	3 × 250 mg	suspension	4.36
Cefoxitin	Mefoxin	3 × 1 g	injection	67.05
Cefuroxime	Zinacef	3 × 750 mg	injection	31.50
Cephalexin	Keflex, Ceporex	4 × 250 mg	capsules	2.75
Cephalexin	Keflex, Ceporex	4 × 250 mg	syrup	2.88
Cephazolin	Kefzol	3 × 1 g	injection	31.80
Cephradine	Velosef	4 × 500 mg	capsules	2.81
Cephradine	Velosef	4 × 500 mg	injection	9.20
Cephradine	Velosef	4 × 500 mg	syrup	2.81
Macrolides and related Antibiotics				
Clindamycin	Dalacin C	4 × 300 mg	capsules	6.64
Clindamycin	Dalacin C	4 × 300 mg	syrup	10.12
Clindamycin	Dalacin C	4 × 300 mg	injection	31.04

Erythromycin	Erythromid Ilotycin Erythrocin	4 x 250 mg	tablets	1.81
Erythromycin	Erythrocin	4 x 300 mg	injection i.v.	25.40
Erythromycin	Erythrocin	4 x 100 mg	injection i.m.	10.80
Erythromycin	Erythroped	4 x 500 mg	suspension	3.11
Erythromycin	Ilosone	4 x 250 mg	capsules	1.72
Lincomycin	Lincocin	3 x 500 mg	capsules	3.84
Lincomycin	Lincocin	3 x 600 mg	injection	9.89
Lincomycin	Lincocin	3 x 500 mg	syrup	5.01
Aminoglycosides				
Amikacin	Amikin	2 x 500 mg	injection	101.40
Gentamicin	Genticin	3 x 80 mg	injection	23.88
	Cidomycin			
Kanamycin	Kantrex	4 x 250 mg	capsules	3.92
Kanamycin	Kantrex	2 x 0.5 g	injection	11.75
Neomycin	Neomin	2 x 1 g	tablets	1.88
Tobramycin	Nebcin	3 x 60–80 mg	injection	26.09
Sulphonamides				
Phthalylsulphathiazole	Thalazole	10 x 500 mg	tablets	0.39
Sulphadiazine	Sulphadiazine	4 x 1 g	tablets	0.20
Sulphadiazine	Sulphadiazine	4 x 2 g.	injection	4.32
Sulphadimidine	Sulphamezathine	4 x 1 g	tablet	0.06
Sulphadimidine	Sulphamezathine	4 x 1 g	injection	2.31
Tetracyclines				
Chlortetracycline	Aureomycin	4 x 250 mg	capsules	2.56
Clomocycline	Megaclor	4 x 170 mg	capsules	1.43
Minocycline	Minocin	2 x 100 mg	tablet	3.94
Oxytetracycline	Terramycin	4 x 250 mg	tablet	1.03

Approved name	Trade name	Average daily dose (adults)	Preparation	Cost (in £) for 5 days (approx.)
Oxytetracycline	Imperacin	4 × 250 mg	syrup	1.46
Oxytetracycline	Terramycin	4 × 100 mg	injection i.m.	12.40
Tetracycline	Achromycin	4 × 250 mg	tablets	0.43
			capsules	0.64
Tetracycline	Achromycin	4 × 250 mg	syrup	2.16
Tetracycline	Achromycin	4 × 100 mg	injection i.m.	14.20
Miscellaneous				
Chloramphenicol	Chloromycetin	8 × 250 mg	capsules	2.30
Chloramphenicol	Kemicetine	3 × 1 g	injection	9.90
Colistin	Colomycin	3 × 2 Mu	injection	30.90
Colistin	Colomycin	3 × 1.5 Mu	tablets	11.70
Cotrimazine	Coptin	2 × 500 mg	tablets	1.33
Cotrimazine	Coptin	2 × 500 mg	suspension	2.36
Cotrimoxazole	Septrin	2 × 960 mg	tablets	1.48
	Bactrim			
Cotrimoxazole	Septrin	2 × 960 mg	suspension	2.09
	Bactrim			
Fusidic Acid	Fucidin	3 × 500 mg	capsules	15.79
Griseofulvin	Grisovin	2 × 250 mg	tablets	0.41
Metronidazole	Flagyl	3 × 400 mg	tablets	2.21
Metronidazole	Flagyl	3 × 500 mg	injection	96.00
Nalidixic Acid	Negram	4 × 1 g	tablets	3.88
Nalidixic Acid	Negram	4 × 1 g	suspension	11.90
Nitrofurantoin	Furadantin	4 × 100 mg	tablets	1.84
Nitrofurantoin	Macrodantin	4 × 100 mg	capsules	1.83
Spectinomycin	Trobicin	1 × 2 g (males) 1 × 4 g (females)	injection	6.18
Trimethoprim	Ipral Trimopan	2 × 200 mg	tablets	1.06
Vancomycin	Vancocin	4 × 500 mg	injection i.v.	133.20

References and Further Reading

Garrod, L. P., Lambert, H. P. and O'Grady, F. (1981), *Antibiotic and Chemotherapy*. 5th edn, Churchill Livingstone, Edinburgh and London.

Keighley, M. R. B. and Burdon, D. W. (1979), *Antibicrobial Prophylaxis in Surgery*. Pitman Medical, London.

Kucers, A. and Bennett, M. C. R. (1979), *Use of Antibiotics*, 3rd edn, Heinemann Medical Books, London.

Lowbury, E. J. L. (1976), Prophylaxis and treatment for infection of burns. *Br. J. hosp. Med.*, 16, 566.

Lowbury, E. J. L., Babb, J. R. and Roe, E. (1972), Clearance from a hospital of Gram-negative bacilli that transfer carbenicillin-resistance to *Pseudomonas aeruginosa*. *Lancet*, ii, 941.

Lowbury, E. J. L. and Ayliffe, G. A. J. (1974), *Drug Resistance in Antimicrobial Therapy*. Charles C. Thomas, Illinois.

Phillips, I. (1979), Antibiotic policies. In: *Recent Advances in Infection* 1 (eds D. Reeves and A. M. Geddes). Churchill Livingstone, Edinburgh, London, New York, p. 151.

Reeves, D., Phillips I., Williams, J. D. and Wise, R. (eds) (1978), *Laboratory Methods in Antimicrobial Chemotherapy*. Churchill Livingstone, London.

CHAPTER THIRTEEN

Immunization and Specific Prophylaxis

Immunization is important in the control of hospital infection (a) for the protection of certain members of staff against poliomyelitis, rubella, diphtheria and some other infectious diseases which could be contracted from patients; (b) for the protection of patients, when a patient suffering from a communicable disease is accidentally admitted to an open ward; (c) for the protection of patients who, because of their illness or treatment, are particularly susceptible to infection; and (d) for the protection of patients with open wounds against tetanus.

For the protection of staff, active immunization with a vaccine or toxoid is the method of choice, and immunity should be established in so far as is practicable before he or she is employed in an area of potential risk, e.g. an infectious diseases ward. Non-immune patients exposed to certain infections can be given immediate protection against the infection by passive immunization with antiserum or immunoglobulin, but not by active immunization, which takes time to develop. The importance of both active and passive immunization in prophylaxis against tetanus is well known, but immunization, antibiotics and surgical techniques must be integrated for the prevention of tetanus in hospital.

Immunization of hospital staff (see also Chapter 14)

General policy

The risks of staff contracting infection vary with the type of hospital, tuberculosis being a special risk in chest hospitals, enteric fever and poliomyelitis in infectious disease units, and a wide range of infections in pathology departments. The person in charge of a unit or department must be responsible for ensuring that measures are taken to avoid infection in staff.

It is neither practicable nor desirable to immunize all members of staff against all diseases for which vaccines are available. This is because the risk may not be great (e.g. cholera in UK), the vaccine may not be very effective or may have serious or unpleasant side-effects (e.g. primary smallpox vaccination and diphtheria immunization in adults). The risks of side-effects from immunization must be balanced against the potential hazard of spread of the infection from patient to staff in a unit at a particular time, account being taken of the fact that the intestinal diseases, in particular, are effectively contained by good hygiene

212

(especially barrier nursing). Secondly, account must be taken of the effectiveness of specific treatment should infection arise (e.g. chloramphenicol is effective against typhoid fever, but there is no specific treatment for poliomyelitis). Thirdly, the usual rapid turnover of nursing and domestic staff makes it virtually impossible to ensure that a stable, well immunized staff is always available; in the average infectious disease unit only the senior nursing staff tend to be permanent. In view of these difficulties, it is impossible to ensure immunity of all staff to meet the chance admission of a patient with unrecognized infectious disease; good hygienic practice is usually a better safeguard for the staff than reliance on an immunity which may not exist. There are, however, circumstances when immunization is useful and necessary; for example, in units dealing with open pulmonary tuberculosis it should always be possible to ensure that only staff who have had BCG or who are tuberculin-positive are in attendance.

Active immunization

Active immunity results from naturally acquired disease or from vaccination. Usually it takes at least 10–14 days for active immunity to develop, and it may take many weeks, depending on the vaccine. To some vaccines (e.g. *Ps. aeruginosa* polyvalent vaccine) immunity develops much more rapidly. Such immunity can be life-long (e.g. naturally acquired immunity to measles), or it may be as short as six months (e.g. cholera vaccination). Immunity may be good and highly protective (e.g. diphtheria) or rather poor in the face of a large infective dose of bacteria (typhoid and cholera).

Smallpox vaccination (see also Chapter 17)

This is required only for nursing, medical and ancillary staff (engineers, domestics) employed in smallpox hospitals. Such persons must have had their primary vaccination in childhood, because of the danger of primary vaccination in adult life. Immunity must be maintained by vaccination every two or three years. *Revaccination* of young adults causes little or no discomfort, gives rise to continuing immunity. However, the WHO smallpox eradication programme has been very successful, so that in May 1980 the WHO was formally able to declare the world free from the disease. Therefore vaccination is no longer necessary for protection of people travelling to countries where smallpox was formerly endemic. Most world states now acknowledge this but a few, at the time of writing, still insist on a traveller having a valid International Certificate of Vaccination. However, a certificate signed, stamped and stating that 'vaccination of the bearer is medically contraindicated' or some similar formula usually meets the requirements. It is *most strongly urged* that travellers are not give unnecessary vaccination for the safety of themselves and others whom they may inadvertently infect (see below), and that only categories of persons mentioned at the beginning of this section are treated.

Smallpox vaccine is now available only in freeze-dried ampoules with diluent in a capillary tube. Enough vaccine may be reconstituted (with difficulty) from each tube to immunise 1–3 persons. The freeze-dried material has a longer storage life (+2 to +10° C) than the glycerolated vaccine formerly available.

213

Persons who reconstitute dried vaccine and those who vaccinate patients are themselves at risk from accidental infection with the live virus, and should have been vaccinated within the last three years. Accidental *primary* vaccination of the eye or of a finger may be dangerous, but accidental revaccination is relatively harmless.

Persons with eczema should *not* be vaccinated, because of the hazard of generalized vaccinia in such patients (eczema vaccinatum); for the same reason *primary* vaccination of adults should not be carried out. If the effects of primary vaccinations are severe, they may be diminished by giving anti-vaccinial immunoglobulin (hyperimmune or convalescent vaccinia γ-globulin). For details of use, see below.

Because of the danger of secondary spread to other patients, recently vaccinated patients must not be admitted to wards for skin diseases.

BCG and tuberculosis

All hospital staff employed either continuously or intermittently in *hazard* (*high risk*) areas (defined below) must have their resistance to infection tested by the tuberculin reaction (Mantoux or Heaf test) *before* being employed in such areas. If tuberculin negative, they must be given BCG vaccine and await tuberculin conversion before taking up duties. If having had a successful BCG vaccination, the individual is tuberculin tested a year or more later and is found to be negative, he/she should be referred to an experienced chest physician for an opinion. BCG should *not* at once be readministered, for this sometimes produces an unpleasant reaction (chronic ulceration at the site, etc.).

Hazard areas are (1) wards of chest hospitals and clinics, where patients with open (i.e. transmissible) tuberculosis are commonly seen (also renal units where patient's urine is occasionally an unrecognized source of tubercle bacilli); (2) bacteriology (and other) laboratories where processing of specimens for isolation and culture of the tubercle bacillus takes place; (3) mortuaries of chest-disease hospitals.

Staff, such as radiographers, physiotherapists, pathology laboratory personnel and others who visit patients in the tuberculosis wards, should be similarly screened and immunized if tuberculin negative. Screening of staff should be the responsibility of a physician with special experience of chest diseases who will keep the necessary records.

Immunization does *not* exclude the necessity for methods of surveillance or for instruction of staff about hazards and how to avoid them, including details of when to seek medical advice, and regular (e.g. yearly) chest X-ray.

Poliomyelitis

Although in this country most young adults will have been immunized against poliomyelitis, it is desirable to maintain immunity by revaccination, as the disease in the adult is often of the paralytic type and because there exists no specific treatment for poliomyelitis. Immunization with the Sabin living attenuated vaccine is easily administered to large populations; it is safe, has minimal side-effects, and is effective. It should be offered to all hospital staff. It is given by mouth, usually 3 drops of the vaccine on a sugar lump. Three doses

214

must be given at intervals of 4–8 weeks. *Note:* Although the vaccine contains strains of the three serotypes of poliomyelitis virus, only one of these generally infects the recipient at a time to produce immunity to that serotype. Thus to confer immunity to all types, 3 doses are required. It is incorrect to assume that 2 doses will confer some degree of immunity to all strains; it will confer immunity against only two of the three strains. Booster doses can be offered every 5 years or more often if thought necessary.

Diphtheria

Most adults born in this country after 1941 will have residual immunity to diphtheria as a result of childhood immunization. Although the vaccine is effective in preventing disease, its administration to adults is not without unpleasant reactions. Adults must be given a Schick test for susceptibility to diphtheria (if occasional unpleasant side-effects are to be confined to those at risk from the disease), and this must be done by a specialist who can interpret the results, which are the converse of the tuberculin test (i.e. Schick + ve = susceptible; Schick − ve = immune). Occasionally unpleasant reactions, such as painful brawny induration of the arm, occur in persons who have received the vaccine. Diphtheria vaccine is therefore not routinely recommended even for staff of infectious disease units; the permanent staff should, however, be Schick-tested to determine their immune state; vaccination of the susceptible should be advised and PTAP (Purified Toxoid Aluminium Phosphate adsorbed) used in preference to PTAH (Purified Toxoid Aluminium Hydroxide adsorbed). PTAP is used for adults and PTAH may be used for children. There is now no place for toxoid-antitoxin preparations (which contain a small amount of horse serum) or for the Moloney test. Vaccine prepared by Swiss Serum & Vaccine Institute, Berne — referred to as 'Di Te Anatoxal Berna for adults' contains adsorbed diphtheria (2Lf) and tetanus (20Lf) antigens. This produces good immunity to diphtheria and tetanus without the side reactions of other vaccines, and therefore preliminary Schick testing is deemed unnecessary.

If diphtheria is diagnosed in a patient in hospital he/she should be transferred immediately to an Infectious Diseases Unit. Staff in close contact should be given a 5-day course of oral erythromycin and placed under surveillance for 7 days after contact. Following the course of antibiotic nose and throat swabs should be taken to detect any possible carriers of *Corynebacterium diphtheriae*.

Typhoid and paratyphoid fevers

It is not essential to immunize staff routinely against typhoid fever, even in infectious disease units. These diseases are not very communicable, are adequately contained by efficient nursing and hygienic techniques and are treatable with antibiotics.

Within hospitals with infectious disease units, engineers and plumbers who may have to clear drains and sewers, and also bacteriology laboratory staff, are at slight risk. Staff in these categories *working in infectious diseases hospitals but not in general hospitals* should be offered immunization. Heat-killed TAB vaccine (Wellcome) may be given intradermally (0.1 ml), as the side-effects are less unpleasant by this route than are the effects of a dose of 0.5 ml given s.c. or i.m. There is also a monovalent typhoid vaccine.

Rubella (German measles)

The Joint Committee on Vaccination and Immunization of the Department of Health has recommended that routine rubella vaccination should be offered to girls between their eleventh and fourteenth birthdays. Women of child-bearing age who are exposed to special hazards of rubella (e.g. those in hospitals caring for children or working in maternity and gynaecological units where contact with clinical or subclinical rubella may occur) should have serological examination for susceptibility to rubella; those who are found susceptible (seronegative) and who are *not* pregnant should be offered rubella vaccination; those who are susceptible and pregnant should be employed in other units. Because of the theoretical possibility (not proven) that rubella vaccine might damage the foetus, pregnancy must be excluded at the time of vaccination and should be avoided for 8 weeks thereafter.

Influenza

When epidemics of influenza are predicted, as occurs almost every winter, those responsible for the health of hospital staff often find themselves under pressure to have the staff vaccinated against this infection. However, the vaccines at present available offer such poor immunity that we are reluctant to advise their routine (yearly) use. When a new strain of virus appears and an epidemic can be expected, it is worth while vaccinating hospital staff if a vaccine which offers even a modest degree of protection is available in time. When better vaccines with greater potency and wider protective powers become available these recommendations may be amended.

Measles

There is no need to offer active immunization to patients or staff in hospitals, except possibly for those working in paediatric or infectious diseases wards. Passive immunization (see p. 219) is available if required.

Rabies

If a patient is thought to be at risk from rabies (e.g. after being bitten by an animal while abroad), the nearest Public Health Laboratory will give advice as to the current procedure (see also Chapter 17).

Other diseases

Active immunization against tetanus should be given to all infants and maintained by booster doses. Tetanus toxoid will, in the event of injury, give good protection to previously immunized patients and make it unnecessary to give antiserum (see section on Tetanus prophylaxis below, page 220).

Passive immunization

Passive immunization is conferred by the injection of human normal immunoglobulin (γ-globulin), hyperimmune human specific immunoglobulin (e.g. anti-vaccinial immunoglobulin) or specific immunoglobulins from animals (usually horse). The purpose is to confer immediate but short-term immunity to certain diseases. In this situation antibodies are not made by the person immunized (hence the term passive), but are provided from other human or animal sources. Pooled human normal immunoglobulin therapy is effective against measles (adult dose 750 mg), and probably also against poliomyelitis (adult dose 1500 mg). It will give a measure of protection for about four months against Virus A hepatitis (adult dose 500 mg); there is no good evidence that it is effective against serum hepatitis, but a specific hyperimmune γ-globulin has been developed for protection against this disease (see Chapter 18). Antivaccinial immunoglobulin is effective against smallpox and complications of smallpox vaccination (vaccinia). Convalescent serum may be used for protection against chickenpox; serum from patients with Herpes zoster (shingles) may be used for this purpose.

Pooled human immunoglobulin is not generally indicated for *adult* contacts of measles, rubella, mumps or chickenpox. Up to date information on the use of these agents is available at the nearest Public Health Laboratory which holds the local stocks; see also notes below.

Documentation

When immunization of staff is mandatory it is essential that a record should be kept in the hospital; it is highly desirable that records of other immunizations should also be held in hospital.

Immunization of patients

There are few circumstances in which immunization of patients against an infectious disease is indicated. When applicable, passive immunization which is immediately effective should be used. Passive immunity conferred by giving human immunoglobulin (γ-globulin) or antiserum of animal origin is applicable to the following diseases in the circumstances mentioned.

Measles

When a case is inadvertently admitted or develops in a paediatric ward, immunoglobulin should be given to those patients on immunosuppressive drugs or to those with debilitating diseases, or those in whom the clinician considers that it is clinically indicated.

Poliomyelitis

If a case is accidentally admitted to or develops on a ward, all persons who have not been immunized with a vaccine (Sabin or Salk) should be given immunoglobulin.

Infectious hepatitis (hepatitis A)

When this disease is imported into units, certain patients (e.g. those with spina bifida and other chronic diseases requiring long stay in hospital) can be treated with human normal immunoglobulin, which may be used to help in the control of an outbreak. Patients who are on immunosuppressive drugs or who have had extensive radiotherapy should also be protected. It may be desirable to protect staff who are especially at risk. Doses are 250 mg for a child and 500 mg for an adult, which gives protection for about four months.

It is not generally possible or necessary to offer immunization to all patients apart from those in the categories mentioned above, because stocks of immunoglobulin have to be conserved. Infectious hepatitis can probably be controlled to some extent by good hygiene.

Chickenpox

Although chickenpox is not a serious disease in the otherwise healthy person, it will occasionally be necessary to attempt to prevent (or attenuate) an attack in the newborn or in persons on immunosuppressive therapy, or in leukaemic patients on cytotoxic drugs. Pooled human immunoglobulin is probably not very effective and rather large doses are recommended, e.g. 750 mg for a neonate and up to 8 g in an immunosuppressed adult.

Recently, limited supplies of hyperimmune antivaricella/zoster (chickenpox/shingles) immunoglobulin have become available for such classes of patients as are mentioned above — the baby born, on rare occasions, of a mother who has varicella will possess no maternally derived immunity and may be given immunoglobulin. Leukaemics who have been in contact with varicella are also at risk, and the MRC Leukaemia Trials at Royal Marsden Hospital, Sutton, Surrey, have access to immunoglobulin for these patients. The nearest Public Health Laboratory should be consulted in case of need.

The prophylactic doses of specific antivaricella/zoster immunoglobulin recommended for various ages are:

Age	mg	Ampoules
Newborn < 1 year	90/100	2 x 0.5 ml
1-5 years	225/250	1 x 2.5 ml
6-10 years	450/500	2 x 2.5 ml
11-14 years	675/750	3 x 2.5 ml
≥ 15	900/1000	4 x 2.5 ml

For treatment of an established case the dose should be doubled.

Diphtheria

As for hospital staff (see p. 215).

Gas gangrene

An immune serum prepared in the horse against the toxins of *Clostridium welchii, Cl. septicum* and *Cl. oedematiens* is available. There is no evidence that this has any value in prophylaxis against gas gangrene when used in patients with open wounds, but the use of a polyvalent antitoxin containing 10 000 u of *Cl. welchii* antitoxin, 5000 u of *Cl. septicum* antitoxin and 10 000 u of *Cl. oedematiens* antitoxin (i.v. or i.m.) has been advocated by some authorities for extensive soiled wounds. In established gas gangrene it may have some value (dose 75 000 u or more i.v.) when used together with the most important measures — wide excision of affected muscle, high dosage of penicillin and hyperbaric oxygen; these are probably of greater value than the antiserum, which carries a risk of allergy, including anaphylaxis (see Tetanus, p. 222).

Other uses to which immunoglobulin (γ-globulin) has been put, to confer short-term immunity

Rubella

Although some protection of experimentally infected volunteers has been demonstrated, it is of no practical value in prevention of rubella in pregnant women exposed to infection.

A clotted blood specimen should be taken from the patient and sent to the laboratory to determine the immune state of the individual. Thereafter the laboratory will advise on any possible course of action.

Infectious hepatitis (hepatitis A)

Good immunity is conferred for up to four months. After this time the subject again becomes fully susceptible. Doses are 500 mg for adults, 250 mg for children. Indiscriminate use of γ-globulin in contacts of cases of jaundice is not justified. It is of no value in prevention of serum hepatitis (hepatitis B).

Measles

Children suffering from cystic fibrosis, chronic suppurative conditions, primary tuberculosis or hypogammaglobulinaemia, or after splenectomy, if not already immune are at risk: immunoglobulin 250 mg, given within 7-10 days of contact, will probably modify an attack of measles. The disease may often be prevented with doses of between 250 and 750 mg depending on age — consult the leaflet accompanying the ampoule. If active immunization of a compromised patient is desired, then the live vaccine may be given together with a small dose of immunoglobulin. This dose is rather critical and special ampoules containing 0.5 ml, 10 mg protein (4-8 i.u. measles antibody) are available. The dose is 0.4 mg immunoglobulin/lb body weight. NB: normal immunoglobulin is NOT suitable for modifying reactions to measles vaccine.

Vaccinia

Vaccination is dangerous and unnecessary (see p. 213) in children and adults suffering from eczema and in those on large doses of steroids or immunosuppressive drugs. There is a slight risk to the foetus in pregnant women being vaccinated for the first time. However, accidental vaccination may occur and in these cases anti-vaccinial γ-globulin (immunoglobulin) prepared from sera of persons recently vaccinated and given at the time of vaccination or shortly afterwards will give some protection to those at risk. It can also be used to treat established cases of eczema vaccinatum, but is useless in postvaccinal encephalitis.

Doses for prevention:	Under 1 year	0.5 g
	1-6 years	1.0 g
	7-14 years	1.5 g
	Over 15 years	2.0 g

Dose for treatment: Repeat these doses after 2 days. For vaccinial lesions of the eye or orbit, half hourly instillation of 1% solution of γ-globulin.

Note: The diagnosis in all cases of eczema vaccinatum should, where possible, be confirmed by electron microscopy.

Mumps

Convalescent mumps γ-globulin may occasionally be available but is in short supply. Human normal immunoglobulin has sometimes been used to modify or prevent an attack of mumps but the efficacy of this measure is doubtful and the adult dose large.

Poliomyelitis (see also above, under Immunization of patients)

Human normal immunoglobulin has occasionally been used to protect non-immune children who have been exposed to contact with poliomyelitis.

Except for close contacts within a family, live polio vaccine is now a much more effective agent for preventing spread in a community.

Severe burns and Pseudomonas infection

Vaccines and antisera against *Pseudomonas aeruginosa* have given promising results in pilot studies and recently in a controlled clinical trial (Jones, Gupta and Roe, 1979). Further development is required before these methods are generally available.

Protection against tetanus

The risk of tetanus varies with the type and severity of wound or injury, the place where the patient was when injured (e.g. there is a special risk to agricultural workers), and with the presence or absence of immunity induced by a course of toxoid. It was formerly standard practice to give all patients with open wounds (apart from superficial abrasions or minor cuts) an injection of antiserum (ATS) prepared in the horse. This practice may be dangerous, because of the risk of anaphylactic shock or serum sickness from injection of foreign protein, and also ineffective, because of the rapid removal of antitoxin from the circulation by antibodies to horse serum. It is, in any case, unnecessary when the patient is known to be actively immune.

The procedure outlined in the chart and notes presented here is based on that which is in use at the Birmingham Accident Hospital; it is a revised version of the chart and notes which had been used there for some years previously. Essential features are: (a) booster doses of adsorbed toxoid (vaccine) for all patients known to be actively immune, unless *known* to have completed a course or received a booster dose of toxoid within the previous year, when they may be omitted; (b) the use of human antitetanus globulin (ATG) for all patients not known to be actively immune; reserves of ATS will be kept, in case of a shortage of ATG, for use in non-immune patients, but the use of ATS will be avoided because of the known risks of anaphylaxis and of inadequate protection of patients who have previously received horse serum; (c) if ATS is used, antibiotic will also be given for reinforcement of protection in patients not known to be actively immune; (d) if ATG is used for such patients, antibiotic will also be given only to patients who have not had prompt and effective treatment, or whose wounds are badly contaminated with soil or faeces, or septic; (e) active immunization with adsorbed toxoid for all patients if there is no evidence that they are actively immune; (f) first dose of *adsorbed* toxoid at same time as ATG (or ATS), but injected separately at another site.

The procedure shown in the chart, *Prophylaxis against tetanus in patients with open wounds* (Appendix 13.1) is similar to that used at Birmingham Accident Hospital and presented as an example.

In the previous edition of this book antibiotic prophylaxis was recommended for less severe wounds, and also for severe wounds if promptly treated and not severely contaminated when ATG was not available. Because of the more reliable supply of ATG and the potential shortcomings of antibiotic prophylaxis (see Lowbury *et al.*, 1978), we have in this edition reduced the recommended use of antibiotic prophylaxis.

Use of toxoid

Active immunity

The patient is considered actively immune (a) for 12 months after the first two injections of an immunizing course of tetanus toxoid (adsorbed) or of diphtheria-tetanus-pertussis vaccine (DTP) started at or after the age of six months; (b) for 10 years after three injections (the full immunizing course) of toxoid or DTP vaccine; (c) for 10 years after a boosting dose of toxoid given to an actively immune individual. Patients with open wounds who by these criteria are actively immune require a boosting dose of toxoid unless they are known to have received a full immunizing course or a boosting dose within the previous year.

Assessment of the state of immunity

If the patient does not know whether he has received tetanus toxoid in the past, consult the patient's general practitioner; if he does not know the patient must, in most situations, be considered non-immune. It is helpful for the Area Health

221

Authority to keep records of active immunization of children and some adults. Where this has been done, it has often been possible to obtain information on the immunity state towards tetanus of patients coming to hospital, by telephoning the Area Health Authority.

Active immunization

(1) Active immunity is induced by three s.c. injections of 0.5 ml of toxoid (adsorbed), the three doses being separated by intervals of 6–12 weeks and 6–12 months respectively.

(2) A patient so immunized should have a booster dose of 0.5 ml toxoid (adsorbed) when wounded, and at intervals of 10 years. In this way immunity is maintained. If a patient with a wound is known to have had a dose of toxoid (the last dose in a course or a booster) less than one year previously, it is not necessary to give a booster dose at the time of injury.

(3) Any patient who is given ATG or antitoxin should be actively immunized, the first dose of tetanus toxoid (adsorbed) being injected into the other arm at the same time as ATG or ATS is given.

(4) Forms. A card is used to record injections of toxoid during the course of immunization; each card has two superimposed flimsy sheets with duplicating backs.

(5) Outpatients.
   (a) If active immunization has been started, the patient is given a card, and told to take it to his doctor for the second toxoid injection in 6 to 12 weeks.
   (b) If a booster dose of toxoid is given, the date of this dose is entered on the card.
   (c) In either case, the flimsy sheets from the card will be placed in the folder. They will be sent respectively to the general practitioner and the Area Health Authority by the Records Office.

(6) Inpatients. Active immunization will be carried as far as the length of stay allows. According to the stage reached at the time of discharge, patients will be given a card suitably inscribed, and the flimsy sheets will be sent to the general practitioner and Area Health Authority. As a general rule former inpatients will not be given their remaining toxoid injections at the hospital.

Use of human antitetanus globulin (ATG)

ATG ('Humotet', Wellcome) is available for prophylaxis of patients not known to be actively immune; an injection of 1 ml (250 u) costs approximately the same as a week's course of cloxacillin. It is safer than ATS and likely to be more effective than ATS or antibiotics. A single dose of 1 ml (by i.m. injection) can give a protective level of antitoxin for 4 weeks.

Tests for hypersensitivity of patients are not required, but ATG should be avoided if patients have had adverse reactions to human gamma globulin; such reactions are very rare.

Use of antitoxin (ATS) prepared in animals

Indications

Tetanus antiserum prepared in the horse (ATS) will be used only when a booster dose of toxoid is inappropriate and ATG is not available; it will be used only when authorized by the Surgeon or Registrar on duty. *It should not be given to patients with a history of anaphylaxis or severe immediate hypersensitivity reactions;* such patients requiring antiserum should when possible be given an injection of ovine (sheep) tetanus antiserum if ATG is not available; this can be obtained from special centres. (See National Health Service Memorandum HM (71) 64.)

Assessment of hypersensitivity state before giving ATS

(1) Patients should be asked if they or members of their family suffer from asthma, hay fever, or other allergies, if they have previously had serum treatment (e.g. ATS, Anti-gas gangrene serum, etc.), and if they have previously had serum reactions.

(2) If there is no history of allergy or previous serum injection, give test dose of 0.2 ml ATS (undiluted), by s.c. injection. If there is no general reaction in 30 min, give 1500 u ATS.

(3) If there is no history of allergy, but patient has received previous serum injections, give test dose of 0.2 ml 1/10 ATS; if there is no general reaction in 30 min, give test dose of 0.2 ml undiluted ATS; if no reaction in 30 min, give 1500 u ATS.

(4) If there is a history of allergy (including serum reaction) give test dose of 1/100, 1/10 and undiluted ATS before giving full protective dose (1500 u).

Have a syringe with 1/1000 adrenaline ready for use when giving ATS or testing for sensitivity to ATS.

Treatment for anaphylactic shock

At the first sign of dysponoea, pallor or collapse, inject 1.0 ml of adrenaline solution i.m. (0.5 ml in children), repeat injection (0.5 ml) every 20 min if recovery is delayed (e.g. systolic BP below 100 mm Hg). Antihistamines* may also be injected if urticaria or oedema develops; also hydrocortisone sodium succinate (100 mg i.v.).

Warn all patients given ATS of the possibility (5 per cent) of a local or general rash, fever and joint pains, generally 7 to 12 days after serum injections, though sometimes sooner. These can be treated with oral antihistamine* preparations.

Use of antibiotics

Patients who cannot be adequately protected with toxoid, because they are not actively immune, or for whom ATG is not available, will rely for protection on

---

*The emergency drug cupboard should contain chlorpheniramine ('Piriton') for injections 1-2 ml (10-20 mg i.v.); by mouth 4 mg thrice daily.

surgical cleansing, ATS and supportive prophylaxis by systemic antibiotics. It is essential that the antibiotic treatment should be started as soon as possible after injury. Patients with badly contaminated wounds and those in whom there has been delay in starting treatment should be given antibiotic prophylaxis *together with ATG (or antitoxin, if ATG is not available).*

The antibiotic used should be one which is highly active against *Cl. tetani* (penicillins, erythromycin estolate, or tetracycline); it is also desirable to give an antibiotic which is not inactivated by penicillinase. Suggested schedules: 7 to 10 days course of oral erythromycin estolate or cloxacillin; for out-patients, the same antibiotics, or i.m. penicillin, followed by oral penicillin V for 7 to 10 days.

Storage and disposal of vaccines

Potency and storage of vaccines

Vaccines are biological products and they have a limited effective life. All conditions of storage are controlled to maintain the potency of the vaccine over the whole of its effective life. Vaccines are normally given a clearly marked expiry date by the manufacturer and all staff involved in immunization programmes should take great care to ensure that the product is not out of date. Rotation of stocks to avoid deterioration is essential.

Temperature is critical for efficacy of immunological products. The optimum storage temperature for most vaccines is between 4° and 10° C (39° F and 50° F). Time at room temperatures is critical and time at freezing temperatures is also a hazard. Modern domestic refrigerators are now used to store immunizing preparations and these are often set at a temperature which is too low for the storage of vaccines, e.g. 2° C (35° F). The thermostat should be reset to approximately 6° C (43° F) to prevent loss of antigenicity.

Disposal of unwanted vaccines and doses

Surplus doses of vaccines should be rendered inactive prior to disposal. Vaccines containing live organisms, i.e. smallpox, BCG, measles, poliomyelitis (oral), rubella, and yellow fever, should be inactivated by autoclaving prior to being disposed of down a sink drain. Residues of vaccine remaining after an immunizing session must be discarded.

Appendix 13.1 Prophylaxis against tetanus in patients with open wounds

Types of wound	Other relevant circumstances	Procedure
1. Superficial wound or abrasion		Cleanse and cover
		No ATS or ATG
		Start active immunization if not actively immune
2. Puncture wounds Deep lacerations Animal or human bites Wounds with devitalized tissue Wounds more than 4 h old Infected traumatic wounds	If KNOWN to be 'actively immune' ⟶	Cleanse toilet and cover
		Toxoid (adsorbed) booster*
	If NOT KNOWN to be 'actively immune' ⟶	Cleanse toilet and cover
		ATG 250 i.u. (or 500 i.u. if 24 h delay). If no ATG available use ATS (1500 or 3000 i.u.)
	Admit to hospital if (a) severe if (b) heavily contaminated	Antibiotic (except for wounds that have had prompt and effective treatment, including ATG, and not heavily contaminated or septic).
		Start active immunization

*Not necessary if last dose of toxoid in course of active immunization or last booster dose was given less than one year previously.

References and Further Reading

Department of Health and Social Security (1972), *Immunisation against Infectious Diseases*; a report by the Standing Medical Advisory Committee of the Central Health Services Council, HMSO, London.

Jones, R. J., Gupta, J. L. and Roe, E. (1979), Controlled trials of polyvalent pseudomonas vaccine in burns. *Lancet*, ii, 977.

Lowbury, E. J. L., Kidson, A., Lilly, H. A., Wilkins, M. D. and Jackson, D. M.

(1978), Prophylaxis against tetanus and non-immune patients with wounds: the role of antibiotics and of human antitetanus globulin. *J. Hyg. Camb.*, 80, 267.

Parish, H. J. and Cannon, D. A. (1962), *Antisera, Toxoids, Vaccines and Tuberculins in Prophylaxis and Treatment.* 6th Edn, Livingstone, Edinburgh.

Tyrrell, D. A. J., Philips, J., Goodwin, C. S. and Blowers, R. (1979), Schedules for routine immunisation, In: *Microbial Disease.* Edward Arnold, London, pp. 305-9.

Department of Health and Social Security (1971), *Supply of Certain Prophylactic or Therapeutic Agents*, Hospital Memorandum HM (71) 64.

Care of Hospital Staff: Infection

CHAPTER FOURTEEN

Hospital Staff Health Services in the Control of Infection

Many commercial organizations have medical services for their staff which help to reduce the incidence of sickness arising from hazards at work and time lost through sickness. It is surprising that hospitals, which are centres of medical expertise, should have been slower to provide a well organized system of medical care for their staff. Transmission of infection, both from staff to patients and from patients to staff, is well recognized in hospitals. Medical care is often available for the nursing staff, but the scope of this service varies greatly in different hospitals. Health services to hospital staff should, of course, include attention to all forms of illness, but the prevention of infection is a major reason for promoting these services.

The establishment of an occupational health service for hospital staff is outlined in a report of a joint committee of the Department of Health and the Scottish Home and Health Department (1968). The Health and Safety at Work Act 1974 (see p. 20) regulates the safety of the work place and applies to hospitals. Stress is laid on the formulation of local rules for each department, and the head of department is responsible for the formulation of such rules. Rules relating to control of infection need to be clearly incorporated into the local departmental rules. Guidelines for drawing up local rules were published by Boucher (1979). The Report of the Howie Committee and subsequent code of practice (DHSS, 1978) contains paragraphs relevant to laboratory and hospital staffs (see also p. 282). This chapter deals only with the infective aspects of health care for hospital staffs.

Risks to the staff from patients

Members of hospital staff are exposed to risks of acquiring many kinds of infection (see Chapter 9), but some infections, notably tuberculosis, meningococcal meningitis, poliomyelitis, infectious hepatitis, enteric fever and other salmonella infections, present special hazards. In the event (now fortunately remote) of admission of a case of smallpox, non-immune staff are likely to become infected. A high incidence of staphylococcal or streptococcal infection among the patients may sometimes lead to outbreaks among the nurses and other members of hospital staff. However, most staphylococci causing infections in hospitals as well as Gram-negative bacilli, such as *Ps. aeruginosa* and *Klebsiella*, are unlikely to infect staff or be transmitted to their relatives. Epidemics of respiratory virus diseases

229

in the community necessitating admission of patients to hospital may lead to outbreaks of the disease in hospitals. Certain infections, such as herpetic whitlow, occur predominantly in members of hospital staff. Head lice and scabies may occasionally be a hazard to staff, the latter especially in mental subnormality units. *Candida* infections may be a problem in maternity and gynaecological units.

In addition to overt clinical infections carrier states may arise. Acquisition of hospital staphylococci in the external nares and of multiresistant Gram-negative bacteria in the bowel flora are common events.

Risks to the patients from the staff

The commonest infections transmitted to patients by hospital staff, apart from upper respiratory viral infection, are staphylococcal sepsis, streptococcal sore throat, and infective diarrhoea. *Candida* spp. may be transmitted to neonates by staff with paronychia. Spread of pulmonary tuberculosis from a member of staff is a rare but important hazard. The likelihood of transmission clearly depends on the activities of the infected person; e.g. a boil on the hand of a surgeon or nurse is a greater risk to a patient than a similar lesion on the hand of a clerk or an engineer. However, these or other workers may well be in contact with patients, and this factor should be considered in deciding when members of staff should be excluded from direct contact with patients.

Symptomless carriers of virulent pathogenic organisms among members of staff are also a potential hazard of infection to patients. Outbreaks of staphylococcal infection in neonatal departments, or of wound sepsis acquired in the operating theatre, may originate from a nasal or less often a skin carrier of a virulent strain of *Staph. aureus*. An important source of infection especially in surgical wards may be a member of staff with eczema colonized by an epidemic strain of *Staph. aureus*. Nose or throat carriers of Group A β-haemolytic streptococci have been responsible for outbreaks of puerperal sepsis in maternity wards, particularly if carried by delivery room staff. Kitchen staff carrying dysentery bacilli or *Salmonella* sp. may also be a hazard, although outbreaks of infection arising initially from staff in hospital kitchens are uncommon.

During an outbreak of infection in the hospital, epidemiological evidence may point to staff members being involved in the occurrence or spread of infection. In these circumstances, a search for carriers or cases among staff may be necessary. Apart from this situation, routine and regular monitoring of otherwise healthy staff members is not required.

Initial screening of staff on appointment

All staff, i.e. medical, nursing, administrative, ancillary (laboratory, physics and other technicians, physiotherapy, X-ray etc.), domestic, portering and mortuary staff, CSSD staff, catering and laundry should be included in the initial screening and immunization programme. Enquiry should be made for diarrhoeal diseases, recurrent sepsis, tonsillitis or chronic skin diseases; it is advisable that applicants suffering from certain chronic conditions (e.g. severe eczema) should not be accepted for nursing or other duties that bring them into close contact with patients. A chest X-ray to exclude tuberculosis or report of a chest X-ray in the previous 12 months is desirable (see HC (78) 3). For those coming into contact with patients, a tuberculin (e.g. Heaf) test for susceptibility to tuberculosis should also be carried out; BCG vaccination should be offered to Heaf-negative persons who have not previously received BCG vaccination and shown conversion of the tuberculin test. Conversion of the tuberculin test to a positive reaction should be demonstrated before close contact with tuberculous patients or laboratory specimens which might be considered to be tuberculous is allowed. (See below, and Chapter 13.)

Bacteriological examination of nose, throat and faeces is not recommended as a routine, but may be indicated in certain special circumstances (see Chapters 2 and 11).

An example of a card which might be used for recording hospital staff immunization is shown in Appendix 14.1.

Immunization of Staff

The principles involved in selecting immunization procedures are discussed in Chapter 13. For most general hospitals the following are suggested:

All staff should be offered protection against tuberculosis and poliomyelitis. Non-pregnant susceptible women of child-bearing age should also be offered rubella vaccination. The Code of Practice (1978) suggests that tetanus toxoid should be given to laboratory staff and to engineering staff who service laboratory equipment; it seems reasonable to offer tetanus immunization to all engineering and gardening staff. Smallpox vaccination should be reserved for staff exposed to special hazard (e.g. in smallpox hospitals).

In general hospitals there is no need for routine immunization against typhoid fever. Rubella vaccination is intended for staff in contact with children, but due to rotation of staff it is usually more practical to offer vaccination to all female members of staff at risk. Rubella-negative women should not work in a maternity unit until they have been immunized. It has been suggested that rubella vaccine should be offered also to non-immune male staff who are likely to come in contact with women in the early antinatal period.

Measles vaccine should be offered to staff in paediatric, infectious diseases or leukaemia wards if they have not already had the disease.

Continuing surveillance

In addition to initial screening, the occupational health service or practitioner and nurse responsible for staff health should be concerned with:

(1) Training of staff of all grades in personal hygiene.
(2) Immunization and vaccination of existing staff at the required time interval.
(3) Organization of special precautions for staff particularly at risk for infection, e.g. chest X-rays every one or two years for medical bacteriology staff. Screening for hepatitis associated antigen of staff of renal dialysis units.

231

(4) Examination of staff returning to work after absence due to diarrhoea or sepsis, to ensure that the infection has cleared.
(5) Arranging tests and possibly treatment for staff with sepsis of hospital origin or who are carriers of pathogens which may be harmful to patients.
(6) Keeping accurate records of infections in the staff.

Where an Occupational Health Department exists, a close working relationship must be established between the Control of Infection Officer and Nurse and staff of the Occupational Health Department. A member of the Occupational Health Department should be on the Control of Infection Committee. In the absence of an occupational health service pressure from the Infection Control Team should be brought to bear on the management to provide one. As an interim measure some of its functions could be met by providing a small centre in the hospital which is open for an agreed time each day. If necessary this could be staffed preferably by a general practitioner or other clinical member of hospital staff. However, if this method is adopted there may be difficulties in maintaining confidentiality of records.

Isolation of staff with, or in contact with, infectious diseases

The recommended periods of isolation for patients with infectious disease (see chapter 9, pp. 136–145) are also appropriate periods of time for members of staff with such infections to be kept away from patients in the hospital. Staff who are in contact — at home or in hospital — with infectious disease need not be excluded, but when they are or have been in contact with cases of typhoid fever, diphtheria, meningococcal meningitis and other potentially dangerous diseases, the Hospital Infection Officer should be consulted for advice. Diphtheria contacts should be given prophylactic erythromycin and kept under surveillance (see p. 146). Poliomyelitis and diphtheria contacts should be offered active immunization. Contacts should not work where there are high infection risk patients unless they are immune or otherwise protected against the infection to which they have been exposed.

Appendix 14.1 Hospital staff immunization record

								Card No.
Name				Department			Date of birth	
Diagnostic tests			Tetanus	Polio	BCG	Rubella	Influenza	Other
Date	Test & Result	Date Amount Batch No.						
		Date Amount Batch No.						
		Date Amount Batch No.						

References and Further Reading

Boucher, B. J. (1979), Guidance on preparing local rules to help implement the Health and Safety at Work etc. Act. *Br. med. J.*, i, 599.

Department of Health, and Scottish Home and Health Department (1968), *The Care of the Health of Hospital Staff*. HMSO, London.

Department of Health and Social Security (1978), Health Circular HC (78) 3: *Health Services Management: Control of tuberculosis in N.H.S. employees: Limitation of X-ray examinations.*

Department of Health and Social Security (1978), *Code of Practice for the Prevention of Infection in Clinical Laboratories and Post-mortem Rooms.* HMSO, London, pp. 5–12.

Health and Safety at Work etc. Act (1974), HMSO, London.

SECTION F

Special Wards and Departments

CHAPTER FIFTEEN

Special Wards and Departments (1)

Intensive care units

Infection is one of the principal hazards to which patients in intensive care (or intensive therapy) units (ICU or, more usually, ITU) are exposed. A patient requiring intensive care may be defined as one who requires support of a vital function until the disease process is arrested or ameliorated; such patients are likely to have poor resistance to infection sometimes due to immunosuppressive or steroid therapy, or due to depression of the immunological response often seen in these patients with multiple organ failure. In addition to being more susceptible, they are exposed in the intensive care unit to greater hazards of contamination and cross-infection than most patients in ordinary wards. This is due to the fact that they receive much more nursing attention and handling, and various forms of instrumentation — in particular tracheostomy, mechanical ventilation, aspiration of bronchial secretions, catheterization of the urinary tract, treatment of open wounds and prolonged intravenous infusion. Special difficulties arise through emergencies, e.g. respiratory obstruction requiring immediate clearing of the patient's airway, and the sudden excessive pressure of work which occurs when several patients are admitted at the same time; in such circumstances it may be difficult or impossible to observe all the recommendations of asepsis. Even so, cross-infection is in many cases probably due to thoughtlessness or staff shortages. Intensive therapy requires what is sometimes considered to be an inordinate number of trained nursing staff, but if such a complement is not available, nurses inevitably have to move rapidly between patients without having time even to wash their hands. The amount of technical assistance and the number of cleaners in ITU is much greater than it is in normal wards, but these are essential if nursing skill is to be used effectively and if meticulous cleanliness of equipment is to be maintained.

The micro-organisms which cause infection in intensive care units include any of those which are associated with hospital infection, but since the patients are often deficient in resistance to infection, many organisms which have little or no pathogenicity for healthy persons and tissues are potentially important as causes of infection in intensive care patients. The commonest infecting organisms in an ITU are *Staph. aureus, E. coli, Ps. aeruginosa* and *Klebsiella* spp., *Proteus* spp., *Enterobacter* spp. and *Bacteroides* spp.; some of the opportunist Gram-negative bacilli, e.g. *Pseudomonas* and *Klebsiella*, are found in the water of humidifiers and other likely sources of contamination. Endogenous infection with coliform bacilli and sometimes with *Bacteroides* and other anaerobic non-sporing bacteria are a hazard in patients with abdominal wounds.

237

Staphylococcal infection may be transmitted by contact or by air, but Gram-negative bacilli when not acquired from the patient's own flora of skin, gut or upper respiratory tract, are most likely to be acquired by contact, and from moist vectors such as solutions and medicaments, food, humidifiers of mechanical ventilators, etc. Airborne infection with Gram-negative bacilli is a remote hazard, except from aerosols produced by a contaminated nebulizer, or from removal of dressings (e.g. of burns) on to which heavily contaminated exudate has dried. Expectoration by patients with tracheostomies or endotracheal tubes may cause heavy local contamination with bronchial mucus, but the air of an intensive care unit has been found usually free from *Ps. aeruginosa*, even when several patients with respiratory and urinary tract *Pseudomonas* infection were in the ward. The suggestion that the expired air of all patients undergoing artificial ventilation in the unit should be exhausted to the exterior seems unnecessary.

Control of infection: general

The general principles of aseptic care and hospital hygiene which are described in Sections B, C and D, must be conscientiously applied and with certain additional precautions relating to special procedures of the Intensive Care Unit.

Design of Unit

Because of the need for quick and unimpaired access of staff to patients, it is usually inappropriate for all the patients to be in single-bed isolation rooms, but one or two isolation rooms are required; e.g. in an 8-bed unit, there could be two 3-bed wards or divisions of a ward, and two isolation rooms. In the 'open' section retractable waterproof curtains between beds may have some value in preventing contamination of adjacent beds with expectorated mucus. There should be adequate space (e.g. 10–12 ft between bed centres) to allow easy access of staff and equipment.

The isolation rooms should be suitable for use either by infected patients (*source isolation*), or by hypersusceptible patients who must be given maximum protection against infection (*protective isolation*), or for combined source and protective isolation — e.g. by plenum ventilation into the room and extraction of air, when required, from the room to the outside of the hospital. It is probably desirable that the open section of the Unit should have mechanical ventilation with a turnover of air (e.g. 10 air changes per hour) sufficient to prevent a build-up of bacteria released by persons in the Unit, and to keep airborne bacteria at a low level. An intensive care unit may, however, be reasonably safe without plenum ventilation, or with a degree of mechanical ventilation compatible with comfort.

Furniture and fittings

Floors and walls should be washable. Furniture should be reduced to a minimum. Monitoring equipment should be wall-mounted on a shelf and sealed; suction apparatus and sphygmomanometers should be wall-mounted but detachable.

Sticky mats at the entrance to the Unit have little or no value in the prevention of infection.

Cleaning of environment
As in wards (see Chapter 7).

Handling of patients
A high standard of aseptic care must be used by nurses, doctors, physiotherapists, radiographers, pathology technicians and others in handling intensive care patients. Hands should be washed with an antimicrobial preparation, preferably disinfection with 70–95% alcohol, which is rapid and effective (see Chapter 7). Plastic disposable (or surgical rubber) gloves should be worn for bronchial and oral toilet and as many as possible of the procedures which involve handling the patients. 'Clean' nursing procedures (e.g. oral toilet) should always be done before 'dirty' procedures (e.g. taking rectal temperature).

Protective clothing (gowns and plastic aprons) should be worn when attending to an infected patient; all members of staff or visitors should wear a gown used for that patient only. A mask should be worn when attending to patients with tracheostomies or extensive open wounds. Overshoes and disposable hats are unnecessary. Non-essential visiting should be discouraged, but relatives or close friends of the patient should be allowed. They must have almost unrestricted access to prevent disorientation of the patient, which can cause severe psychological disturbance, one of the major problems for those who survive. Furthermore, there is good evidence that infection is more likely to be acquired from a member of the hospital staff who attends to other patients than from a (healthy) visitor who visits only one patient in the ward.

Procedures

Tracheostomy and endotracheal intubation
The benefits of tracheostomy, by which exudates can be aspirated and mechanical ventilation established, are offset by hazards of infection. Colonization of the trachea, which may sometimes lead to the development of bronchopneumonia, can be caused by various organisms, including *Staph. aureus* and *Ps. aeruginosa*; the bacteria may be introduced into the respiratory tract at the time of aspiration of exudate or during mechanical ventilation or humidification, or (*Staph. aureus*) from the inspired air. The tracheostomy wound may become infected, and pressure of the tracheostomy tube against the tracheal lining may cause abrasion leading to local wound infection and ulceration. Because of these drawbacks tracheostomy has, to a large extent, been superseded by the long-term use of endotracheal tubes. These also may be a channel of contamination, but they have the advantage of avoiding an operation, with possible infection of the operation wound; there is usually no difficulty in re-intubating patients, and secretions can be aspirated as easily from an endotracheal tube as from a tracheostomy particularly if a mucolytic agent is used.

The control of infection through tracheostomy or endotracheal tubes is difficult; when any patient in the Unit has *Pseudomonas* infection (of the

239

respiratory tract or of a wound) it is common for the infection to spread to other patients in the Unit. Aseptic techniques for aspiration of bronchial secretions should reduce the incidence of infection of patients with tracheostomies and endotracheal tubes. Nurses carrying out the bronchial toilet and aspiration should wear plastic aprons, gloves, and also masks if desired. This procedure should not be carried out immediately after wound dressing and after colostomy or rectal care. It must be emphasized that the natural habitat of Gram-negative 'opportunists' is often the human gastro-intestinal tract. Bacterial culture and sensitivity tests on sputum should be done frequently (if possible daily).

Injections

Only the most essential injections should be given through intravenous cannulae.

Ventilatory equipment

Prevention of infection from this source is very important. Various methods of sterilization are available (see Chapter 7). Of importance in the design of all modern lung ventilators is the ability either to isolate the ventilator completely from the patient by bacterial filters, or for the patient's circuit and humidifier to be easily removed for autoclaving, or both.

Even if bacterial filters are employed to isolate the ventilator it may still be advisable to decontaminate the ventilators themselves at either one or two monthly intervals, depending upon the frequency of their use.

Urine drainage

See techniques of catheter drainage in the section on Urological departments in this chapter.

A fluid balance is required as part of management of patients in the Intensive Care Unit. Drainage bags must be changed or emptied twice daily under aseptic conditions, and the collected urine for 24 hours analysis must not be stored at the bedside. Collected urine can be preserved with formalin, which does not affect electrolyte or nitrogen values.

Equipment

All equipment used in intensive care units should be kept meticulously clean and dry. In a study on sources of infection, washing bowls used by patients in an intensive care unit were often found to be contaminated with *Ps. aeruginosa* in residues of moisture; individual bowls, heat-disinfected or at least thoroughly washed and dried after use, are desirable. Shaving brushes should be avoided; electric razors used for one patient and then for another are also potential vectors of infection. Individual shaving kit is desirable. (See Chapter 7 for details on disinfection of ventilators, nebulizers, humidifiers and suction equipment.)

Antibiotic therapy

Prophylaxis with broad spectrum antibiotics should be avoided. There is no evidence that it helps to prevent infection of patients receiving intensive therapy and it is likely to lead to the selective growth of multiresistant opportunist organisms for which, if they cause clinical infection, effective antibiotics may not be available. The prevalence of Gram-negative infections in ITU work is to some extent probably a result of the greater effectiveness of the antibiotics against Gram-positive organisms and to the prophylactic use of antibiotics. Restriction of certain antibiotics (e.g. gentamicin) may sometimes be necessary (e.g. in an outbreak due to resistant strains). Mere identification of a Gram-negative organism in a tracheostomy wound or in sputum is not an indication for treatment, which should be given only if there is good evidence of a significant clinical infection.

Relationship to Recovery Units

After major surgical procedures patients may go to a recovery unit or area; after a short stay for initial treatment and assessment, they are transferred to the ITU. During their time in the recovery area such patients are cared for by nursing staff who, either because of lack of training or because of the large numbers of patients passing through the unit per day, may possibly not practise the meticulous techniques and barrier nursing procedures necessary to prevent infection; such patients may later spend long periods in the ITU. Furthermore, the close proximity of such potential ITU patients in the recovery unit to other patients who have infected or potentially infected surgical wounds often requiring attention may well lead to cross-infection. If patients, after major surgery, are considered to need intensive therapy, it is probably wise to transfer them directly from the operating theatre to the ITU.

Paediatric departments

Special problems of infection

Many children are admitted to hospital with (or incubating) community-acquired infections and consequently the proportion of infected patients in a children's ward is usually considerably higher than in adult wards. Some of these infections, such as respiratory virus infections, severe gastro-enteritis and infected skin lesions, are difficult to keep under control and may spread rapidly. Children are also more susceptible to community-acquired diseases than adults and they may not have developed an immunity to the common infectious fevers. Most children's wards also contain a few patients who are particularly susceptible, for example those with blood disorders or receiving steroids. Patient discipline is understandably rather lax in children's departments and care must be taken to avoid the escape of children from isolation cubicles and misplaced generosity in sharing of toys, dummies etc. Food is often prepared in the ward and provides a further potential hazard.

The organisms which may be involved in cross-infection are many, including viruses such as respiratory syncytial virus, measles virus and gastro-enteritis viruses such as Rotavirus, bacteria such as β-haemolytic streptococci, enteropathogenic *E. coli*, *Campylobacter* spp., fungi such as *Candida albicans*, dermatophytes

241

affecting the scalp, and even skin or intestinal parasites. *Ps. aeruginosa* and *Staph. aureus* are likely to infect children with cystic fibrosis. Chapter 9 (on isolation and barrier nursing) is particularly relevant to paediatric departments, and procedures are suggested for management of children admitted with community-acquired infections.

Prevention of infection (see also section on Maternity departments)

The numbers of nursing staff and the quality of their training are major factors in controlling the spread of infection. It is helpful for senior nursing staff to have some experience of practices in a communicable disease ward.

Isolation facilities are needed for between one in five to one in ten of the patients in the unit, depending on the type of patients admitted. Because of the risk of gastro-enteritis, no more than four infants should be in any one ward and they should preferably be in cubicles with one or two cots only. No ward should be exclusively occupied by infants. Adequate washing facilities must be available in each cubicle and each cubicle should have its own weighing machine. Older children should not be in wards with adults. Each ward should have a play room and a separate examination room. There should be one or two special beds available in each ward to allow a parent to sleep in the hospital. Ideally, a separate block for isolation is desirable. Screening the faeces of all children admitted to paediatric wards, for the presence of *Salmonella* spp., has been found useful by some pathologists, though generally not considered practicable or worthwhile.

There is evidence that frequent and prolonged visiting by parents to their own children does not have any effect on infection rates, but some protection may need to be provided for parents. For example, gowns or plastic aprons should be worn by parents nursing children with gastro-enteritis, and hand-washing facilities must be available to them, together with instructions on how to avoid acquiring the infection. Visiting of children with dangerous infections, e.g. diphtheria, poliomyelitis and (for the first 48 hours) meningococcal meningitis, should be restricted to parents and preferably to those who are immune, when this is possible.

Visitors should avoid contact with other children.

For preparation of feeds see below (p. 247); for treatment of incubators, suction equipment, thermometers and other equipment, see Chapters 5 and 7. Crockery and cutlery need be only domestically clean, but washing in a machine at 70-80° C (158°-176° F) is preferred.

Oxygen tents should be washed and thoroughly dried before being used by the next patient. In an emergency, tents may be disinfected with 0.1% chlorhexidine (see also Chapter 7).

Toilet arrangements

Because of the common occurrence of intestinal infections in children, special precautions are necessary for toilet areas and bedpan handling. The toilet areas require a high standard of domestic cleanliness, especially the toilet seat, which should be washed at least daily and more frequently if this is necessary. Washing

the toilet seat frequently with a phenolic or hypochlorite disinfectant may be
required during outbreaks of gastro-enteritis, but attention to hand-washing and
use of paper towels is of greater importance. A steam supply capable of destroy-
ing vegetative forms of bacteria should be fitted to bedpan washers (see Chapter 7).

Laundry

Napkins are treated as 'foul' linen and are sealed in plastic or alginate bags.

Personnel

Communicable diseases may be acquired by staff from patients if they are not
immune. One of the most important of these is rubella, and all female staff of
child-bearing age should have rubella HAI titre assessed and be vaccinated if
necessary before working on paediatric wards. The acquisition of *Salmonella* and
Shigella by nursing staff can have disastrous effects and most outbreaks of infection due to these organisms have been associated with the infection in the nursing
staff. *Herpes simplex* infection in attendants may produce a variety of lesions
and may cause severe infections in children. Staff with herpetic lesions should
not handle babies.

Surveillance systems

A list of patients with infection admitted to the ward or acquired in the ward is
useful in the investigation of spread of infection. The infections which are most
usefully recorded are those due to *Salmonella*, *Shigella* and enteropathic *E. coli*,
staphylococcal and streptococcal infections and non-bacterial acute enteritis (as
indicated in laboratory reports), and the common infectious diseases (obtained
from ward notes).

Maternity departments

In the maternity department there are three types of patients who can acquire
infection. *The antenatal patient* is at particular risk only if the foetal membranes
have ruptured, allowing access of organisms to the foetus and liquor amnii. *The
post-natal patient* has a large endometrial surface with thrombosed blood vessels
which is vulnerable to invasion by many organisms. Wound infection may follow
a Caesarian section. Thirdly there are problems of *the neonate* who has very little
natural immunity to infection and has come from a sterile environment and met
bacteria for the first time. Premature or damaged babies are particularly vulnerable to infection.

Almost any organism may give rise to dangerous disease in maternity departments, even those, such as coliforms, enterococci, Group B streptococci or
bacteroides, which are often of low pathogenicity, while more invasive organisms,
such as Group A haemolytic streptococci, *Staph. aureus* or *Clostridium welchii*,
are particularly dangerous. Theinfant may be infected by organisms derived from
the mother either *in utero* (rubella, syphilis, tuberculosis) or during delivery
(gonococcal ophthalmia, chlamydial eye infections, salmonellosis) and may be

243

highly infectious. Mothers known to be hepatitis antigen carriers may, from time to time, be admitted for delivery. For them special precautions are required (see below).

Colonization of the child with bacteria begins shortly after birth. The intestinal tract and often the throat are colonized by antibiotic-sensitive coliforms which may be rapidly replaced by resistant strains if the baby is treated with antibiotics. In susceptible infants, these may cause respiratory tract infection, meningitis and septicaemia. Within seven days of delivery, *Staph. aureus* may be found particularly in the flexures and on moist areas of skin (axillae, groin and napkin area) and on the umbilical stump. *Staph. aureus* is found in the throat or nose of many newborn infants after a few days. The carriage of this organism is usually inconsequential but may be associated with minor skin pustules or eye infections. Occasionally invasive disease may supervene: a septicaemia, which perhaps gains entrance from the umbilical stump, or that now rare skin disease, pemphigus neonatorum. The epidemic strain may cause breast abscess in the mother some weeks later. *Candida albicans* is also common, causing oral and skin infection, and can produce serious disease in weaker babies.

The infant must be guarded as far as possible from acquiring a heavy load of pathogenic organisms, for it will in its turn disseminate these into the environment. Poor standards of hygiene may be followed by heavy contamination; good hygiene lowers the risk. Infants are apt to get sticky eyes within a few days of birth; a variety of organisms may be isolated from these and it seems likely that the conjunctivitis is often of chemical origin, caused by the antiseptics used during labour. The staphylococci, coliforms and other organisms are then thought to have caused the infection. Rough handling of the child or damage by nurses' rings and watches may produce excoriations and allow access of bacteria. Napkin rash is due to the action of bacteria (chiefly coliforms) which produce ammonia and other substances which damage the wet skin.

Spread of infection after delivery is mainly by contact, usually on attendants' hands, with some additional spread of Gram-negative bacilli by way of apparatus or disinfectants, and, less commonly, of staphylococci in the air.

Prevention of spread

Isolation facilities are necessary for both mothers and babies. Maternal diseases requiring isolation include puerperal sepsis, which may be due to a Group A β-haemolytic streptococcus, gastro-intestinal infections, breast abscess, and staphylococcal skin sepsis. Infected neonates should also be placed in isolation as soon as an infection is suspected. It may be necessary to separate infants from their mothers if the latter are infected, particularly in cases of maternal pulmonary tuberculosis and skin sepsis. Infant nurseries should be small and contain not more than four beds. Overcrowding is responsible for cross-infection in the nursery. Cross-infection may also be reduced by rooming-in, i.e. keeping the baby in the mother's room. If there are insufficient numbers of small rooms, cohort nursing is a particularly useful routine measure for prevention of infection or for ending an outbreak; babies born over a period of 24 to 48 hours are kept in one nursery; when all these babies are discharged from hospital the room is cleaned if necessary and another batch of babies admitted.

Babies with gastro-enteritis should be immediately isolated. If an infection is severe or more than two cases occur, the ward should be closed to further admissions. The other infants should be screened and all carriers kept in one nursery. If possible, separate nurses should attend babies in the infected and non-infected nurseries. Nurses preparing feeds should not handle infected babies or their contacts.

As the main method of spread of infection is by way of attendants' hands, these require special care. Hands should be washed after any procedure involving handling of a baby or its immediate environment. Washing with soap and water is usually adequate, but an antiseptic preparation should be used for hand-washing by staff in premature baby units and in outbreaks of infection; povidone-iodine solution, or chlorhexidine detergent preparations are equally suitable, but washing with ethyl alcohol (see Chapter 7, p. 73) is an even more effective method. In overcrowded nurseries or during outbreaks of staphylo-coccal infection, hexachlorophane or chlorhexidine powder should be used (see Chapter 9) on the babies. This should not be continued after the baby leaves hospital. Masks are unnecessary in nurseries, but separate gowns or aprons should be worn for attending each baby in the premature baby unit. In the general nursery, gowns or aprons should be worn and changed regularly, but not necessarily after attending each baby. Specific procedures requiring standardization are napkin changing and disposal, bottle feeding, tube feeding and bathing. Napkins should be disposed of into a bucket lined with a plastic bag which is sealed when full. Alginate or hot water-soluble bags may also be used. Disposable napkins should be considered during outbreaks of infections. Separate sterile catheters should be used for each tube feed and discarded after use. If not disposable, catheters should be processed in the CSSD and autoclaved. If it is necessary to leave the tube *in situ* for feeding (e.g. nasal catheters), it should if possible be replaced every 24 hours. Bathing of neonates should be limited to essential times only and usually not more than twice in one week. Addition of disinfectants to the bath is not necessary and is best avoided because of potential toxicity, but washing with a chlorhexidine detergent preparation may be advised during outbreaks of staphylococcal infection. The bath itself, however, should be thoroughly cleaned and disinfected between patients (see Chapter 7).

Although the administration of antibiotics may be necessary as soon as infection of a neonate is suspected, the widespread use of chemoprophylaxis is not recommended. The use of antibiotics selects resistant strains of bacteria, and in particular use of ampicillin-cloxacillin mixtures, as a prophylactic, encourages the appearance of ampicillin-resistant *Klebsiella* or *Pseudomonas aeruginosa.* The prevalence of resistant bacteria in nurseries should be determined from time to time as a guide in the choice of antibiotics for treating undiagnosed infections arising in the unit.

The CSSD can provide much of the equipment needed in maternity departments. Delivery packs, episiotomy sets, dressings and sterile sanitary pads are routine supplies in most hospitals. In addition, as far as possible the CSSD should sterilize equipment for preparing special feeds on the wards, and the containers and teats and tube feeding equipment for neonates. Cleaning and disinfection of incubators and suction equipment is also best carried out in the CSSD if conveniently near. If incubators must be processed in the maternity department, space must be set aside for this purpose and procedures similar to those used in CSSD (see Chapter 5) followed.

Disinfection of teats and bottles on wards should be regarded as second best to presterilized feeds or CSSD processing. Milk kitchens and infant feeds are discussed below.

Female personnel working in the department should be immunized against rubella, as neonates with congenital rubella are highly infectious. Another disease of which they should take special care is gonococcal ophthalmia.

The risks of infection spreading from workers in the unit to the patients are similar to those in other wards, but two special infections, herpes (facial lesions or herpetic whitlow of the fingers) and candida paronychia, are readily spread to neonates; attendants with these lesions should be excluded while infected.

Colonization of the genital tract with group B streptococci occurs in up to 40% of pregnant females. Many are carriers early in pregnancy whilst others only become colonized immediately preterm, making screening logistically difficult. Antibiotics make little difference to the spontaneous loss of the carrier state. Not all babies become colonized by their mother and less than 1% of these develop overt infection. For these reasons we do not recommend routine screening. Group B infection must be borne in mind in any sick neonate, particularly the low birth weight or premature, and in those with respiratory distress.

Some maternity units require nose and throat swabs from new members of staff before starting work, to exclude carriers of staphylococci and streptococci, but most units have abandoned these procedures without ill-effect. Other routine screening systems have been suggested, including that of mothers for carriage of *Salmonella* or *Shigella* before admission to the unit. These suggestions followed the occurrence of several outbreaks of gastro-enteritis in maternity departments, but are impractical as a routine procedure. *Salmonella* may not be detected even if present; the organisms may be acquired after the faeces have been examined and some infected patients are unbooked. Furthermore, most laboratories could either not offer such a service without its detracting from more essential services, or if they did, the examination would be of poor quality and without significant value. However, if there is reason to suspect a patient of having a gastro-intestinal infection or of being a *Salmonella* or *Shigella* carrier, her faeces must be examined and she must be immediately isolated. After delivery of a patient with enteric fever, careful follow-up of other patients in the unit is necessary.

Surveillance of infections is particularly important in neonatal wards, so that immediate action may be taken to prevent extension of an outbreak.

Management of delivery of mothers who are carriers of hepatitis virus

The Blood Transfusion Service is currently screening the blood of pregnant women for the presence of hepatitis antigen $HB_S Ag$, and women found to be

246

HB$_s$Ag positive are now being delivered in hospitals. The recommended precautions are described in Chapter 18 (see p. 301).

Preparation of infant feeds and milk kitchens

Milk is an excellent growth medium for most pathogenic or potentially pathogenic bacteria and contamination of feeds is a particular hazard in neonatal nurseries. Although there is little published evidence that contaminated feeds have caused outbreaks of infection, it seems likely that such outbreaks have occurred more commonly. Many organisms, sometimes in large numbers, have been isolated from feeds, e.g. *Salmonella* spp., enteropathogenic and other strains of *E. coli*, Group A and other groups of β-haemolytic streptococci, *Candida albicans*, *Proteus* spp., *Klebsiella* and *Pseudomonas* spp., *Staphylococcus aureus* and many other organisms.

Contamination of a feed can occur due to faulty disinfection of bottles, teats, dispensing and mixing equipment. Milk, water or other additives may be contaminated prior to use. Recontamination or additional contamination can occur at any time during the preparation process or when feeding the baby. This may be from the air, from the hands of preparation room or ward staff or from the mother.

Usually the initial contamination of the feed is low, and the main hazard is storage at room temperature for a sufficient time to allow organisms to grow. An additional hazard is warming the feed in a contaminated sink or container immediately before administration.

All feeds must be free from intestinal pathogens. The greatest hazard is from these organisms, but other bacteria (e.g. *Proteus* and *Klebsiella* spp.), may cause infection if abundant. The hazard of a major outbreak is much increased if one milk kitchen supplies feeds for all babies in a large unit.

Preferred methods

Commercially supplied pre-sterilized or, if locally produced, terminally sterilized or heat-disinfected feeds should be used in all of the larger maternity units (e.g. over 50 beds with a single milk kitchen). The choice of methods must be made on the basis of effectiveness, economy, availability of staff and space.

Where possible, one of these methods should be introduced into all maternity units. When feeds are sterilized or disinfected by heat, controls to ensure exposure of the feed for the required time at the correct temperature are necessary. Charts showing this information should be regularly inspected by the head of the department. Disinfection by heat, including pasteurization, in a specially designed machine is satisfactory if the processes are adequate; in these instances bacteriological tests should also be made at intervals (e.g. monthly). Commercially prepared presterilized feeds should be bacteriologically safe, provided their control and testing process is satisfactory. Bottles and caps should be inspected before use for obvious damage, and if any doubt exists the bottle should be discarded. Commercially supplied presterilized feeds with the teat already attached to the bottle and adequately protected from contamination are preferable. Single-use teats packed separately are almost as satisfactory, if put on (preferably by the mother) immediately before giving the feed. If teats are used repeatedly, they should be thoroughly cleaned and autoclaved after each use.

Other methods

Chemical disinfection of bottles and teats (by hypochlorite) is reliable if correctly performed but more difficult to control than those methods already described and more susceptible to individual staff errors. The hypochlorite method of disinfection is suitable for use in small units and at home. The hazard of infection in large, well controlled units using chemical methods is not very great if dispensing equipment involving taps which can be easily taken apart and autoclaved are used and if disinfection is well supervised. Bottles and teats should be thoroughly cleaned before disinfection or sterilization by any method, but particularly prior to chemical disinfection. The disinfectant solution should be made up to the correct strength (Hypochlorite — 125 ppm available chlorine). All equipment should be completely immersed, with removal of air bubbles, and should be left for at least the recommended time. Autoclaving of bottles and teats is preferable to chemical disinfection because of the greater reliability of the process. Boiling, correctly performed, should also be more reliable than a chemical method, but the boiling of bottles and teats in an open container is difficult to control and is not recommended.

Paediatric feeds

The recommendations are similar to those for maternity units. Commercially prepared feeds are often not suitable, since a number of babies may require special feeds. Arrangements for terminal sterilization, or autoclaving of bottles and teats, are still necessary in these units.

Milk kitchen and staff

For hospitals where commercially prepared presterilized feeds are used a clean store-room is all that is required. In small units, a kitchen which is used only for preparation of feeds is required. In all milk kitchens, washing up of used bottles, teats and other equipment should be carried out in a room separate from that used for preparing feeds. A hand-washing basin should be available immediately adjacent to the milk kitchen. Staff should be trained in techniques of feed preparation, and in personal hygiene. The training should include methods of preventing contamination, e.g. thorough cleaning of equipment, and the reduction of airborne and contact transfer by hands to a minimum. The preparation of feeds should, if possible, be carried out by staff not handling babies and supervised by a senior member of the nursing staff. After preparation, feeds (unless sterilized) should be placed in a refrigerator (4° C; 39° F) preferably within 30 and not more than 60 min. Non-sterile feeds should be discarded after 24 hours. Supplements should be added to the feed immediately before use.

Newborn infants will usually accept a feed at room temperature and, if possible, warming before use should be avoided. If the feed is warmed, a special container should be used and kept for this purpose only. The container should be filled with boiled water, or with fresh water and boiled for 5 min. The bottle with intact teat cover should be placed in the container at body temperature,

248

and the water level should be well below the neck of the bottle. After use the container should be immediately emptied, cleaned and dried.

Human expressed breast milk

Human milk contains antimicrobial factors which are believed to provide some protection to premature infants against infection. These factors may be heat-labile, although the inactivating effect of pasteurization at relatively low temperatures, e.g. 63–65° C (145–149° F) remains to some extent uncertain. Inadequately collected or stored milk may be heavily contaminated with potential pathogens such as *Klebsiella* spp., *Ps. aeruginosa* and *Staph. aureus*. Unless microbiological tests are made on all samples, pasteurization is required.

Careful attention must be paid to hygienic methods of collection, to ensure milk of an acceptable microbiological standard. These high standards are more easily attained in hospital than in the home. Potential donors should be free of infection, not excreting drugs in the milk, and able to produce sufficient milk to make collection worthwhile. They should be trained in aseptic practices and supplied with suitable equipment for disinfection. The home conditions should be hygienically acceptable. In addition, several samples should be tested microbiologically before the donor is accepted. Instructions on collection and storage should be clear and precise, and should include hand-washing, care of the breast, and methods of cleaning, disinfection and storage of the pump. Whenever possible, sterilized equipment should be supplied. The first 5–10 ml of milk should be discarded and the remainder transferred to a sterile bottle which is labelled with the time of collection, storage time and temperature. It must be placed in a refrigerator as soon as possible at 4° C (39° F) and the temperature during transport should not be allowed to rise above 10° C (50° F). The time out of the refrigerator should not exceed 2 hours, and refrigerated transport or insulated containers may be required for transport.

In most units, pasteurization will also be necessary, but excessive heating should be avoided. Exposure at 65°C (149° F) for 10 min is recommended. The process must be carefully controlled and temperatures checked with a thermometer initially and at regular intervals afterwards. A standard volume of milk should be treated, and should be cooled rapidly. As well as temperature checks, microbiological tests should be made on setting up the process and at regular intervals afterwards. Milk should be deep frozen (−28° C; −18° F) as quickly as possible after collection, and repeated heating and freezing avoided.

Microbiological standards. Since the numbers of organisms required to infect the infant, as well as the role of relatively non-pathogenic organisms, remain uncertain, proposed standards are variable. The resistance of the infant to infection is also variable and the possible deleterious effect of pasteurization is uncertain. It is generally agreed that Gram-negative bacilli should be absent, but the acceptable numbers of *Staph. aureus* or of the normal skin flora are controversial. Some authorities accept the presence of normal flora up to 10^8/ml (Carroll *et al.*, 1979), but we prefer higher standards and suggest the following: total counts should not be above 10^5 organisms/ml, *Staph. aureus* should preferably be absent and not above 10^2/ml, and no Enterobacteriaceae, pseudomonas, other

249

Gram-negative bacilli or groupable streptococci should be present. Although there is little evidence of infection occurring from milk containing much larger numbers of normal flora or *Staph. aureus*, it seems illogical to have lower standards than would be acceptable for milk feeds for normal infants (Ayliffe *et al.*, 1976). Until raw milk can be shown to be more effective than pasteurized in preventing infection in premature infants, it is obviously safer to pasteurize all breast milk before use. An exception would be freshly expressed milk which is given to a woman's own infant.

Burns and open traumatic wounds

Burns are at first free or virtually free from bacteria, which have been killed by the heat, but soon the layer of dead tissue and exudate becomes heavily colonized by bacteria unless effective measures are taken to keep them out. In small superficial burns and in many deeper and more extensive burns the bacteria cause no apparent ill effects, though this depends on the types of bacteria present and on the patient's resistance. In more extensive burns bacterial infection is the most important cause of illness and death.

Strep. pyogenes, when present, will usually cause the complete failure of skin grafts and delay healing; today it rarely causes invasive infection, though it may cause fever. Of the other bacteria, *Ps. aeruginosa* has proved to be the most important cause of septicaemia and toxaemia; it can also cause the failure of skin grafts, but to a smaller extent than *Strep. pyogenes*. Other Gram-negative bacilli (*Proteus* spp., *Klebsiella* spp., *Serratia*, etc.) and *Staph. aureus* are less important pathogens, though they can occasionally cause septicaemia in severely burned patients; rarer pathogens are *Candida albicans* and other fungi, gas gangrene and tetanus bacilli and *Herpes* virus.

Ps. aeruginosa and other bacteria are usually acquired from the burns of other patients in the ward, transmitted on hands of nurses, various fomites and by air; air is a less important route, especially for Gram-negative bacilli, but may be important if dressings are changed in an open ward.

In addition to the burn, the urinary tract, the respiratory tract and intravenous infusion sites are important portals of entry and sites of infection.

Open wounds resemble burns, but there is usually less necrotic tissue in which small numbers of bacteria can multiply. Contaminants acquired at the time of injury, including tetanus and gas gangrene bacilli, are more likely to play a role in infection of open wounds than of burns, but hospital-acquired infection, both exogenous and endogenous, is potentially more important than contamination at the time of injury.

Prevention of infection

The bacterial flora of all burns should be examined on admission and at all changes of dressings for *Strep. pyogenes*, *Ps. aeruginosa* and other common aerobic bacteria. If *Strep. pyogenes* is present, the patient must be treated with systemic erythromycin or cloxacillin, and grafting operations must be postponed until the organisms are removed from the burn; benzyl or phenoxymethyl

250

penicillin are not suitable for this purpose, because they are likely to be inactivated by penicillinase from other bacteria, especially resistant *Staph. aureus*
colonizing the same burn.

First line of defence (i.e. methods of protecting the patients against microbial
contaminants) includes (1) primary excision and skin grafting (only suitable for
relatively small burns of full skin thickness); (2) antisepsis: i.e. application of
antibacterial substances to the burn; for extensive burns 0.5% silver nitrate compresses and 11% mafenide acetate cream with exposure have proved effective,
but require laboratory controls of electrolyte balance; mafenide has been
rejected in some centres because it causes pain which may be severe; creams containing 1% silver sulphadiazine or 0.5% silver nitrate with 0.1% chlorhexidine are
also effective and more convenient; silver sulphadiazine cream has been widely
adopted as a standard prophylactic application, but a preponderant flora of
sulphonamide-resistant Gram-negative bacilli has been found to emerge, with
associated resistance to antibiotics, in one centre where silver sulphadiazine cream
had been in regular use for some years; when this occurs it is important to change
the routine topical prophylaxis (e.g. to silver nitrate-chlorhexidine cream); monitoring of sensitivity of burn flora is an important routine procedure in a burns
unit; (3) asepsis: dressing of burns in ventilated dressing room, barrier nursing,
source and protective isolation of patients and good ward hygiene contribute to
control of infection (see Chapters 8 and 9). For patients with burns in hospital, a
dressing technique with two nurses should be carried out if possible in a room
with combined source and protective isolation (e.g. plenum ventilation with an
exhaust-ventilated air-lock). Exposure treatment, which is clinically desirable for
many burns of the trunk and the face, provides some protection by the development of a dry eschar on which bacteria cannot grow (but which may cover a
zone of heavy growth and suppuration); exposure treatment is better than moist
applications with no antibacterial activity.

The second line of defence (i.e. methods of preventing invasion of the tissues
and blood-stream by bacteria growing on the burn) includes *antibiotic therapy*
and *active* or *passive immunization*. Systemic treatment of all *Strep. pyogenes*
infections with an appropriate antibiotic (e.g. erythromycin or cloxacillin) protects all patients in the ward by eliminating reservoirs of infection. Severely
burned patients who have acquired heavy growths of *Ps. aeruginosa* may be given
protection with systemic gentamicin (and/or carbenicillin) (though resistant
variants are likely to emerge if such treatment is often used). A more promising
procedure may be the use of a polyvalent *Pseudomonas* vaccine which has been
found to give early protection and reduced mortality in patients with severe
burns; hyperimmune globulin prepared from immunized human volunteers has
also proved valuable. Prophylaxis against tetanus, by use of a 'boosting' dose of
toxoid when the patient is known to be actively immune, or by antiserum
(human ATG), if there is no evidence of active immunity, should be given to all
patients with burns admitted to hospital (see Chapter 13).

Special problems of sterilization and disinfection

The principles of sterile supply outlined in Chapters 5 and 7 are relevant to patients with burns. The electric dermatome and the bone saw can be sterilized by dry heat in a hot air oven at 160° C (320° F) for 1 hour. The outside of electrical equipment, cardiac monitoring equipment, portable lights, diathermy and X-ray machines, suction apparatus and respiratory ventilator must be cleaned after use, because of the possibilities of heavy contamination.

For disinfection of respiratory ventilators and anaesthetic apparatus, see Chapter 7. Water circulating mattresses may be disinfected with a clear soluble phenolic, and body temperature recorders with 70% alcohol. Mattress covers may be damaged by repeated application of phenolic disinfectants or by silver nitrate treatment of patients (e.g. burns); gram-negative bacilli are then likely to grow in the mattress.

Dermatological wards

Most patients with skin diseases are not physically very 'ill', but their condition often causes them some mental stress. When it is considered necessary to use source isolation procedures, it is important that it should be explained to the patient that the underlying skin condition (e.g. eczema or psoriasis) in itself is not infectious and will not spread to the rest of the family or to visitors. The risk is of the transfer of bacteria capable of causing infection in susceptible patients in hospital (e.g. patients undergoing surgery), and that healthy people will not become infected from them even when in close contact. This does not apply to certain septic lesions, e.g. impetigo, where there is a definite risk of transfer to healthy subjects.

Patients in dermatological wards often have generalized desquamating lesions which are heavily colonized with *Staph. aureus*. These patients are often heavy dispersers and cross-infection is frequent, but clinical sepsis is rarely caused by these staphylococci. However, such a patient admitted to a surgical ward may be responsible for widespread nasal colonization and wound sepsis. These strains of staphylococci are commonly resistant to two or more antibiotics. Children admitted with clinically apparent staphylococcal infections (e.g. impetigo) not only spread infection, but cause similar septic lesions in other children and sometimes pyogenic lesions in the staff. These strains are often resistant to penicillin only and are initially acquired outside hospital. Some of these infections are caused by β-haemolytic streptococci (often associated with *Staph. aureus*) and may similarly spread to other patients. Cross-infection with Gram-negative bacilli (e.g. *Ps. aeruginosa* and *Proteus* spp.) is also common in dermatological wards and these organisms are usually found in varicose ulcers, but clinical sepsis is unusual.

Candida infection may also occur, but owing to problems of typing, good evidence of cross-infection is difficult to obtain. Patients with dermatophyte infections are not usually admitted to hospital, but the risk of cross-infection exists (e.g. tinea corporis and pedis, which may not be clinically obvious). Transmission of *Tinea capitis* between children occurs readily in schools and could similarly spread in paediatric wards.

The spread of virus infection is not a particular hazard of dermatological wards apart from vaccinia (see page 137 and page 214).

Control of infection

Staphylococcal infection spreads both by contact and by air. Environmental contamination is so heavy that prevention of cross-infection is difficult, but some potentially effective measures are possible, especially the following:

(1) Children with clinical sepsis must be isolated in single rooms, whether in general or dermatological wards.
(2) Patients with desquamating lesions must be kept in single rooms, if admitted to *general* hospital wards.
(3) General hospitals should have wards kept solely for dermatological patients.
(4) When isolation is required, it must be complete; i.e. patients should not leave the ward to visit other patients.

Dressing techniques

Open lesions (e.g. ulcers) and wounds should be treated as in a general surgical ward, using CSSD packs and a no-touch technique. A special room should be provided if possible for carrying out surgical techniques (e.g. biopsies). The dressing of patients with non-surgical lesions is rather different, since it is often necessary to apply creams with the hands, but the following points should be observed.

(1) Dressing rooms should be immediately adjacent to the bathroom and should have an extractor fan.
(2) Couches in dressing rooms should be covered with paper covers which are changed between patients.
(3) Dressing materials in contact with broken skin should have been sterilized.
(4) Large bags should be provided for disposal of contaminated dressings.
(5) Gloves or instruments should be used for carrying out dressing techniques whenever possible; creams and ointments should be applied when possible with the gloved hand. Staff should wash their hands thoroughly with soap or an antiseptic detergent preparation and water after handling each patient.
(6) Staff should wear plastic, disposable aprons, which should be discarded at the end of a dressing session; wiping or spraying the front with 70% alcohol after each dressing should reduce the hazards of cross-infection.

Additional precautions

(1) Disposable toilet-seat covers and bath-mats may be of some value; patients should be instructed in their use.
(2) Floors should be cleaned with a vacuum-cleaner, never with a broom.
(3) Special attention should be paid to the disinfection of baths and wash-bowls after each use. In general, cleaning methods and techniques are similar to those recommended for rooms containing infected patients (see Chapter 7).
(4) Because of the danger of eczema vaccinatum, recently vaccinated staff and patients should be excluded from dermatology wards.

253

Antibiotic treatment

Emergence of resistance is especially likely to occur in patients with skin disease because of the large populations of bacteria on the skin. Antibiotic treatment (especially topical) should be avoided whenever possible and other antimicrobial agents should be used if available or suitable (e.g. silver nitrate, chlorhexidine). Resistance emerges particularly readily to erythromycin, lincomycin (or clinda-mycin) and fucidin and their use should be severely restricted. Topical prepara-tions of fucidin should not be used in hospital. Neomycin and bacitracin are useful topical antibiotics, although resistance of *Staph. aureus* and hypersensi-tivity to neomycin are uncommon. Gentamicin is a useful systemic antibiotic and should not be used topically in hospital. The combination of neomycin with chlorhexidine in a topical preparation may reduce the likelihood of resistance emerging. When possible, patients receiving treatment with antibiotics on the 'restricted' list (see Chapter 12) should be given source isolation.

Ointments and other medicaments

Since patients with widespread skin lesions are particularly susceptible to infec-tion and large amounts of topical medicaments are often applied, the application must be free from pathogenic bacteria. Tubes should be used whenever possible for creams and ointments. Jars or bottles should be thoroughly cleaned (or preferably disinfected) and dried before refilling, and occasional bacterial checks should be made on preparations and distilled water in the pharmacy. Topical preparations supplied by manufacturers should also be checked, unless the manu-facturer's system of preparation and testing is known to be satisfactory. In the wards, ointments or creams should be supplied for the individual patient and if jars are used the ointment should never be removed with the fingers.

Ophthalmic departments

Problems of infection

The eye is particularly susceptible to infection with Gram-negative bacilli, fungi, adenoviruses and *Herpes simplex* virus, organisms which are often or always resistant to antibiotics sometimes used for prophylaxis. Traumatic wounds and surgical operations increase or determine the risks of severe infection with these organisms.

Extra-ocular and orbital surgery

Control of infection in extra-ocular and orbital operations presents problems which are, in general, similar to those in any other branch of surgery. Many of these operations are performed for cosmetic reasons, so any unsightly scarring due to infection is a serious complication.

There are special considerations when implants are used in the orbit, either on the scleral surface to produce infolding in retinal detachment surgery, or when enucleation implants are used to impart movement to an artificial eye. Any

254

contamination during such operations carries a graver risk of inflammation and possible extrusion of the implant.

Intra-ocular surgery

The greatest dangers from contamination occur in intra-ocular operations, and also in patients who have corneal injuries or ulceration. The transparent ocular media have no direct blood circulation and are deficient in antibodies; they are, however, well oxygenated and provide good culture media for exogenous microorganisms (in particular, *Ps. aeruginosa*).

Control of infection

(1) Operating theatre techniques

(a) Sterility of the conjunctival sac: disinfection of conjunctiva. The conjunctival sac is more likely to be sterile than any other part of the body surface. In one Eye Hospital about 25% of patients coming to operation were shown to have no detectable organisms from conjunctival samplings: of the remainder about 55% had saprophytic or commensal bacteria, and about 20% had organisms classified as pathogens. It may be necessary to use pre-operative antibacterial medication in the form of eye-drops to remove potential pathogens, and such medication will certainly be required after operations. Sterility is especially important for intra-ocular operations. Because antiseptics which are tolerated by the skin cannot be applied to the conjunctiva, it is usual for antibiotic drops such as chloramphenicol 0.5% or neomycin 0.5% to be used for pre- and postoperative disinfection of the conjunctiva.

(b) Bacterial sampling of conjunctival sac. Admission of patients from a waiting list for operation is commonly conditional on the satisfactory results of the clinical examination of the conjunctiva. Before the operation, a conjunctival swab is taken, the result of which may be available before the operation and at least at the time of the first dressing; should infection be suspected at that time, the culture may provide confirmatory evidence and data for selection of an appropriate antibiotic. When conjunctival swabs are taken great care must be exerted to avoid contamination of the swab from the margin of the lid. The value of pre-operative conjunctival swabs is obviously limited because bacteria may appear in the conjunctiva between the time of sampling and operation. Critics of the system prefer to rely on disinfection by pre-operative antibiotic eye-drops; but such disinfection does not always eliminate the bacteria from the conjunctival sac, and the complications of an intra-ocular infection make it worthwhile to use the extra precaution of pre-operative sampling.

(c) Solutions, eye-drops and ointments. The greatest risks of intra-ocular infection are associated with the use of contaminated fluids; contamination may be due to inadequate sterilization or failure to sterilize (possibly associated with poor supervision and checking of the sterilizing procedure), and to recontamination of sterile fluids due to inadequate methods of supply, handling and multiple use of solutions from one container. The greatest possible care must be taken in the preparation of solutions for intra-ocular use; not only must microbial contaminants be excluded, but also chemical irritants which may cause irreparable damage. Pharmaceutical preservatives which are acceptable for other purposes may lead to loss of vision when used for preservation of ophthalmic solutions. The precautions to ensure sterility which apply to solutions and ointments are, of course, especially important for intra-ocular implants, such as intracameral lenses and keratoprostheses.

(d) **Corneal grafts.** In one centre the method is as follows. Prior to the removal of the donor eye, a conjunctival swab is taken. The eye is then enucleated with sterile instruments and put into a sterile container with normal saline and antibiotics such as neomycin and benzyl penicillin. On return to the centre, a second culture is taken and then the whole cornea, together with a few millimetres of surrounding sclera, are excised and placed in a medium containing gentamicin and proteins: the material is then stored at 4° C. The medium is derived from the McCarey Kaufman solution (McCarey and Kaufman, 1974) based on M199 and Rheomacrodex. This method allows the operation to be planned and carried out in about thirty-six hours, and the result of microbiological sampling to be known.

As an alternative method, the eye is left in the original saline/antibiotic solution until required, when the cornea is removed by trephine, at the time of the keratoplasty: this procedure is still in use in certain cases but allows less time in planning the operation as, especially for a penetrating graft, the material should be used within about twenty-four hours. In all cases the donor material must be removed as early as possible from the cadaver, preferably within two to three hours, the corneal endothelium being the most delicate structure to be preserved by these methods; the viability of this thin layer is crucial to the success of a penetrating keratoplasty. The partial thickness, or lamellar, graft is not so critical in this respect.

In both cases the final surgical step consists in fitting the corneal disc (removed by a trephine matching another used for removing the patient's diseased cornea), to the recipient site, and fixing it there by appropriate suturing.

(e) **Other transplants.** These are mostly autogenous and carried out at operation; they are therefore under direct surgical control. The tissues are taken from the skin around the eye, the back of the ear, or other sites, e.g. buccal mucosa (for conjunctival grafts), teeth (odontokeratoprostheses) and plantaris tendon.

(f) **Implants.** In general these are plastic devices, to be used intra or extraocularly. Examples of intra-ocular implants are intracameral lenses, fitted to replace a cataractous lens removed surgically (usually in one stage) and keratoprostheses. Extra-ocular implants, described as straps and sponges, composed of silicone materials, are frequently used in retinal detachment surgery. The 'sponges' may be porous, so that cells

256

and even blood vessels may grow into the spaces of the implant; sterilization is obviously of the utmost importance, and reliance is often placed on radiation, the material being packed in suitable containers for subsequent surgical use.

(2) Sterility of ophthalmic preparations

Recommendations on the preservation of sterility in fluids used for treatment of the eyes were published in the Hospital Memorandum HM(69)86 of the Department of Health and Social Security (1969). They have been considered unnecessarily stringent, and a revised set of recommendations is given in Health Service Circular HSC(75)122, March 1975, which supersedes HM(69)86; the following notes are based on the new Report. Various recommendations are also given from time to time in the British Pharmaceutical Codex.

(a) **General requirements.** All ophthalmic preparations should be supplied sterile. They should be provided in individual supplies for each patient. Where the dangers of infection are high, single-application packs which cannot be reclosed should be preferred, e.g. in accident and emergency departments and clinics for external eye disease. If single-application packs are not available, multiple-application packs may be used on a single-application basis (e.g. glass bottles with droppers incorporated in a screw cap, or glass screw-cap bottles to be used with a single-use glass pipette or plastic squeeze-containers with dropper caps). Ointments should be contained in single-application packs or small collapsible tubes which meet the accepted criteria of freedom from particles.

(b) **Closure of containers.** Cork stoppers or screw-cap liners made of cork or card must not be used on the closure of containers of eye-drops or eye lotions; the suitability of a cap liner must be established before it is used — closure should be covered with a seal that can be readily broken to show that the container has been opened.

(c) **Labelling.** The label should show the name and concentration of the active ingredients, the total volume contained, issue and expiry dates, batch number, also the name and concentration of antimicrobial preservative if present, and the words 'Sterile until opened'. The patient's name, whether left or right eye, and number of applications per day, should be written on the label or, if there is not enough room on this, on the outer container. A separate labelling procedure may be envisaged for in- and for out-patients.

(d) **Methods of use of eye drops**
    (i) In operating theatres: use single-application packs without preservatives. These should have sterile overwraps so that the outer surface of the container may remain sterile. In the event of single-application packs not being available, use previously unopened multiple-application packs (with dropper in screw cap or separate single-use pipette) *for single use only.*
    (ii) In the wards: a multiple-application bottle with dropper incorporated in the screw cap may be used but a Blind cap and separate

257

sterile dropper are generally preferred. Each patient should be given a previously unopened bottle (a separate bottle for each eye if both require treatment); the bottle should contain no more than 10 ml of liquid and be used for no longer than seven days. Eye-drops used before an operation should be discarded at the time of the operation, and be replaced by fresh supplies prescribed for use after the operation.

(iii) In out-patient departments: single-application packs are now available for almost all purposes, so that there should be no need for the use of multiple-application bottles, with a dropper; these are collected and discarded at the end of the clinic session.

(iv) In external eye disease clinics, accident and emergency departments: there is a special risk here of transferring epidemic kerato-conjunctivitis and other virus infections. Little is known about the rate of inactivation of the highly transmissible type 8 adenoviruses and conjunctival picornaviruses by antimicrobial preservatives. For this reason, and also because there is a risk of contaminating and transferring the infection from the outsides of multiple-application bottles and screw caps, it is desirable that single-application packs should be used in these clinics; the pack (whether of single- or multiple-application type) should be discarded after a single use. Sterile overwraps are not necessary, but hands should be thoroughly washed before and after examination of each patient.

(v) Fluorescein preparations: whenever these are used they should be provided in single-application packs; individually wrapped sterile impregnated strips are convenient.

(e) **Methods of use of eye lotions.** Use single-application containers, containing the volume required for a single treatment (e.g. 25 ml or 200 ml); discard the container after use. Label the container 'Sterile until opened; use immediately after opening, then discard.'

(f) **Methods of using eye ointments.** If a single-application pack is used, open with a sterile instrument if possible and apply ointment directly to the eye. If a multiple-application pack is provided, squeeze a small portion from the tube and discard; then apply the ointment to the eye with a sterile applicator (which should be provided in a peel-type pack, and used for one application only).

(g) **Education of staff and patients in the use of ophthalmic preparations.** Staff in ophthalmic departments must be instructed on the hazards and on the methods of preventing contamination by ophthalmic preparations (in particular the necessity of discarding single-application packs after a single use). Patients should also be given instructions on the safe use of eye-drops and other preparations: leaflets may be made available for the patients.

(3) Sterilization of instruments and appliances

While autoclaving provides satisfactory sterilization, some instruments (e.g. cataract knives) may suffer damage to their delicate cutting edge if sterilized in this way. Some authorities accept sterilization by dry heat at 160° C (320° F) for 1 h, or at lower temperatures for longer periods, as being satisfactory (see *Trans. ophthal. Soc.*, 1973). As this method is much slower than autoclaving, a stock of sterile instruments must be held to replace an instrument at short notice, as when an instrument is dropped or otherwise contaminated. Gamma-sterilized disposable knives, and autoclaved diamond knives are solving some of these problems. Ethylene oxide has a particular application in the sterilization of cryothermy leads, a complex apparatus containing a gas duct and electrical leads inside a PVC envelope; the epoxy resin used to assemble the leads has not been found to react with ethylene dioxide. As the gas must be allowed to escape for at least 24 hours from the sterilized pack before use of the equipment on patients, this method requires multiplication of essential apparatus to cover the 'turnover' of sterilization, especially where transport to another centre adds further delays. Vitrectomy and other aspiration/infusion apparatus also require careful sterilization, as the vitreous provides an ideal nidus for colonization by micro-organisms.

The adjustment of the operating microscope and other equipment by the surgeon requires special precautions; the provision of dry sterile guards is usually considered satisfactory; most microscopes can now be adjusted by the foot or by other methods not requiring direct handling by the surgeon. The equipment must be kept meticulously clean, as cleaning during the operation is out of the question.

(4) Surgical technique

During operations instruments are held in such a way that the part which comes in contact with the eye is not touched either primarily or secondarily with the fingers that control them. This is a standard part of the discipline of the surgical team.

Instruments are more effectively controlled when regularly used with an operating microscope, which is also an effective mechanism for excluding foreign material from the operating area. Some surgeons prefer to use the ungloved hand, because of the finer control which they believe they can attain in this way. If it can be assumed that the hands are dry and never touch the operation area or the operating ends of instruments, this may involve little risk; regular and repeated use of an effective detergent antiseptic, such as the 4% chlorhexidine detergent preparation ('Hibiscrub'), is a particularly important precaution if gloves are not worn. Risk of infection from the ungloved hand may occur through accidental contact or from dry epidermal scales which are likely to drop from the hands during the course of a long operation. Most surgeons now prefer to accept the slight disadvantage of wearing gloves, when weighed against the disastrous results of a postoperative infection. If the edges of the wound are carefully apposed, the wound is secure and there should be little risk of intra-ocular contamination from the exterior from about 48 hours after the operation. During the 48 hours before and the 48 hours after the operation it is essential that all eye drops or other topical medication should be provided in single-dose containers, with contents sterilized in the container.

(5) Wards

Dressing packs from the CSSD are used; also individual droppers, which are provided by the CSSD, and eye-drops sterilized in their final containers, individual to the patient and renewed each day. Eye-drops may be preserved with benzalkonium chloride (0.01% w/v) or, for short-term use by patients, phenylmercuric nitrate or acetate (0.002% w/v); also chlorhexidine (0.01% w/v).

(6) Out-patient and casualty departments

Fluorescein drops have been found on many occasions to be contaminated. The use of single-dose applicators is a method of eliminating this hazard. Epidemics of keratoconjunctivitis associated with the use of tonometers have been reported. Schiøtz tonometry, which almost inevitably causes some damage to the cornea, carries a special hazard. The prism used in applanation tonometry must be cleaned before and after use with an antiseptic such as phenylmercuric acetate (0.002% w/v). A dry, clean prism is probably safe, but if a virus or other transmissible infection is suspected, the prism should be sent for ethylene oxide sterilization before being returned to general use.

(7) Contact lenses

Hard lenses are difficult to contaminate, and simple personal hygiene is sufficient when they are used. With soft lenses there is a greater risk of contamination with infective and chemical agents, which may seriously damage the cornea. Low water content soft lenses can be satisfactorily disinfected by heating to 80° C (176° F) for 20 min daily. The saline solution used for storage should also be changed daily. High water content lenses may deteriorate on heating and require chemical disinfection.

Surveillance

The infection control team must keep a close watch on the incidence of infection in ophthalmic wards. Any outbreak must be reported immediately to the Control of Infection Committee, and an appropriate investigation for the causal microorganism and its source should be made (see Chapter 2).

Ear, nose and throat departments

Patients in ENT departments may be divided into two groups with different problems with regard to hospital-acquired infection. Short-stay patients who are admitted for operations such as tonsillectomy are vulnerable in the postoperative period to endemic hospital organisms, such as staphylococci, but also to β-haemolytic streptococci and other community-type organisms which are brought into hospital by patients. Viruses such as measles and poliomyelitis which are spread by droplet infection are also especially hazardous in the operative period.

Long-stay patients usually are suffering from more severe illness, such as carcinoma of the larynx where the tissues are more susceptible to infection and where, in addition, operative procedures such as tracheostomy provide an

260

alternative route for colonization and ultimately infection by hospital strains of *Pseudomonas aeruginosa*. The mode of spread in these cases is usually by contact; medical apparatus, such as suction tubing or ventilators, may also be important.

Apart from these, many patients with community-acquired infections may be admitted to the wards adding to the hazards. These include patients with tonsilitis, quinsy or acute otitis media (due to streptococci, pneumococci, haemophilus or staphylococci) and patients with chronic external otitis (often heavily colonized with Gram-negative bacilli, staphylococci, yeasts or fungi).

Prevention of infection

Isolation facilities are essential in ENT departments both to isolate infected cases coming into hospital and to protect those particularly susceptible to infection. Long-stay patients with tracheostomy should ideally be nursed in separate rooms. Patients with streptococcal infections, if admitted at all, must be in a room separate from patients requiring operations. Children admitted for tonsillectomy and found to be pyrexial are best isolated, or, as is common practice, sent home. Patients with chronic ear disease do not generally merit isolation, although the organisms present are often highly resistant to antibiotics and care should be taken to prevent contact spread, particularly by fomites; most of these patients are, however, treated as out-patients. Children and adults should preferably be in separate wards.

Operations on the ear, throat and sinuses require incision through colonized mucous membranes and surface disinfection provides considerable difficulties. Some agents damage the membranes or may lead to fistula formation if they gain access to the middle ear. Patients requiring operation on the middle ear may require intensive out-patient treatment of infection, if present. At the time of operation many surgeons use 1% aqueous cetrimide as a membrane disinfectant, but this agent has poor activity against *Ps. aeruginosa*, and an alternative (e.g. an aqueous solution of iodine (or iodophor)) should be considered. Care of tracheostomy is dealt with under the section on Intensive care units (see above). The hospital hygiene problems associated with ENT wards do not differ from those in other wards. CSSDs should be able to supply sterile apparatus for examination of patients and for minor procedures. Nasal and aural specula should be used only on one patient before being treated in CSSD. Many units without immediate access to CSSD may need to decontaminate these small items in the clinic or ward. This may be done by boiling in water for 5 min or by 5 min immersion in 0.5% alcoholic chlorhexidine solution. In each case the specula should be allowed to dry and stored covered in the dry state. Tracheostomy tubes, suction catheters and similar apparatus must be supplied sterile either from CSSD or in commercial presterilized packs. Most laryngoscopes are capable of withstanding autoclave temperatures and should be so treated. Fibre-optic bronchoscopes are usually disinfected with glutaraldehyde (see Chapter 7). The light carrier components must be removed and may be sterilized. A less satisfactory alternative is immersion for 3 h in 2% glutaraldehyde (see page 86). Operating microscopes present some difficulties; wiping with 70% ethyl alcohol is probably the most effective method of disinfection.

Particular risks to and from personnel in the department are similar to those in other wards, but emphasis should be placed on two infections: (1) streptococcal disease is especially hazardous in ENT departments, so staff with sore throats should be excluded; (2) tuberculous laryngitis can lead to dissemination of many tubercle bacilli into the air, so that a tuberculin test and chest X-ray are mandatory for nurses and doctors working in the unit; tuberculin negative staff must not be employed (see Chapter 13).

Problems in the Community

Although this book is mainly concerned with infection in hospital, improved collaboration between medical and nursing staff working in hospital and the home is necessary. Patients are often discharged earlier than in former times and a continuity of care at a high standard is important. This applies particularly to hygienic and aseptic techniques.

Hospital nursing procedures are based on the known availability of equipment, linen, sterile supplies, lotions and antibiotics (all at no direct cost to the patient), which are delivered to the ward or unit. The environment is controlled by the hospital authorities. The community nurse has such supplies and equipment as can be carried in the nursing bag or in her car, or which the patient can buy or loan. As a guest in the home, she has limited control over the environment, and laundry and refuse must be dealt with in the home by the patient or his relatives.

Changing patterns of hospital care have influenced domiciliary practice; e.g. early discharge of postoperative patients (possibly with infected wounds or urines, or developing an infection shortly after leaving hospital); early discharge of mothers who are sometimes carriers of HB_sAg or *Salmonella typhi*, or babies carrying hospital-acquired organisms; use of disposable sharps and single-use packs (often bought on prescription, not supplied by an HSDU); disposal of used dressings from discharging wounds in the absence of coal-burning fires; disposal of colostomy bags and their contents. Although laundry and refuse collection services are available, there may be long waiting lists for them. Equipment supplied on loan may be difficult to disinfect adequately, e.g. commodes with fabric-covered seats. In addition, family practitioners will have their own views on methods of treatment, both in the home and in health centres or group practices. Both community nurses and family practitioners are often more aware than their colleagues in hospital of the cost to the patient of procedures or treatments which they may recommend.

However, the patient at home has certain advantages over the patient in hospital. He is isolated and 'barrier-nursed' in his own home; care is given by a limited number of trained nurses who tend to use the same methods.

The structure of the community nursing service is such that it is difficult to lay down procedures which can be universally applied. It is, therefore, important for community nurses to be able to apply principles of hygiene and asepsis wherever the patient may be, even in an isolated farm supplied with well water, or an inner city slum with no water at all.

The use of equipment which cannot be readily dried should be avoided, e.g.

cotton hand towels, dish cloths for wiping surfaces, or soap dishes. Paper towels should be used to dry hands, and to clean and dry work surfaces. Soap should be stored dry. Failing this, washing-up liquid containing a preservative can be used. In either case, running water must be used, not static water in a washing bowl. Provided the hands are physically clean, an alcoholic hand disinfectant (see Chapter 7) containing an emollient rubbed on to the skin until it is dry is effective and should be particularly useful in domiciliary practice. The addition of an emollient is necessary to prevent chapped hands in winter.

Sterile packs should ideally be supplied by an HSDU, although this is not always possible. HSDU managers may be able to supply special packs to meet specific nursing requirements.

Disposable gloves are convenient for carrying out dressing techniques; plastic bags, subsequently inverted and sealed, are useful for removing dressings. Dressing packs containing these items are available (see Chapter 5).

Many Areas do not supply disposable insulin syringes and needles. Glass and metal syringes are stored in surgical or methylated spirit and may be rinsed with boiled water before use. There is some indication that organisms may survive in the lumen of the needle after this treatment. Disposable needles are therefore preferable. However, disposal of sharps may be a difficulty. Small plastic bottles may be recycled and used for the disposal of needles and stitch-cutters. These should be returned to a central point for collection and disposal by the hospital authorities.

Disinfectants are seldom required for inanimate surfaces in the home. Washing with soap and water and thorough drying will usually be adequate, even when a sterile pack is to be opened on the surface. Freshly drawn tap water, i.e. collected in a clean, dry container after allowing the water to run for 30 s, may be used for wound cleaning, catheter toilet, inflating catheter balloons and rinsing insulin syringes. Sachets containing antiseptics (e.g. 'Savlodil') for cleaning dirty wounds are convenient.

Notes on the use of disinfectants are given in Chapter 7. Metal instruments, generally scissors or forceps, may need to be disinfected in the home. Although boiling is effective in killing *Staph. aureus* and other non-sporing bacteria, instruments should preferably be supplied in sterilized packs. Scissors not used for aseptic procedures should be washed, dried and then wiped with an alcohol-impregnated swab. A disposable plastic cover may be used for thermometers or, alternatively, the thermometer can be disinfected by wiping with an alcohol-impregnated swab.

A disposable plastic apron should be worn to protect the nurse's uniform. The apron should be longer than those normally used in hospitals, because working heights tend to be lower in the home, e.g. divan beds, arm chairs. Often the nurse can work comfortably only when kneeling on the floor; it is then the area immediately above knee height which is likely to be contaminated rather than the waist area. The apron should either be discarded immediately, or left in the home, with the outer surface marked so that any organisms surviving on the apron will not be transferred to the uniform of the next nurse to use it.

The early discharge of mothers who are carriers of *Salmonella typhi* or HB_sAg presents particular problems for community midwives. Salmonella carriers should be careful with their personal hygiene, especially with hand-washing before food preparation and after using the toilet. Simple isolation methods, e.g. hand-washing and wearing of aprons, are described in Chapter 9, and are equally applicable in the home.

If an outbreak of gastro-enteritis occurs, hand-washing under running water is again the most important measure. Toilet seats, chamber pots etc., may be washed with a reliable disinfectant, but disinfectants are unnecessary as a routine in the home. Many disinfectants sold to the public are mainly of use as a deodorant, and should not be required if cleaning is satisfactory. Linen from patients with hepatitis or intestinal infection should be laundered in the home at the highest temperature the material will withstand. Cotton or cotton/polyester fabrics should be ironed when dry, using the heat of the iron to destroy any surviving pathogens. Nylon fabrics should be thoroughly dried, preferably out of doors and stored dry for 48 hours before re-use.

Outbreaks of boils or other superficial sepsis in a family may be caused by strains of *Staph. aureus* brought home from a hospital. Patients should be treated with antiseptic nose creams and baths (see Chapter 7). It may be necessary to sample and treat all members of the family (Leigh, 1979). Bed linen and underclothes should be laundered at as high a temperature as possible soon after treatment has commenced (see above), and this should be repeated after completion of treatment.

Antibiotic policies are not commonly used in domiciliary practice, but care is particularly required in the use of topical agents, e.g. gentamicin or fusidic acid, which should not be used except in very special circumstances in hospital. Varicose ulcers and pressure sores are particularly likely to be colonized with antibiotic-resistant *Staph. aureus* and Gram-negative bacilli. If it is thought necessary to use a topical antibiotic, the length of treatment should be no more than seven to ten days.

Care is necessary in collection of specimens (see Chapter 8) and transport to the laboratory should be as rapid as possible. Urines kept at room temperature for more than three hours may be useless due to growth of contaminants; haemolytic streptococci may die on dry swabs, and sputa are also rapidly overgrown with contaminating Gram-negative bacilli or yeasts.

Further guidance on aseptic and hygienic methods can be obtained from the Infection Control Nurse or Infection Control Officer at the nearest district general hospital.

Disinfection of loaned equipment

A variety of equipment is available on loan, including hospital beds. Contamination during the period of loan appears to present few practical difficulties. Generally a deodorant/disinfectant is used, since unpleasant smells are the worst problem.

Decontamination should be done in the home before returning equipment to the central stores. Careful washing, using a detergent such as washing-up liquid, followed by thorough drying is usually adequate, even when the patient was infected. If water cannot be used, alcohol or methylated spirit is effective.

Fabric-covered commodes are widely used and are difficult to disinfect adequately. If the fabric is soiled though not contaminated with known pathogens, a carpet cleaning solution, used in accordance with the manufacturer's instructions, may be effective in improving the appearance of the fabric. If it is contaminated, then it should be replaced by the central stores.

Some warning of specific infection risks, e.g. enteric infections, should be given so that equipment can be collected and decontaminated by the hospital. Whenever possible, equipment supplied for home use should be as easy to decontaminate as that used in the hospital.

An area within the central stores of the hospital should be set aside for decontamination of loaned equipment. Adequate sinks and drainage should be available. A member of staff should be properly trained in equipment decontamination techniques.

References and Further Reading

Ayliffe, G. A. J., Collins, B. J. and Davies, J. (1976), Contamination of infant feeds in hospitals. *Midwife, Hlth Visitor and Commun. Nurse*, 12, 18.

Carroll, L., Osman, M., Davies, D.P. and McNeish, A. S. (1976), Bacteriological criteria for feeding raw breast milk to babies on neonatal units. *Lancet*, ii, 732.

Department of Health and Social Security (1969), *Preservation of Sterility in Ophthalmic Preparations in Hospitals*, Hospital Memorandum HM(69)86.

Department of Health and Social Security (1975), *Preservation of Sterility in Ophthalmic Preparations in Hospitals*, Health Service Circular HSC(75)122.

Feldman, S. A. and Crawley, B. E. (ed.) (1977), *Tracheostomy and Artificial Ventilation in the Treatment of Respiratory Failure*, 3rd edn, Edward Arnold, London.

Gaya, H. (1976), Infection control in intensive care, *Br. J. Anaesth.* 48, 9.

Leigh, D.A. (1979), Treatment of familial staphylococcal infection. *J. antimicrob. Chemother.*, 5, 497.

McCarey, B.E. and Kaufman, H. E. (1974), Improved corneal storage. *Invest. Ophthalm.*, 13, 164.

Transactions of the Ophthalmic Society of the United Kingdom (1973), The sterilization of surgical instruments, 92, 539.

CHAPTER SIXTEEN

Special Wards and Departments (2)

Neurosurgery departments

The meninges are particularly susceptible to infection, and clinical infection may be caused through contamination occurring at operation or during a lumbar or ventricular puncture by Gram-negative bacilli of low pathogenicity, as well as by the usual organisms causing wound infection. Infections caused by these opportunistic organisms, e.g. *Ps. aeruginosa*, *Serratia marcescens* and flavobacteria, have occurred because of inadequate sterilization or maintenance of sterility of instruments or water applied topically. Organisms normally present on the skin (e.g. coagulase negative staphylococci) which are usually of low pathogenicity may also cause low grade infections, particularly in association with Spitz–Holter valves. Infections may be transmitted on the hands of staff from infected patients or following the use of contaminated nail-brushes, hand-creams, soaps or detergents. Inadequate disinfection of the patient's skin pre-operatively, or use of contaminated shaving equipment, may also be followed by infection. As regards other types of infection, neurosurgical units have the same problems as other departments, and some neurosurgical patients are in hospital for long periods. They may have indwelling catheters; tracheostomy or endotracheal intubation is sometimes necessary, and patients with ear infection may be admitted to the unit. Unconscious patients are apt to acquire chest infections or bedsores. Although cerebral abscesses are usually endogenous in origin, hospital strains of Gram-negative bacilli and *Staph. aureus* are likely to spread in the ward and be acquired in the nasal and intestinal flora to become a potential source of endogenous infection unless effective control measures are employed.

Prevention of infection

Isolation and barrier-nursing of infected patients, particularly of patients with pseudomonas infection, are important in neurosurgical units. Dressings of wounds exposing the meninges should, if possible, be changed in the operating theatre or, if not, in a plenum-ventilated dressing room; the patient's own single-bedded room, if the facilities are adequate, may be suitable for many of the routine procedures. Special wards are required for intensive care treatment, including patients with tracheostomies (see section on Intensive care units, Chapter 15). Other procedures, e.g. lumbar puncture and catheterization, may be carried out in non-specialized wards; the relevant precautions are described elsewhere (see below under Urology units and Chapter 8). Pre-operative shaving should be carried out on the day of operation, to avoid the possibility that small scratches or excoriations which sometimes occur might become heavily colonized. Shaving either of head hair or of pubic hair for vertebral angiography should be completed before disinfection of scalp or skin. Shaving brushes should not be used; razors should be sterilized or adequately disinfected and individual sterilized gauze swabs should be used for applying shaving cream. If shaving cream is used, it should contain an antiseptic which prevents the growth of organisms that might cause infection. A povidone-iodine shampoo or chlorhexidine detergent may also be used before shaving. Subsequent skin preparation in the operating theatre is carried out with 0.5% alcoholic chlorhexidine. Equipment for aseptic procedures should be autoclaved, and CSSD packs supplied whenever possible, e.g. for lumbar puncture, catheterization, wound-dressing and tracheostomy toilet. Particular care is required to avoid contamination of lotions. If aspiration of an effusion of a craniotomy wound is required, insert the needle through intact skin and not through the suture line. Organisms may enter the bloodstream from monitoring equipment and set up an infection at the operation site. This equipment should be regularly disinfected or sterilized, preferably by heat.

Urological units

Urinary tract infection is the commonest type of acquired infection in hospitals. Many patients already have urinary infection when they enter the unit, but instrumentation and operations on the urinary tract can lead to infection either by introducing organisms into a previously uninfected tract or by replacing the existing organisms with hospital strains which are more resistant to antibiotic therapy.

Although some patients acquire urinary tract infections without having had instrumentation, most infections follow catheterization, cystoscopy, drainage or more extensive operative procedures. In particular, the indwelling catheter can be hazardous, and if precautions are not taken to prevent contamination, the incidence of bladder infections in patients on continuous drainage approaches 100% after a few days.

Routes of contamination

The entry of bacteria into the bladder may occur either through the lumen of the catheter or between the catheter and the wall of the urethra. Both routes are important and effort is needed to close both.

The organisms most likely to be found in urological patients with urinary tract infection vary. If there has not been any manipulation of the urinary tract the organisms are usually *E. coli* or *Proteus mirabilis* sensitive to many common antibiotics, such as sulphonamides, ampicillin and nitrofurantoin. In hospital-acquired infections *Klebsiella* spp., indole-positive *Proteus* spp., *Ps. aeruginosa* and *Strep. faecalis* are commoner. Less frequent are *Acinetobacter* spp. and *Providencia* spp. These organisms are usually resistant to many antibiotics and may prove difficult to eradicate. In order to prevent ascending infection of the urinary tract the following points must be considered: (1) management of patients; (2) selection of apparatus and materials; (3) sterilization and disinfection of materials.

Management of patients

Patients who require long-term bladder drainage are usually managed by continuous rather than intermittent catheterization. By a carefully painstaking technique patients can be kept free from infection for many weeks using intermittent catheterization, but the method is time-consuming, more painful for the patient and not widely used outside special centres. Surgical patients after operations on the urinary tract are usually managed with continuous drainage.

Catheterization should be performed with no-touch technique with adequate disinfection of the urethra using a local anaesthetic combined with an antiseptic. Packs for this purpose should be available from the CSSD; 50 ml of 1/5000 aqueous chlorhexidine ('Hibitane') can be instilled into the bladder, before the catheter is withdrawn. Some surgeons use 1% Noxythiolin solution for this purpose, but this substance releases formaldehyde on hydrolysis and may prove irritating to the bladder mucosa.

Selection of apparatus and materials

It has been demonstrated that with closed drainage infection could be prevented from reaching the bladder for several days (Gillespie *et al.*, 1964 and 1966; Kunin, 1974). A continuous unbroken connection is required extending from the urethral catheter to the receptacle. If a glass bottle is used a disinfectant such as 1% formaldehyde is placed in the bottom. When the bottle is replaced, the drainage line is clamped externally — not closed with a spigot — and the stopper transferred to a clean bottle already to hand. Such simple precautions prevent the spread of infection through the lumen of the catheter.

Bottles have to a large extent been replaced by plastic bags of which there are two main types: those with a mechanism for removing urine by means of a tap and those without a tap. Bags with a tap are now most frequently used, but great care is necessary in handling and emptying. Most of the so-called 'non-return' valves allow bacteria to ascend from the bag into the tubing above, particularly if the bag is tipped upside down or sat on by the patient. The bag should be kept below bladder level. When emptying the bag, the nurse's hands are often heavily contaminated with Gram-negative bacilli (e.g. over 10^6 organisms) which are not easily removed by routine hand-washing. Wearing of disposable gloves is recommended, one pair for each patient, and the use of alcohol for hand disinfection after emptying each bag. The bag should be emptied into a separate disinfected or sterilized container for each patient. Some Gram-negative bacilli, such as *Klebsiella*, may survive better than others in a dry environment and on hands (Casewell and Phillips, 1977). Bags should not be allowed to stand or drag along the floor. Similar care is necessary for changing bags without a tap; an external clamp should be used and not a spigot. Specimens for culture should be removed with a sterile syringe and needle after cleaning the special sleeve with 70% alcohol.

Contamination by bacteria ascending to the bladder between the catheter and the urethra can be reduced by instillation of chlorhexidine (with local anaesthetic) into the urethra before catheterization. However, even when full precautions are taken with an indwelling catheter, infection is likely after about a week.

268

Long-term catheter care is a major problem. Anchoring the catheter with a sponge soaked in 1/5000 chlorhexidine has been successful in females, but is not entirely satisfactory. Daily or twice daily cleaning of the catheter-meatal junction is often recommended, with the possible application of chlorhexidine or povidone-iodine cream. There is, however, some evidence that repeated cleaning of the catheter-meatal junction during the day may be associated with a higher risk of infection. There is also some evidence to suggest that silastic catheters are associated with less infection than others and preferable for long-term catheterization, but this is uncertain.

Although some patients with in-dwelling catheters remain free from bacteriuria for long periods, an optimal catheter-care routine has not been defined. Catheters should be removed as soon as possible.

Sterilization and disinfection

For sterilization and disinfection of cystoscopes, see Chapter 10.

Catheters for insertion into the ureter should be disposable or sterilized by autoclaving.

Most apparatus associated with bladder drainage is now disposable and is discarded after use. All non-disposable items, e.g. bladder syringes, require autoclaving.

Other problems

Urine from patients with renal tuberculosis contains tubercle bacilli and should be disposed of with care. The bottle used for collecting the urine must be disinfected (see Chapter 7). The patient should have his own urine bottle.

Apart from the hazard of infection from tuberculous patients, the risk of ward staff acquiring infection from urological patients is negligible.

Collection of specimens for laboratory examination should be made directly into a sterile universal container. The use of the urine bottle as an intermediary container has often given false results, because of failure to decontaminate the bottle between patients.

Outbreaks of infection

Widespread cross-infection with antibiotic-resistant *Klebsiella aerogenes* has been reported in many hospitals. The emergence of gentamicin-resistant strains is particularly worrying as they may spread to other patients and limit the available treatment in a unit. These organisms are commonly associated with indwelling catheters and their mode of spread is thought to be mainly on the hands of staff (Casewell and Phillips, 1977). Nevertheless, some attention should be given to the environment, e.g. disinfection of bedpans and urinals by heat (not a tank of disinfectant), correct drying and stacking of wash-bowls, disinfection (by heat) of containers used for emptying urine-bags, and urine-testing equipment, and adequate disinfection of baths, etc. Although microbiological monitoring of the environment is not routinely recommended, a survey in an epidemic situation will

269

serve a useful educational function and may bring to light defects in cleaning
and disinfection schedules. Single-room isolation is not usually recommended
for Gram-negative infections, but this may be advisable to eradicate a gentamicin-
resistant strain from a hospital. Restriction of certain antibiotics may also be
desirable.

Wards of psychiatric, geriatric and subnormal patients

Many of these patients are incapable of understanding the principles of personal
hygiene or of carrying out normal hygienic procedures; some may be incontinent
of faeces or urine or both. Gastro-intestinal and skin infections or infestations
and hepatitis are likely to spread rapidly in these units.

Methods of control are similar in principle to those used in other wards of the
hospital, but there are special problems. Surveillance and immediate action is
particularly important. New patients should be admitted to a special ward and
screened for skin infection and infestation; faeces should be examined if there is
any history of diarrhoea. Patients with diarrhoea should be isolated, and if more
than one case occurs in a ward, the faeces of other patients and staff should be
examined. New patients should not be admitted until the ward is clear of infection. Skin infections and infestation should be promptly treated; all patients
(and staff when on duty) should use antiseptic soaps and other appropriate
treatment (see Chapter 7) if there is evidence of an outbreak of skin sepsis. Staff
should maintain as high a standard of hygiene as possible, e.g. washing hands
(patients' and their own) before eating, prompt cleaning up of excreta and regular cleaning of toilets and baths. 'Communal' towels and flannels should be
avoided. Floor, walls and furniture should be washable. It is desirable that
patients should wear clothes that can be disinfected; where psychiatric considerations require that a patient should wear his own clothes, it must be recognized
that some risk of infection exists.

Out-patients and casualty departments

Since many of the patients who attend out-patient departments have recently
been in hospital wards, their wounds and other lesions are likely to be infected
with antibiotic-resistant Gram-negative bacilli and *Staph. aureus* which they
acquired in hospital. Patients with skin diseases may have been treated with a
variety of antibiotics and are also likely to be carrying antibiotic-resistant
strains. Most patients with infections are either carrying or infected with
antibiotic-sensitive strains, which are usually less transmissible than hospital
organisms; the risk of cross-infection with Gram-negative bacilli and *Staph. aureus*
in out-patient or casualty departments is less than in wards, but owing to the
large number of patients attending out-patient departments, the risk of spread of
community-acquired infections, e.g. measles, influenza etc., is high. The conse-
quences may be severe if a case of undiagnosed Lassa fever is brought into the
department.

Many patients are also particularly susceptible to infection, e.g. those with
immunodeficiency diseases, and they may come into close contact with infected
patients. The range of surgical procedures carried out in out-patient theatres is

270

increasing, and clean operations may alternate with incisions of abscesses. Diagnostic procedures, such as endoscopy, are also now more frequently done in outpatient departments. Endoscopy instruments are often difficult to disinfect or sterilize (see Chapter 7).

Prevention of infection

Surgical procedures should, when possible, be carried out in a mechanically-ventilated operating theatre; aseptic and cleaning techniques should correspond to those used in the main operating theatres (see Chapter 10). These recommendations are particularly applicable to the types of operation which previously required admission to hospital for several days, though the wearing of masks and caps is not essential for incision of abscesses. The risk of airborne spread of infection after drainage of abscesses to patients subsequently undergoing operation in the same operating room is not great, especially if the theatre is mechanically ventilated, but precautions against contact spread, e.g. adequate cleaning of operating tables, are necessary. The general principles of prevention of infection are similar to those which apply in other areas in the hospital and a few reliable techniques will reduce the risk to a minimum. Facilities for minor surgery and for dressing wounds should be adequate, with rooms for laying-up of trolleys and disposal of contaminated dressings and linen.

Sufficient hand-washing basins and disposable paper towels should be provided for the staff. Hand-washing by the staff between handling patients and before and after procedures is one of the most important measures. Wearing of a gown or plastic apron when handling infected patients and covering of couches with paper or a cleanable plastic material when examining potentially infected patients are also useful measures. Linen should be changed after use on an infected patient, and at least daily. Gowns for patients to wear during examination should preferably be disposable, but owing to expense and since the risk of transfer of infection is usually not great, it may be necessary to use gowns for a whole morning or afternoon session. A separate gown should be provided for patients with infections or with a skin disease in which heavy skin colonization by potential pathogens is likely. Some segregation of patients is also advisable; in particular, hypersusceptible patients should not be mixed with those who are likely to be infected, e.g. chronic bronchitics with leukaemics, or dermatological with surgical cases. A separate clinic for patients with varicose ulcers may also be advisable.

Facilities should be provided for examination of patients with communicable disease. A room, which can be fumigated, is required for isolation of cases of suspected viral haemorrhagic fevers or other dangerous infections; and a routine for management of these cases must be available (see Chapter 17). Plentiful supplies of specula and other instruments, either disposable or provided by the CSSD, should be available in the departments. If not available, such equipment should be sterilized in a small autoclave. Disinfection by chemicals or by boiling should be avoided, if possible; although disinfection by immersion of a clean instrument in 70% alcohol, with or without 0.5% chlorhexidine, or by boiling water for five minutes, is effective (against vegetative organisms), it should rarely be necessary to do without proper sterilization. Instruments and needles should be stored in a dry state and not in chemical disinfectants. They should be disinfected by heat immediately before use, or, if possible, sterilized in the CSSD and supplied in packs. A routine for disinfection of endoscopes and other instruments which are heat-labile and of emergency equipment should be known and always followed in the department (see Chapter 7).

Radiology and radiotherapy departments

Radiography

Patients are brought to this department from all parts of the hospital and from the community. Patients coming from different wards may be responsible for spread of infection between wards. The radiographers also visit patients in the wards and may transmit infection on their hands or clothing or on equipment. The principles of control are similar to those which apply in other areas of the hospital. The staff should be informed of any patient with communicable disease sent to their department, or if an X-ray is required on such a patient in the ward. In the ward, the radiographers should follow the recommended barrier-nursing routine, paying particular attention to hand-washing and gowning techniques. Similar procedures may be necessary if the patient is brought to their department, and it may be necessary to cover the X-ray table with disposable paper, or to disinfect it after use. X-ray equipment is not an important source of infection, and routine cleaning with a detergent and allowing it to dry will usually be sufficient. Cleaning the equipment between patients is not necessary, except when a patient is known to be infected. Disinfection by wiping over with 70% alcohol is quick and fairly effective and it may be necessary after X-raying an infected patient, or on taking the equipment into the operating theatre; wiping with other disinfectant solutions is rarely necessary. For cleaning of the environment, see Chapter 7.

Many procedures involving aseptic techniques are now carried out in the X-ray department, and facilities should be adequate, including a hand-washing basin. The room used should be well ventilated and unnecessary equipment excluded; it should, if possible, be reserved for procedures involving aseptic techniques. As few people as possible should be in the room during the procedure, particularly if a catheter remains *in situ*. Good surgical techniques are as necessary for these procedures as they are in operating theatres. Instruments and dressings should be supplied by the CSSD. The use of patients' gowns is described in the section on Out-patient departments.

Radiotherapy

Patients treated in this department may be particularly susceptible to infection, e.g. immunosuppressed patients, or those with low natural immunity; if in wards, these patients should be nursed in single-bed cubicles with full protective isolation precautions (see Chapter 9). Special skills are often necessary in nursing these patients, and suitably trained staff should be available. Other patients, e.g.

272

those with fungating carcinoma or with thrush, may be sources of infection. Isolation of these patients and techniques to prevent contact infection, such as hand-washing and wearing of plastic gowns, are necessary. The protection of examination couches and provision of patients' gowns are discussed above (see section on Out-patients and casualty). Equipment used is often difficult to sterilize or disinfect. Whenever possible it should be autoclaved and supplied in packs by the CSSD. If the equipment is heat-labile, ethylene oxide or low-temperature steam formaldehyde is preferred to chemical solutions. Immersion in glutaraldehyde for 3 h should kill spores if the item is initially clean. The methods described below are in use and probably satisfactory, but every effort should be made to replace them with physical methods of sterilization or disinfection.

If surface disinfection of equipment is required, wiping with 70% alcohol is rapid in action and preferable to aqueous disinfectants. If an item is likely to contact the conjunctiva, mucous membranes or skin, immersion in 0.5% aqueous chlorhexidine for 15 min should adequately disinfect; it should be rinsed off in sterile water before the item is used. Gold grains and gold guns are supplied ready packed and sterilized, and the gun may be wiped with 70% alcohol between cases. Needles, ovoids and stocks are cleaned ultrasonically and immersed in 0.5% chlorhexidine solution. Other radioactive sources, radium moulds, oral moulds and strontium plaques may also be disinfected in 0.5% chlorhexidine and should be rinsed in sterile saline before use. Lead eye shields (contact lenses) and mouth inserts may be similarly treated. Lead screening materials, plastic shells and after-loading devices may be wiped with 70% alcohol, or, if this is not suitable, with aqueous chlorhexidine.

It is essential that the X-ray staff are trained in aseptic techniques and control of infection, and that the system for warning the radiological department of infection hazards is effective.

Physiotherapy departments

Physiotherapists treat many ill or infected patients and move from one patient to another and from ward to ward. Infected wounds are exposed during certain treatments. Patients are handled and the opportunities for contact transfer of infection are high. Patients attend the physiotherapy department from all parts of the hospital and from outside. Infection from patients with wounds or skin lesions may readily be transferred on couches, equipment, other fomites and on the hands of the staff. Treatment with wax or water baths and in hydrotherapy units may aid the spread of infection. Fungal infection of the feet may be spread in the gymnasium, particularly if patients exercise with bare feet or wear communal shoes.

Prevention of infection

The physiotherapy department should be informed of patients known to have a communicable disease or hospital infection which could spread to other patients. Meticulous care in hand-washing before and after handling any patient, and wearing a plastic apron when treating an infected patient, are important. This applies both to wards and to the physiotherapy department. Infected wounds should be effectively sealed whenever possible during treatment and contaminated dressings should only be handled with forceps or plastic gloves. The department should have adequate facilities for dressing wounds and lesions, a complete CSSD supply and an effective disposal system for contaminated linen and dressings. Recommended aseptic dressing techniques should be used. Other facilities are described in the sections on wards and out-patients, but, in particular, treatment couches should be covered with paper or cleaned after each infected patient. Bedding should be changed after use by an infected patient and at least daily.

The skin of the hands of patients undergoing paraffin wax treatment should be inspected, and any patients with an infected lesion should not be treated until healed; if this is not possible they should wear polythene gloves. Patients should wash their hands before and after treatment and used wax should be heated to disinfect before being returned to the wax bath.

The hydrotherapy unit

(1) (a) All persons entering pool area should wear plastic overshoes on top of their outdoor shoes (e.g. workmen, porters, etc.);
   (b) staff and patients should wear special sandals kept only for hydrotherapy.
(2) Patients' feet and skin should be inspected for infected lesions.
(3) Patients should take showers before entering the water and after leaving it.
(4) Everyone entering the water must step through a foot-bath containing hypochlorite or an iodophor solution. Use of a mycostatic powder after bathing might have some value.
(5) Patients should keep the same swimsuit for the duration of their course of treatment, and the suit should be laundered after each attendance.
(6) The water is continually circulating and is tested daily for adequacy of chlorination. Periodically, bacteriological tests should be made on the water.
(7) The floors should be washed down each evening.

The gymnasium

(1) All patients should be inspected for skin infections, especially of the feet (e.g. athlete's foot).
(2) Patients should be issued with a pair of shorts which are kept by them for the course of treatment and sent to the hospital laundry upon completion of treatment.
(3) Staff should wear special training shoes which are kept only for the gymnasium.
(4) Patients should wear preferably their own or disinfected gym shoes when entering the gymnasium.
(5) The gymnasium, patient toilet and changing room floors should be cleaned each evening.
(6) Equipment should be washed at regular intervals.
(7) Patients should be encouraged to take a shower after their classes and be supplied with towels.

Training

Physiotherapists should be trained in aseptic methods and control of infection.

Pharmaceutical department

The Pharmaceutical Department issues medicinal products, disinfectants and other related preparations to wards and departments and sometimes to other hospitals; it has an important responsibility for preventing hospital infection caused by the use of contaminated supplies of these products.

Medicinal products for injection into blood or for instillation into tissues or viscera which are normally sterile must be provided sterile. Though sterility is not essential for preparations which are ingested or applied to surfaces which have a normal microbial flora (skin, mouth, vagina), pathogens must be excluded and large numbers of any micro-organisms must be avoided in these products. Contamination may occur due to inadequate sterilization of preparations required sterile, or to the subsequent acquisition of micro-organisms by sterilized or aseptically prepared medicaments through inadequate storage or handling. Safeguards to prevent contamination by either of these channels are necessary. Aqueous solutions, which may allow bacterial growth during storage, present a special hazard. Unlike human tissues, pharmaceutical preparations cannot protect themselves against small numbers of bacteria, so the degree of environmental cleanliness in areas where aseptic dispensing is carried out must be very high. Areas where fluids are being prepared for sterilization do not demand such a high standard of environment as those used for aseptic preparation of medicaments which are not to be sterilized. Nevertheless, strict measures are currently in force as an insurance policy against unforeseen hazards.

Sterile pharmaceutical products

Sterile medicinal products and pharmaceutical preparations are produced in pharmaceutical departments having specialized facilities as described in the Guide to Good Pharmaceutical Manufacturing Practice (1977) (known as GMP). The manufacture of medicinal products is controlled by the application of the Medicines Act 1968 to Health Authorities (DHSS, 1975), and manufacturing activities are inspected by the Medicines Inspectorate and approved by the Medicines Division, DHSS.

Products to be terminally sterilized are prepared under standard 'clean room' environmental conditions to Class 2 specifications of BS 5295 (1976) Parts 1-3. Other sterile preparations are produced in aseptic rooms which contain laminar airflow work stations providing Class 1 environmental conditions. These are solutions to be sterilized by filtration, admixtures of sterile solutions, and radiopharmaceuticals.

Pharmaceutical production now has quality control built into its procedures, so that the quality, safety and efficacy of the manufactured product is assured. Final product analysis and testing of samples for sterility completes the quality control procedure before the product is released for use in the hospital. Sterility testing of samples must not, however, be regarded as providing guarantees of

275

sterility — nothing short of tests on the whole batch could provide that. It can, of course, provide evidence of gross or moderate contamination; but since bacteria can grow rapidly from very small numbers in many solutions, the value of sample testing, though cumulative, is uncertain, and the main emphasis in producing sterile pharmaceuticals must rely on other criteria.

Sterile production units concentrate on the non-commercially available sterile preparations required to treat patients in hospital, e.g. sterile topical solutions, antiseptic solutions, solutions for irrigation and injections.

Further details of the requirements to produce sterile pharmaceuticals are set out in the GMP (1977) where guidelines are given for personnel and training, documentation, work flow systems, changing rooms, preparation and filling rooms, sterilizing, and product quarantine area. Equipment should be designed, located, and maintained to suit the processes and products for which it is to be used; e.g. autoclaves should have planned operational and maintenance programmes as recommended by the DHSS (1980).

Sterile pharmaceuticals are also prepared as a dispensing service for named patients. This specialized service is available for injections, creams, powders, and sterile medicinal products required for the treatment of patients without undue delay.

A back-up service of drug information is provided by the pharmaceutical department. Whenever possible, pharmaceutical preparations are supplied in unit-dose packs, to minimize bacterial contamination of the preparations; e.g. eye-drops may be supplied in single-dose applicator packs, tablets in unit-dose strip packs, injections in single-dose glass containers, and oral mixtures in small volume containers for use by a single patient. As pharmaceuticals are good media for bacterial growth, opened containers should be exposed for a minimal period of time. As a rough guide, injections should be administered at once and any residue discarded, oral mixtures may be kept for up to 10–14 days after opening, whilst tablets can be kept for a longer time, if properly stored for an indefinite period, or until the activity of the drug diminishes or alters. A practicable storage time of 28 days for tablets has been suggested.

Work of the pharmaceutical department

The work in pharmaceutical departments is segregated into a number of specialized areas. Sterile products are manufactured in controlled production areas with those terminally sterilized by heating in an autoclave being prepared in Clean Rooms. Thermolabile preparations are produced in Aseptic Rooms which have a very high standard of cleanliness. The prepacking of tablets takes place in rooms provided with dust extraction facilities to minimize contamination. Oral mixtures and ointments are prepared in manufacturing areas maintained to the requisite standards laid down in the GMP (1977).

It is of greatest importance that an efficient work flow pattern should obtain in manufacturing areas so that every product is subjected to the full quality assurance procedures before it is released from quarantine for administration to patients.

The work flow in the pharmacy should not permit 'dirty' returned containers

276

from wards intermingling with 'clean' supplies to be issued to the wards. Re-use of containers is an economical part of the pharmaceutical service and such containers must be thoroughly washed and dried prior to recycling. Containers which are damaged or cannot be satisfactorily cleaned and disinfected or sterilized are destroyed. Staff are provided with the appropriate clean clothes, suitable for the purpose, which are worn only in specific areas in the pharmacy department, and the staff must observe a high standard of personal hygiene.

Storage and handling

Pharmaceutical products require special conditions of storage and handling (see also Chapter 7). Directions as to storage, e.g. in a refrigerator or protected from light, should be noted and adhered to. Ampoules and vials should be kept in their outer containers or wrappings to protect them, as far as possible, from external contamination.

(1) Parenteral solutions

(a) **Ampoules.** The contents of the opened ampoule must be withdrawn into a syringe immediately, and any surplus discarded. Ampoules of solution for intrathecal injections should be sterilized by autoclaving inside a sealed container. Some solutions are not thermostable and therefore will not withstand this process, so before subjecting injections to this procedure the Pharmacist's advice must be sought (see Chapter 7).

(b) **Multidose vials.** The cap or diaphragm must be swabbed with an antiseptic solution that acts rapidly, e.g. chlorhexidine 0.5% in ethyl alcohol (70%) or a spirit-impregnated swab (available in sachets) of the type commonly used for preparing the skin before injection.

On no account should an injectable solution be transferred to a gallipot before it is drawn into a syringe. This increases the risk of contamination and also introduces the more dangerous risk of administering the wrong injection.

Multidose containers do not keep indefinitely and must be inspected routinely for opalescence before use; such containers must not be held over for subsequent use after a clinic.

(c) **Rubber-capped vials of dry powder for preparing injections.** The cap should be swabbed with an antiseptic solution, e.g. ethyl alcohol (70%) or a spirit-impregnated swab, before injecting the vehicle into the vial. Most of these are intended for single doses, but some may be used for several doses provided that the solution is stable enough to retain its potency and that it is used within 24 hours of being reconstituted. The pharmacist will give advice on particular preparations.

(d) **Intravenous infusion solutions and emulsions** (see also Chapter 8). Solutions for infusion are supplied in glass bottles with rubber plugs or in PVC bags. The rubber plug or diaphragm must be swabbed with, for example, ethyl alcohol (70%) or one of the spirit-impregnated swabs available in sachets before the cannula is introduced or drug solutions are injected into the container.

277

(2) Topical preparations

It is desirable that antiseptic solutions used on open wounds or normally sterile areas should be issued as sterile, ready-to-use dilutions. This ideal situation can only be approached as closely as facilities will permit and many chlorhexidine and chlorhexidine/cetrimide solutions are issued in sterile, concentrated form which need to be diluted immediately before use. Alternatively, they may be issued in clean and disinfected bottles with an appropriate preservative added, such as isopropanol 7% w/v. Such solutions need to be diluted as appropriate.

Liquids and powders applied to larger open wounds and major burns. Once the container is opened, sterility cannot be assured. The contents should be used as soon as possible and any surplus discarded. NB: This does not apply to semi-rigid 'puffer-packs'. Where small volumes of liquids (up to 20 ml) are required the preferred containers are ampoules.

(3) Bladder irrigation solutions

(a) **Commercially available solutions.** These are currently supplied in 1 l or 3 l plastic containers and the irrigation sets for use with these solutions are purchased separately.

(b) **Hospital manufactured solutions.** These should be isotonic and pyrogen free, and are currently issued in the DHSS Winchester type bottles, the necks of which are designed to take the DHSS pattern of sterile irrigation set. Catheter lubricants should be sterile.

(4) Irrigation solutions for the eye, wounds, and body cavities

These are sterile solutions diluted ready for use, and they should be used on one occasion only.

Pathology laboratories

In recent years much attention has been focussed on transmission of infection associated with hospital and research laboratories and several committees have considered and made recommendations in this regard. The two major areas of concern are firstly the escape of dangerous organisms from laboratories to hospital patients, other workers in the hospital or institute and to the public at large, and secondly the acquisition of infection by laboratory and other hospital workers as a result of handling biological materials derived from patients. Both these problems, which are matters of legitimate public concern, have received not only review by the scientists involved but also social and political consideration. One of the two areas of concern has been highlighted by events such as the acquisition of laboratory strains of smallpox by patients or staff in London and Birmingham. These occurrences require, and have received, careful study and control to prevent further escape of highly dangerous pathogens. The number of laboratories in the UK working with such organisms is very small and likely to be reduced still further. The organisms included in the 'extremely hazardous' category A are all viruses — smallpox, rabies, and related haemorrhagic fever or encephalitis producing viruses.

The requirements for handling these viruses are now extremely strict and work on them requires the endorsement and supervision of the Dangerous Pathogens Advisory Group (DPAG) of the Department of Health and Social Security. Should any isolation of these organisms occur from clinical specimens immediate transfer to a specialised laboratory is necessary. At present only four or five laboratories in the UK are recognized as sufficiently safe for this work.

The second area which has to be considered is that of infection from category B organisms such as *Salmonella typhi* and *Myco. tuberculosis.* Although these organisms are not classified as 'extremely hazardous' the number of laboratories handling them is large and many laboratory workers are therefore at risk. Our main attention is given to organisms in this category.

The passing of the Health and Safety at Work Act 1974 and the report of the Working Party into the *Laboratory Use of Dangerous Pathogens* (the Godber Report) which recommended production of a code of practice for the use of those handling 'category B' pathogens has stimulated extra concern about laboratory safety, in particular about the prevention of laboratory acquired infection. Accordingly the Government set up a Working Party under the chairmanship of Sir James Howie, charged with the task of preparing a Code of Practice for preventing infection in laboratories, including a recommendation for safety in post-mortem rooms. This Code has now been published. In so far as it refers to hazards of infection it supersedes the publication *Safety in Pathology Laboratories*, published by the DHSS in May 1972, but that publication also gives information and advice about chemical hazards, electrical hazards, control of inflammable substances, mechanical hazards and the handling and disposal of radioactive material. The Howie Code of Practice was deliberately written in mandatory terms, and its requirements, after revision and redrafting, may well become legal requirements in the future. Circumstances and techniques, however, change and a Committee has been set up in the Department of Health to revise and keep up to date the recommendations of the Howie Code of Practice. Some changes have already been suggested.

The recommendations of the Code are extensive and demand much from the laboratory worker and also from those who design or direct laboratories. They comprise all the sensible and feasible precautions which need to be taken in diagnostic clinical (and research) laboratories. No code of practice, however, can prevent infections due to negligence or poor technique of the laboratory worker. Everyone who works in a pathology department must develop habits of safe and careful technique. However, precautions against laboratory-acquired infection should be reasonable and be based, whenever possible, on scientific or clinical evidence. Useless rituals should be discouraged, and those remaining in the Report should be removed as soon as possible.

Special risks of infection

There are several ways in which the pathology department may be involved in the spread of infection in hospital. The patients are at risk from infection carried from the laboratory by laboratory staff collecting specimens in the wards or out-patients, and may also be infected by procedures carried out by the technician involving transfer of microbes from one patient to another. The laboratory staff are at risk both from the patients and from the specimens of biological material and cultures examined in the laboratory. This last involvement, i.e. the risk to laboratory staff from biological specimens, is in practice the most important. Many of the hazards are well known and precautions are taken to prevent spread, but infections can also arise from unsuspected sources, such as a request form contaminated by faeces and handled by clerical staff, or from serum containing hepatitis virus examined in the biochemistry department.

There are many ways in which infections are acquired in pathology departments, e.g. infected aerosols or sprays generated when pipetting or pouring liquids in the laboratory may be inhaled by workers; enteric infections may be acquired by ingestion of infected particles; hepatitis virus or other agents may enter through skin abrasions. Tuberculosis and serum hepatitis have been particularly important in hospital and laboratory infections in the UK, less in microbiological than in biochemical and haematological laboratories; in recent years such infections have become less frequent, through better training in safe working. It is usually not the specimen which is already known to be infective that causes the trouble but a specimen not suspected as being dangerous. Nevertheless, it is not necessary or cost-effective to treat every specimen as though it contained a highly dangerous pathogen. Some areas of the laboratory, such as animal houses, tuberculosis laboratories and hospital mortuaries, are especially hazardous and require special precautions.

Prevention of infection

The methods of collecting specimens to minimize infection risks are described in Chapter 8. The ward staff should identify high risk specimens to protect the laboratory staff. Laboratory specimens should be sorted and distributed from a central area — not general office — by staff who know the risks and have been trained to handle such specimens safely. Laboratory staff involved in specimen collection should use materials prepared by or supplied from CSSD for this purpose. Single-use lancets should be used for finger-prick specimens of blood and there should be adequate skin preparation before puncture. The use of separate white coats in laboratory and wards is recommended. Infective illnesses such as boils, sore throats and diarrhoea which exclude nursing staff from the ward apply with equal force to laboratory staff who visit wards. Cuts and abrasions on the hands must be covered with a waterproof dressing. Laboratory staff attending the wards should be trained in barrier-nursing techniques and must follow carefully the instructions for handling infected patients.

Transportation of specimens

Attention should be given to the containers used to transport specimens from the patient areas to the laboratories. The specimen containers should be leak-proof, robust and transported in trays or boxes which will hold the specimens upright. Some laboratories heat seal all specimens for the laboratory in plastic

280

bags with a pocket to keep the forms from contamination. Simple clear rules need to be formulated for staff involved in transporting specimens. The Code of Practice (1978) recommends that metal boxes used for transporting specimens should be autoclaved weekly.

Procedures within the laboratory

Details of hazards and their avoidance are given in several publications (DHSS, 1972; DHSS, 1978). In handling specimens, particular attention should be given to centrifuges and other possible sources of infective aerosols. Infected materials such as slides and pipettes should be discarded into jars containing a phenolic disinfectant which is replaced daily. A hypochlorite solution should be used if viruses are handled, e.g. where hepatitis is a risk; formaldehyde or glutaraldehyde may be used for this purpose (see Chapters 6, 7 and 18). Plastic petri dishes involve problems of disposal; they should be made safe before removal from the laboratory, and this is best achieved by autoclaving in a suitable container or in stainless steel buckets. Polypropylene boxes are particularly suitable (WCB Containers Ltd). The resultant lumps of polyethylene can be handled by the refuse collectors, but should be kept in sealed plastic bags. Difficulties have arisen when plates have been discarded without treatment and subsequently appear on local refuse sites. Incineration of plastic plates in bulk may lead to an unacceptable smoke hazard and should be discontinued unless a satisfactory incinerator is available. Used glass petri dishes should be autoclaved by trained staff before handling by domestics. Other glass containers, such as bijou bottles containing infective material, should be similarly autoclaved before leaving the laboratory, whether they are going to be reprocessed or disposed of.

Immunization procedures which should be offered to laboratory staff include tuberculosis, poliomyelitis, tetanus, and, where appropriate, smallpox. Female staff should also be offered rubella vaccination, preferably after testing the immune state. None of these procedures are mandatory, except for BCG protection of Heaf-negative technicians, who must be excluded from work with tuberculous material until conversion has taken place. The other protective measures should be strongly urged on all staff on joining the laboratory (see Chapter 13).

Training of staff in aseptic procedures and in methods of handling infected material is part of routine education in microbiology departments. In many hospitals the various branches of pathology recruit their own staff and there may be no opportunity for biochemists or technicians to acquire experience in bacteriology departments. In these cases some basic instruction should be given on methods of spread of infection, aseptic procedures and handling of potentially infected biological material. The DHSS Code of Practice should be readily available for consultation but in addition other warning signs should be available at points of particular hazard, e.g. 'no mouth pipetting' signs in serology laboratory; exhaust protective cabinets should have a chart attached indicating the results of airflow monitoring; hazard labels for specimens from renal units (see Chapter 18) to be available where specimens examined, etc. In addition a short list of the most important rules should be on visual display, for example:

Precautions against laboratory infection

Any specimen entering the laboratory may be infectious. Some will certainly contain the agents causing hepatitis, typhoid, tuberculosis, and other infections. Your safety, your family's safety, and your colleagues' safety depend on observing the following instructions:

General

No smoking, no eating, no drinking in the laboratory. Keep your bench clean and tidy.

Wash your hands thoroughly
>   on leaving the laboratory;
>   before taking food or drink, or handling personal possessions;
>   after handling specimens;
>   after changing tubing or dialysers or diluters in the autoanalysers.

If you think you have contaminated them:
>   use plenty of soap and water; if contamination with bacterial cultures has occurred and in 'high risk' laboratories use an antiseptic hand-washing method. (*Hand-washing is your most important safeguard.*)

Cuts and abrasions

Wash well in running water.
Cover with waterproof protective dressing.
If you splash your eye with serum or culture, wash it out with saline or tap water.
Report to Chief Medical Laboratory Scientific Officer or deputy at once.
Enter in Accident Book (even needle-pricks must be entered).

Spilt specimens: treatment of contaminated area

Swab with plenty of clear soluble phenolic solution, or hypochlorite solution containing 0.5% available chlorine where hazard of virus contamination exists; on metal surfaces, use glutaraldehyde. Rinse well with water and discard swab into incinerator bag.

Pipettes

Use automatic pipettes, or rubber bulbs, or teats.
Discard all Pasteur pipettes and graduated pipettes into enough clear soluble phenolic or hypochlorite solution containing 0.5% available chlorine to cover them completely.

Other equipment

Plastic tubes, pilot tube segments and other plastic disposables should be incinerated. Slides should be autoclaved in the discard jars in which they have been placed. Syringes and needles should be discarded into a receptacle such as a Burn Box and incinerated.

Centrifuging

Use only closed centrifuges, with wind-shields if possible, and preferably with sealed buckets which should be opened only within a protective exhaust cabinet when dangerous pathogens are involved.

Swab out the centrifuge bowl with a clear soluble phenolic or, for virus infections, an aldehyde disinfectant (formalin 10% or glutaraldehyde 2%) weekly. Wear disposable gloves for this.

If a breakage occurs, autoclave the bucket and its contents. Swab out the bowl as above.

White coats

A plentiful supply is necessary. Coats must be changed immediately if contaminated; all coats should be treated as infected linen in the laundry; coats known to be contaminated with dangerous pathogens must be autoclaved in the laboratory autoclave.

Don't wear your lab. coat to visit the wards.

Don't wear *any* white coat to visit the coffee room or rest room.

Tuberculosis laboratories

The report *Precautions against tuberculosis infection in the diagnostic laboratory* (DHSS, 1970) gives a detailed account of precautions to be taken to prevent tuberculosis in laboratory staff; the report was prompted by the high incidence of this disease among laboratory workers, although this has now been reduced.

It is highly desirable that a separate room should be available for tuberculosis work. Because of the dangers of handling cultures and the need to standardize further tests on these cultures, it is advisable in most routine laboratories to limit the procedures to staining and primary isolation of the organism which is further examined at a reference laboratory.

Protective equipment must include a hood with exhaust ventilation with an air flow of at least 100 f/min. Adequate filters must be used and the exhaust system disinfected with formalin vapour before maintenance work is carried out. The centrifuge must have a wind-shield (Newsom, 1980).

Protective clothing is advisable; a gown or plastic aproh should be worn and rubber gloves for more dangerous manipulations. Staff must be adequately trained in the use of aseptic measures in addition to providing this protective clothing; otherwise a false sense of security may lead to simple errors which would not arise if gloves were *not* being worn. An annual chest X-ray should be performed on all members of staff exposed to these hazards.

Fungi

Cultures of fungi causing communicable systemic infection should be processed in a ventilated cabinet, as recommended for tubercle bacilli.

Post-mortem room and mortuary (see also DHSS, 1972; 1978)

The body, whether previously infected or not, may be a source of infection and the mortuary and post-mortem staff are at risk. As in the ward, bacteria may spread by air or by contact, but there are special hazards when a post-mortem examination is being made. Contaminated aerosols or splashes may be released through squeezing sponges, cutting tissues such as lung or incising abscesses, and the sawing of bones may also release small contaminated chips into the air. Cutting or pricking a finger with a contaminated instrument or ragged bone edge is one of the commonest modes of infection. Although most organisms in the dead body are unlikely to infect healthy people with intact skin, there are some particular hazards. Tubercle bacilli may be spread in large numbers in aerosols. *Salmonella*, *Shigella* and other intestinal pathogens may be transmitted from the intestinal tract, and smallpox or anthrax may spread to members of staff by air or contact. Following a break in the pathologist's or technician's skin, large numbers of *Staph. aureus* or *Strep. pyogenes* may be introduced, and unless he receives treatment with appropriate antibiotics this may cause a severe local infection and sometimes septicaemia; hepatitis virus introduced by a cut or needle-prick may cause severe infection for which no chemotherapy is available. The conjunctiva may be infected by splashes or aerosols, and a severe local infection may follow; the hepatitis virus may also enter the body by this route (see Chapter 18).

Prevention of infection

The risks of infection are not high if adequate precautions are taken. Cleanliness of mortuary, refrigerator, post-mortem room and good personal hygiene of members of staff are essential.

The post-mortem room should be mechanically ventilated and designed so that cleaning can be readily carried out. Fly-proofing arrangements in the mortuary and post-mortem room should be efficient. A shower with soap and towels supplied should be available for the post-mortem room staff. When performing post-mortem examinations the pathologist and mortuary technicians should completely change their outer clothing and a plastic apron and rubber boots should be worn. Clean white trousers, vests and jackets should be supplied daily if possible, or at least several times a week. Visitors not in close contact with the body should wear a gown and overshoes. A wash-basin with disposable paper towels and an antiseptic hand-washing preparation (povidone-iodine or chlorhexidine detergent, or 70%–95% ethanol (see Chapter 6)) should be available in the post-mortem room.

Staff should wash their hands after handling any contaminated surface or material irrespective of whether gloves are worn, and always on leaving the post-mortem room. If hands are likely to have become contaminated, they should also be washed before handling case notes or any other clean items. Gloves should be washed thoroughly and immersed in disinfectant before removal.

If the skin or eye is splashed it should be thoroughly washed. An eyewash bottle containing sterile saline should be available. Any cut or finger prick should be immediately reported to the pathologist, after thorough washing under running water and application of an antiseptic (e.g. 0.5% alcoholic or aqueous chlorhexidine or 1% iodine in 70% alcohol). All cuts or open lesions on the hands should be covered with a waterproof dressing. Open injuries, other than minor ones, should be treated in the casualty department.

Instruments used on bodies known to have suffered from a communicable infection should be immersed in a disinfectant (e.g. 2% 'Stericol', or glutaraldehyde if the infection was hepatitis) for at least 1 h (see Chapter 7, page 82) before cleaning and sterilizing or terminally disinfecting. Others may be washed in cold water before disinfection, and all instruments should be autoclaved if possible; boiling or immersion in 2% 'Stericol' or 1% 'Sudol' are less satisfactory alternatives to autoclaving. After treatment with a disinfectant, instruments should be rinsed and dried. The room and other equipment should be thoroughly cleaned after use with a phenolic disinfectant (e.g. 1% 'Sudol', 2% 'Stericol'), or with 1% hypochlorite if hepatitis or poliomyelitis was diagnosed in the patient before death.

Linen should be sent in a sealed bag and treated as infected by the laundry. Dressings, waste materials and body tissues should be sealed in plastic bags and preferably incinerated on site. Aprons and gloves should be autoclaved if possible after washing, or alternatively immersed in a phenolic disinfectant solution. Boots should also be thoroughly washed and dried after use.

Special precautions should be taken with certain infections. Aerosols and splashing should be particularly avoided in post-mortem examination of patients with tuberculosis, and filter masks should be worn by operators. Post-mortems on patients with known or suspected serum hepatitis, or if HB_sAg positive, should be avoided unless absolutely essential (for general precautions see Chapter 18). Special care is necessary to avoid cuts and needle pricks. In the event of any such mishap, specific immunoglobulin should be given.

Viruses causing spongeiform encephalopathy (Creutzfeldt–Jakob disease) and other slow virus infections are believed to be relatively resistant to heat and chemical disinfectants, especially aldehydes. Instruments should be autoclaved at $121°$ C ($250°$ F) for 1 h and the environment disinfected with a strong hypochlorite solution (containing 0.25% available chlorine); blood should be mopped up with a solution containing 1% available chlorine.

Formaldehyde used for the preservation of tissues is an effective anti-bacterial agent, but thorough penetration should be ensured before handling, particularly if lesions caused by dangerous infections, such as tuberculosis, typhoid or hepatitis, are present.

It is most important that the mortuary staff should be informed about the bodies of patients who have died from or were suffering from a communicable disease, and a warning label could usefully be attached to them in the ward. Training of mortuary staff in prevention of infection is also necessary.

Immunization should be offered as for laboratory staffs (see p. 280).

References and Further Reading

British Standards Institution (1976), *Environmental Cleanliness in Enclosed Spaces*. BS 5295; Part 1: Specification for controlled environment, clean

285

rooms, work stations and clean air devices; Part 2: Guide to the construction and installation of clean rooms, work stations, and clean air devices; Part 3: Guide to operational procedures and disciplines applicable to clean rooms, work stations and clean air devices. BSI, London.

Casewell, M. and Phillips, I. (1977), Hands as route of transmission for Klebsiella species. *Br. med. J.*, ii, 1315.

Department of Health and Social Security (1980), *Pressure Steam Sterilizers.* Hospital Technical Memorandum HTM 10. HMSO, London.

Department of Health and Social Security and Welsh Office (1970), *Precautions against Tuberculous Infection in the Diagnostic Laboratory.* Hospital Memorandum HM(70)60.

Department of Health and Social Security and Welsh Office (1972), *Safety in Pathology Laboratories.*

Department of Health and Social Security (1975), *Application of Medicines Act to Health Authorities.* Health Circular HSC(IS)128.

Department of Health and Social Security (1978), *Code of Practice for Prevention of Infection in Clinical Laboratories and Post-mortem Rooms* (Howie Report). HMSO, London.

Gillespie, W. A., Lennon, G. G., Linton, K. B. and Slade, N. (1964), Prevention of urinary infection in gynaecology. *Br. med. J.*, ii, 423.

Gillespie, W. A., Linton, K. B., Miller, A. and Slade, N. (1966), The diagnosis, epidemiology and control of urinary infection in urology and gynaecology. *J. clin. Path.*, 13, 187.

Guide to Good Pharmaceutical Manufacturing Practice (GMP) (1977), HMSO, London.

Kunin, C. M. (1974), *Detection, Prevention and Management of Urinary Tract Infection.* Lea and Febiger, Philadelphia.

Medicines Act (1968), HMSO, London.

Newsom, S. W. B. (1980), Safety cabinets encounter the British Standard. *J. hosp. Infect*, 1, 11.

Report on Prevention of Microbial Contamination of Medicinal Products (1973), HMSO, London.

Miscellaneous Problems

CHAPTER SEVENTEEN

Diseases Caused by Dangerous Pathogens

Smallpox

Variola major/variola minor

The World Health Organization's vaccination programme has resulted in the apparent eradication of smallpox. However, the virus is still retained in a small number of reference laboratories and, from time to time, patients with undiagnosed vesicular rashes will continue to raise a suspicion of smallpox. Further, monkey-pox, an infection of primates, is similar in appearance to smallpox and is also communicable from monkey to man in whom it can be fatal. So far as is known, it does not spread from man to man.

The action which must be taken to prevent the spread of smallpox in hospital provides an example of the extreme measures which are necessary to control life-threatening infections which can be transmitted by the airborne route. Smallpox vaccination for *routine* purposes should be abandoned except for staff of smallpox hospitals.

Cases arising in hospital (out-patients and in-patients)

The hospital doctor dealing with a suspected or confirmed case of smallpox will take the following action:

(1) Transfer the patient to a side room or similar accommodation.
(2) Where the diagnosis is not made by a consultant physician (or in the case of children by a consultant paediatrician), immediately obtain, wherever possible, in consultation with the Hospital Control of Infection Officer, the opinion of a consultant physician/consultant paediatrician.
(3) In addition it is imperative to notify immediately the Medical Officer for Environmental Health by telephone in order
  (a) to request the Medical Officer for Environmental Health to see the patient *in hospital* in order that he will make the necessary arrangements for the confirmation or otherwise of the diagnosis by a member of the Special Panel of Smallpox Opinion:
  (b) for the Medical Officer of Environmental Health to make arrangements for the removal of the patient by special ambulance to the smallpox

289

hospital, acting on the advice of the member of the Special Panel of Smallpox Opinion:

(c) to obtain advice on the precautionary measures to be taken both as regards patients and contacts in the hospital, in consultation with a senior member of the medical staff, a senior nursing officer, the administrator of the hospital concerned, and the Infection Control Officer, who will form the Emergencies Committee for the duration of the incident.

In no circumstances should a suspected case seen in the out-patient department be sent home to await a visit by the Medical Officer for Environmental Health or a general practitioner. (Detailed information for hospital medical staff is set out below.)

Action in general hospitals in dealing with confirmed or suspected cases of smallpox

(1) The principles of control enunciated in the *Memorandum on the Control of Outbreaks of Smallpox* (DHSS, 1975) are equally applicable when a case of smallpox is first diagnosed in a general hospital, but there are certain special considerations which might be overlooked. All Area Medical Officers should make plans for dealing with such a situation before it arises.

(2) As soon as the diagnosis of smallpox is entertained it is essential to inform the Medical Officer for Environmental Health and to invite him to see the case in hospital. He in turn is free to call upon the services of a member of the Panel of Smallpox Opinion. Meanwhile, all unessential movement to and from the vicinity of the affected ward or department should cease until a decision has been made.

(3) If it is decided by the Medical Officer for Environmental Health that the patient must be dealt with as though suffering from smallpox, he will give advice as to the best route from the department to the ambulance, the protection of the attendants by vaccination, the use of protective clothing and the terminal disinfection of the stretcher trolley and any blankets not removed in the ambulance.

(4) All persons who have entered the department or ward since the patient there was deemed to have been infectious should be regarded as known or probable contacts, immediately offered vaccination and placed under formal surveillance for 17 clear days.

(5) There are certain persons in whom vaccination carries an additional risk of complications, and attention is drawn to the following paragraphs from the *Memorandum on Vaccination Against Smallpox* (DHSS, 1974).

Vaccination procedures (paragraphs 14 and 15 of Memorandum)
Pregnancy. It is wise to avoid primary vaccination at any stage of pregnancy unless it is necessary to confer protection against smallpox; when this occurs human specific immunoglobulin given into the opposite limb at the time of vaccination may help to prevent this complication.

The possibility of pregnancy should be remembered when offering vaccina-

290

tion to any woman of child-bearing age and the nature of the risk to the foetus explained to her. There is no evidence that vaccination against smallpox during pregnancy is associated with congenital malformation and the inadvertent vaccination of a woman subsequently found to have been pregnant is not an indication for deliberate termination of the pregnancy.

Specific contra-indications (but see paragraph 22). These are:
(a) a history of or the presence of eczema. *Eczema is an extremely important contra-indication to vaccination. Primary vaccination should not be performed on any person with eczema or a history of eczema unless there is a risk of exposure to smallpox. Moreover, any infant or person with eczema should be kept away for at least 21 days from any recently vaccinated member of the household.* Neglect of this advice may give rise to eczema vaccinatum and the risk of death therefrom;
(b) immune deficiency states;
(c) leukaemia, lymphoma and other malignancies;
(d) corticosteroid and immunosuppressive treatment.

Revaccination (paragraph 19)

Contra-indications. The caution as regards primary vaccination during pregnancy (see paragraph 14) and the specific contra-indications to primary vaccination see paragraph 15) apply also to revaccination. *A history of postvaccinal encephalitis or other serious postvaccinal complication is an additional contra-indication to revaccination.*

Vaccination in the presence of smallpox (paragraph 22)

Contra-indications. In the presence of suspected smallpox there are no absolute contra-indications to the immediate vaccination or revaccination of all close contacts. (But see paragraph 23 below.)

Use of human specific immunoglobulin and methisazone (paragraphs 23 and 24)

When it is essential, because of a possibility of exposure to smallpox, to vaccinate a pregnant woman or a person with any specific contra-indication, human specific immunoglobulin should be given into the opposite arm at the time of vaccination. The dosage recommended for this purpose is:

Under 1 year	250 mg
1 to 6 years	500 mg
7 to 14 years	750 mg
15 years or more	1 g

In addition, when it is considered desirable to provide passive immunity to known close contacts of smallpox who have been previously unvaccinated or who have not been vaccinated for many years, the dosage recommended is:

Under 1 year	0.5 g
1 to 6 years	1.0 g
7 years or more	1.5 g

Human specific immunoglobulin is in short supply and therefore it is essential that stocks remain centralized at the Epidemiological Research Laboratory, Central Public Health Laboratory, Colindale, London NW9 5HT. Small amounts are also held at Public Health Laboratories in Birmingham, Bristol, Cambridge, Cardiff, Leeds, Liverpool, Manchester, Newcastle, Oxford, and Sheffield. In Scotland this material is available from Regional Blood Transfusion Centres.

The use of the antiviral drug, methisazone, should also be considered as a measure additional to, but not in substitution for, vaccination in the protection of known and probable contacts of a case of smallpox.

(6) The responsibility for this vaccination and surveillance of persons within the hospital may be designated to senior medical members of the staff, but wherever possible the Medical Officer for Environmental Health, or a person designated by him, should be seconded to assume the duties of an Outbreak Control Officer. In this case direct liaison between this officer and the Medical Officer for Environmental Health should be maintained.

(7) Special accommodation should be provided in an appropriate part of the hospital for the temporary isolation of patients or staff who, whilst under surveillance, fall sick. They should remain there until their final disposal is determined. Plans must be made for the protection of staff who deliver food and who remove refuse and soiled linen from this isolation accommodation.

(8) It will be necessary to identify all visitors to the affected ward during the period when the patient was considered to have been infectious. The appropriate Medical Officer for Environmental Health must be told so that these individuals can be vaccinated and placed under formal surveillance.

(9) If the patient was first diagnosed in a casualty or out-patient department the building should be closed for terminal disinfection after the contacts have been identified and vaccinated. Thereafter it may be re-opened and work may continue (but see paragraph 12 below).

(10) If the case is first diagnosed in a ward, it is advisable to place the patients and staff in quarantine whilst they remain under observation.

(11) The Hospital's Control of Infection Committee in consultation with the Medical Officer for Environmental Health will give consideration to the need to vaccinate some or all of the remaining patients or staff of the hospital in otherwise unaffected departments (see paragraph 5). The need to curtail visiting will depend on local circumstances, but in general visiting should be limited to close relatives of the seriously or dangerously ill patients and to religious advisers, all of whom should be offered vaccination.

(12) Beyond the domestic arrangements already discussed, the Area Medical Officer, in consultation with the Regional Medical Officer, will need to determine with the Medical Officer for Environmental Health whether all or part of the hospital should be closed to new admissions until the period of surveillance is complete. It would seem reasonable, if the affected block or department can be adequately policed, for the rest of the hospital to be re-opened after all patients have been vaccinated and placed under surveil-

lance. However, if a common ventilation system is shared by the whole hospital, serious consideration must be given to discontinuing admissions during the surveillance period.

Viral Haemorrhagic Fevers (VHF)

Lassa fever, Marburg disease and Ebola virus diseases

These virus infections are endemic in West and Central Africa. All have a significant mortality and there is no vaccine or treatment available at the time of writing. Lassa fever, the commonest of these infections, is contracted by man from a rodent, *Mastomys natalensis*, which is widely distributed in Africa but not in Europe. Human-to-human transmission of infection is probably uncommon and has never been known to occur outside Africa; it occurs only on very close contact with the patient or with his body fluids. The incubation period of these infections is usually from 7 to 10 days with a range of 3 to 17. For control purposes a period of up to 21 days is usually taken.

The *Memorandum on Lassa Fever* (DHSS, 1976) describes the control of these infections.

Control measures depend on:

(1) Early identification of known or suspected cases

A medical practitioner suspecting that the patient might be suffering from a viral haemorrhagic fever (pyrexial illness, occupation and residence in endemic area) should *not* refer the patient to hospital but immediately seek the advice of a consultant in communicable or tropical diseases. If the patient is already in hospital he should be confined in a single room until seen by the consultant. If a suspected case arrives in a casualty department, the Infection Control Officer should be informed, and the patient should be placed in a room specially designated for this purpose, where a box containing special protective clothing is available. There is considerable urgency in making contact with the appropriate expert not only for epidemiological purposes but also to exclude *Plasmodium falciparum* malaria, which can be rapidly fatal, as a cause of the illness.

In practical terms, the above advice applies to any patient with a pyrexia of unknown origin during a period of 21 days after arrival from West and Central Africa. It is the duty of the medical practitioner who first sees the patient and/or the second opinion to notify the MOEH at the earliest possible opportunity.

(2) Isolation of cases or suspects using special units designated for the purpose

Confirmation of diagnosis of VHF may take several days, and if it proves impossible to make an alternative diagnosis, such as malaria, it usually becomes necessary to transfer the patient to a designated High Security Unit. At the time of writing there are five such Units in England, one in Wales and one in Scotland. The patient is usually conveyed to the Unit in an ambulance containing a Trexler Transit Isolator.

293

(3) Surveillance of contacts

Close contacts of the case should be placed under medical surveillance for a period of 21 days from the last possible date of exposure to infection. Surveillance is the responsibility of the MOEH.

(4) Control in hospitals (confirmed or highly suspect cases only)

(a) An Emergencies Committee should be set up (p. 290).
(b) An Outbreak Liaison Officer should be appointed.

Notes:
   (i) Protective clothing (cap, gown, surgeon's shirt and trousers, mask, gloves and boots or overshoes) should be worn by attendant staff and ambulance personnel.
  (ii) Laboratory specimens from suspected or confirmed cases of VHF should *not* be examined in routine laboratories but only in category A pathogen laboratories. If malaria is likely, a blood film must be examined without delay.
 (iii) Terminal disinfection of wards, departments or ambulances must be carried out using procedures recommended for smallpox (see p. 79).
 (iv) Particular care should be taken in the disposal of stool and urine specimens which should first be treated with a virucidal agent such as a hypochlorite solution (see Chapter 18).

Rabies

Human-to-human transmission of rabies has never been reported and the strict precautions recommended for the prevention of transmission are therefore unnecessary. However, the disease has emotive connotations for hospital staff, while the intensive medical and nursing care which is essential if the patient is to have any chance of survival increase the possibility of exposure to infection.

The following precautions are recommended:
(1) The patient should be isolated in a single room, preferably in an Intensive Therapy Unit.
(2) Attendant staff and other close contacts, e.g. anaesthetists, should be offered immunization with human diploid cell vaccine (4 intradermal injections of 0.1 ml given on the same day).
(3) Staff should wear protective clothing including goggles, mask and gloves.
(4) Mouth-to-mouth resuscitation should not be used.
(5) Pregnant female staff should not attend the patient.
(6) Specimens from the patient should not be sent to routine diagnostic laboratories but only to Category A pathogen laboratories.
(7) Equipment soiled by secretions or excretions must be destroyed or autoclaved.

Further information is contained in the *Memorandum on Rabies* (DHSS, 1977).

294

References and Further Reading

Department of Health and Social Security (1974), *Memorandum on Vaccination against Smallpox*, Memo 312 Med. (Revised), HMSO, London.

Department of Health and Social Security (1975), *Memorandum on the Control of Outbreaks of Smallpox*, HMSO, London.

Department of Health and Social Security and Welsh Office (1977), *Memorandum on Rabies*, HMSO, London.

Department of Health and Social Security and Welsh Office (1976), *Memorandum on Lassa Fever*, HMSO, London.

CHAPTER EIGHTEEN

Control of Hepatitis in Hospital

Several viruses may attack the human liver, but three are relevant here: (1) hepatitis A virus; (2) hepatitis B virus; (3) the virus of 'non A–non B' hepatitis.

Hepatitis A (infectious hepatitis)

The infective agent is a small RNA virus about 26 nm in diameter. Infection is contracted by swallowing the virus. After an incubation period of about three weeks a febrile, undifferentiated disease develops. During this stage, virus is excreted in the faeces in quantity. After a few days of this illness jaundice appears; by that time virus excretion in the faeces is either undetectable or at a very low level. By the time patients have been admitted to hospital they are usually no longer infectious. At this stage antibodies are present in their blood. A transient viraemia occurs in the pre-icteric stage of the disease, but this is of such short duration that infection is not likely to be transmitted parenterally by injection of blood or blood products.

Laboratory diagnosis

This can be made by radioimmunoassay of IgM (macroglobulin) antibodies to the virus in a single sample of serum taken in the acute phase of disease. Virus can be detected in the faeces, especially in the prodromal stage of the illness, by electron microscopy of faeces, but this is not as sensitive nor as reliable a technique as the radioimmunoassay for IgM antibodies which appear by the time the patient is in hospital with jaundice. IgG antibodies can also be determined; their presence without IgM antibodies indicates not a recent but an earlier infection by the virus. There is only one serological variety of the virus, and the presence of antibodies indicates full immunity.

Protection against hepatitis A

About 30% of the population of the United Kingdom appear to have some antibody to hepatitis A virus in the circulation; γ-globulin extracted from pooled donors' serum therefore confers good protection upon those who are likely to be exposed, as are, for example, travellers to tropical countries where the standards of hygiene are low and the chances of infection are considerable;

296

particularly at risk are those who work in the countryside, while undertaking voluntary service overseas. The globulin, present in the blood after injection, decays with a half-life of about a month, so that one injection will not confer protection for more than about three or four months, after which the subject can again become susceptible. To confer continuing protection an injection of gammaglobulin is needed about every three months.

Hepatitis B (serum hepatitis)

This disease has an incubation period of about 40–160 days, often about 90 days. It is usually transmitted by the parenteral route, but can be transmitted in other ways. The disease is often subclinical; it is usually a mild infection, but often more severe or lethal than hepatitis A; indeed, one strain of the virus has caused a death rate of over 15%, but this was a unique episode. Individual cases of serum hepatitis cannot be distinguished from infectious hepatitis on clinical grounds alone, though associated arthritis suggests serum hepatitis.

Laboratory diagnosis

Different serotypes of hepatitis B virus occur. Five antigenic determinants on the hepatitis B surface antigen (HB_SAg) particles are known (a, d, y, w, r), and the antigens can be typed. Typing is of value in epidemiological studies. Subtype *ay* has caused most incidents of hospital-transmitted infection, but blood containing any subtype must be regarded as potentially dangerous. Another antigen known as '*e*' is often found in the blood of HB_SAg carriers. There is some evidence that the presence of this *e* antigen indicates that the blood is more likely to be infectious than the blood of carriers whose serum does not contain it; but the distinction is not absolute, and blood which does not contain *e* antigen may also be infectious. All blood donations in the UK are nowadays tested for HB_SAg. The test used in most centres at present is reversed passive haemagglutination of sensitized turkey erythrocytes, but it is likely that all blood transfusion centres will soon adopt a more sensitive test, e.g. radio-immunoassay; some are already using this method, especially in Scotland. But no test, even the most sensitive, can be guaranteed to exclude all infective donations. Serum hepatitis is a potential hazard in general wards, especially when patients with the disease are being treated, or in operations upon immunosuppressed patients who are known carriers; but provided the rules of safe-working are observed (see below, and Chapter 19) the risk is small.

Carriers of hepatitis B virus

About 1:800 of the population in the UK continuously carry serum hepatitis virus in their blood. In most other parts of the world, the proportion of the population who carry the virus is much higher; the nearer they live to the equator and the humbler their status in the social scale, the more likely people are to carry the virus. Men are more likely to be carriers than women. High carrier rates are found among certain members of the community, in the UK

297

especially among inmates of prisons, drug addicts, mental defectives (in institutions rather than those living at home) and immigrants from tropical countries. Healthy carriers in the general population usually carry virus in comparatively low titre in their blood, but certain patients, if infected, may carry the virus in very high titre and for that reason their blood is much more likely to transmit infection than blood from most carriers. The patients who, if infected, constitute a special hazard, are those who are immunosuppressed through their illness or as a result of treatment, e.g., patients with chronic renal failure (this condition in itself is immunosuppressive), patients with inborn immunodeficiency and patients immunosuppressed as part of the treatment (such as after kidney grafting or for certain diseases such as leukaemia). Before blood from these patients is put through other laboratory investigations it must be tested to make sure that it does not contain HB$_S$Ag; if found negative, such blood is no more dangerous to handle than normal blood. It is prudent to test these patients every three months; it is not necessary to test every sample from them.

Because the damage to the liver in hepatitis B patients is immunologically mediated, those with chronic renal failure and those who are immunosuppressed when they become infected usually do not show characteristic features of the disease; if they are in dialysis units, however, they may very easily transmit infection to other patients or to the staff of the unit. Infection in the past has entered dialysis units by transfusion of blood from a carrier and has been spread from patient to patient by shared dialysis machines or possibly by other mechanisms also. Infection may be spread to staff by spilt blood getting into a scratch or into the eye, or by a prick from a contaminated needle. It may be transmitted by acupuncture. Patients with serum hepatitis or patients who are carriers, even high titre carriers, do not transmit the infection as an aerosol. To acquire infection from them one has to get their blood or possibly other tissue fluids under one's skin. Medical procedures are by no means the most important ways of acquiring serum hepatitis. It may be transmitted by sexual intercourse, by sharing a razor with a carrier, by insect bites, by tattooists, or by scratching oneself on a twig or thorn which has previously scratched a hepatitis carrier.

Non A–non B hepatitis

Now that laboratory diagnosis of hepatitis A and of hepatitis B can be made, it has become clear that some cases of hepatitis are caused by a virus which is neither hepatitis A nor hepatitis B virus and which has been present in transfused blood, or more commonly in injected blood products, especially cryoprecipitates and other antihaemophilic preparations. There is at the moment no laboratory test for this infection; it is diagnosed by exclusion. There is certainly one and there are probably at least two such viruses that can be isolated, but so far this has been achieved only by inoculation of chimpanzees.

Measures designed to prevent accidental transmission of hepatitis B (see below) should be equally successful against accidental transmission of 'non A–non B' hepatitis, as both these viruses are transmitted by the same route. It is not known whether there is a carrier state for the 'non A–non B' viruses, but the evidence available suggests that this is quite likely.

Isolation of hepatitis viruses in the laboratory

Hepatitis B virus has not yet been successfully grown in tissue culture, but there has recently been a report of successful isolation of hepatitis A virus (Provost and Hilleman, 1979).

Prevention of hepatitis B transmission

The main hazards are due to contamination of small skin wounds, conjunctiva or mucous membranes with blood from patients with serum hepatitis or from immunosuppressed carriers of hepatitis B virus (e.g. those with chronic renal failure or grafted kidneys), in which it is likely to be present in high titre; healthy carriers usually have a relatively low titre and therefore present a much smaller hazard. The persons most likely to acquire hepatitis B infection in hospital are therefore members of staff working in renal units, where contamination of the skin or of the environment with blood during dialysis, as well as the presence of high titres of virus in the blood, provide maximum opportunities for transmission. The principles and procedures for preventing transmission of hepatitis virus in renal units are described in Chapter 19.

Risks of infection with the virus obviously exist also in other hospital departments where blood is handled, especially in operating theatres, maternity departments, dental departments, laboratories and mortuaries. Recommendations for protection of patients in these areas are presented in this chapter. Although the same basic principles apply wherever a special hazard exists, there are practical features peculiar to each area, and these will now be considered.

Laboratory staff

(1) General precautions (see DHSS, 1972; 1978).

(2) Staff must be trained to work safely. This is the responsibility of the Director of the Laboratory usually exercised through his Safety Officer or a senior member of the technical staff.

(3) Specimens from *high risk areas* such as the Renal Unit must be marked to indicate that they may carry a hazard, and handled with surgical or disposable gloves. Blood should be sent in screw-topped rubber-washered glass bottles (Bijous, McCartneys, Universal Containers) and specimens should be transported from the Renal Unit in sealed impermeable plastic bags.

Blood specimens must either be discarded into a strong hypochlorite solution or, preferably, placed in a bucket and autoclaved. The time and temperature reached by the autoclave must be carefully checked. Urine may also contain $HB_S Ag$. Winchester glass bottles should not be used for urine because they may break. We recommend the use of screw-capped disposable plastic containers with a rubber washer incorporated in the screw cap.

(4) Before centrifuging samples of blood from high risk areas, bottle tops should be wiped with 2% buffered glutaraldehyde or with hypochlorite containing 0.1% available chlorine.

(5) Centrifuges used for blood, urine and faeces must be closed.

299

(6) Auto-analysers — surgical or disposable plastic gloves must be worn when changing dialysers or tubing. Plastic cup trays should be disinfected in hypochlorite solution.

(7) Blood or serum specimens should be tested for presence of HB_SAg before being included in the 'laboratory pool' of test sera.

(8) Staff collecting blood from HB_SAg-positive patients must wear gloves and place the patient's arm on a piece of disposable plastic sheeting before collecting the specimen. It is commonly recommended that containers should be filled from the syringe with the needle still attached; some prefer to separate the needle carefully with forceps or disposable gloves before discharging the contents. Syringe and needle must be disposed of by placing them in a box with a lid (e.g. 'DRG' Box), which must be available on the ward.

Surgical operations on patients known or suspected of being HB_SAg positive

(1) All staff in the theatre must wear gloves during the operation and when cleaning the theatre afterwards.

(2) 'Disposable' linen should be used wherever possible — including gowns if these are available, and a disposable plastic apron should be worn by the scrubbed team under their gowns.

(3) Special care must be exercised to avoid accidents with needles or sharp instruments. If someone pricks or cuts himself he must stop what he is doing and attend to the injury by making it bleed if possible and applying tincture of iodine. Special immune γ-globulin will be made available should the subject wish it.

(4) Those taking part in or assisting at the operation should wear goggles or a vizor. If conjunctival contamination occurs, the eye should be washed out with saline or tap water and special immune γ-globulin offered. Blood-splashed surfaces should be disinfected with 10% hypochlorite (1% available chlorine).

(5) All disposable items must be discarded in impermeable plastic bags and sent for incineration — this will include endotracheal tubes.

(6) Those surgical instruments and other tools used in the operation which cannot be autoclaved must be placed in a bucket of 2% glutaraldehyde and soaked for at least 2 hours before being cleaned and returned to service. If possible, autoclave. For treatment of endoscopes see Chapter 7.

(7) The theatre walls (if visibly soiled) and floor should be wiped down with hypochlorite (0.1% available chlorine) at the end of the operation. The table should be wiped down with 2% glutaraldehyde, or by hypochlorite which should be rinsed off after application.

(8) 'Non-disposable' linen used for the operation must be autoclaved or transported to the laundry in impermeable polythene bags labelled 'Hepatitis, take special care' (see Chapter 11).

(9) Blood of organ donors should, if possible, be tested for HB$_S$Ag before the transplant is done.

Dental departments

Dentists run the same risk of infection as their medical and nursing colleagues when treating HB$_S$Ag-positive patients, especially those who are regarded as 'high risk' patients. The same precautions should be taken as are listed under *surgical operations*. In addition, the following precautions relating to dental equipment are appropriate. Conventional low speed hand-pieces of a sterilizable type and the traditional methods of scaling should be used. High speed hand-pieces and ultrasonic scalers can contribute to considerable splashing of blood and particulate matter which increases the risk of infection to the dentist and his staff. When working in the mouth, dental surgeons and their assistants should wear suitable gloves, and so should any of the staff of the theatre or dental room when cleaning instruments, benches or other surfaces, or preparing materials for sterilization or disposal.

Certain categories of patients, unless they are known to be HB$_S$Ag negative, should be treated in hospital dental departments rather than by general dental practitioners; these include (a) patients with chronic renal failure who are receiving or are likely to receive regular dialysis treatment, and patients who have had a renal or other organ transplant; (b) patients who are receiving long-term immunosuppressive therapy; (c) patients with haemophilia and others with haematological disorders who receive multiple transfusions of blood or blood products; (d) patients from institutions for the mentally handicapped (mentally handicapped patients living at home do not constitute a special risk); (e) known drug addicts; (f) patients suffering from jaundice which is thought to be infective in nature, and those who have suffered from such jaundice within the previous six months.

This list is taken from *Recommendations of an Expert Group on Hepatitis in Dentistry* (DHSS, 1979). Such patients are likely to be referred to hospital dental departments by general dental practitioners.

If possible, the patient should be tested for HB$_S$Ag before treatment. If found negative, treatment can proceed in the usual fashion. If found positive, the precautions which have been detailed above should be adopted. Precautions as for positive patients should be adopted if the hepatitis carrier state of the patient is not known, or cannot conveniently be determined.

Maternity departments: delivery of carriers of hepatitis B virus

Hepatitis has not been a noticeable hazard among midwives and obstetricians, but when a mother is known to be a carrier of hepatitis B virus it is reasonable to take precautions against infection of staff and of other patients. The following measures are advised:

(1) Delivery should be carried out with standard aseptic technique, taking special care to disinfect blood splashes with 10% hypochlorite (1% available chlorine). Disposable articles should be incinerated. Case notes should be

marked to indicate that special precautions are required; certain hospitals use a special coloured star or label for this purpose.

Some authorities recommend that deliveries should be carried out in the isolation unit or in an isolation cubicle, and that a notice should be displayed outside the room, denying entry to unauthorized staff; those expressly invited in should be warned not to touch anything.

The working team should wear rubber gloves during the delivery and while handling blood-stained materials. A disposable plastic apron should be worn under the sterile (preferably disposable) gown; a mask should be worn, and glasses (either one's own or disposable safety spectacles) may be worn to give the delivery staff protection against conjunctival splashes. When cutting instruments or needles are being used the point or cutting edge must always be directed away from the hands. It is convenient for the patient to lie on disposable paper sheets laid on an impervious rubber or plastic sheet.

(2) Blood specimens for laboratory investigation must be marked with a BIO-HAZARD label for identification, and the container enclosed in a sealed plastic bag. The request forms must be similarly marked and attached to the outside of the bag.

(3) After the delivery, the labour room should be thoroughly cleaned with 1% hypochlorite (0.1% available chlorine). Disposable sharp instruments should be placed in a suitable box for autoclaving or incineration; other disposables should be bagged for incineration. Non-disposable instruments should be immersed in 2% glutaraldehyde and allowed to stand for at least two hours before being sent to the CSSD; glutaraldehyde should be used for decontamination of metals, because of the corrosive effects of chlorine, which is appropriate for other virus-contaminated surfaces. Spilt blood should be disinfected before it dries, using plenty of disinfectant; if it is allowed to dry it will be harder to clear up, and the dust may be infectious.

(4) The mother should be reassured that she is not a hazard to her child and can be allowed normal visiting.

(5) If a woman contracts clinical serum hepatitis during pregnancy, a dose of immunoglobulin should be given to the infant within ten days of birth. The globulin is also available for staff members who become injured by sharp instruments during delivery; consult the Blood Transfusion Centre or the Regional Virus or Public Health Laboratory for information about supplies.

(6) Women delivered by caesarean section require similar precautions. They should be last on operating lists, and the theatre floor should be disinfected with hypochlorite (0.1% available chlorine) following operation; blood-stains and spillage should be cleaned with hypochlorite (1.0% available chlorine).

(7) During the puerperium nurses should wear gloves or use forceps to handle dressings.

Mortuary staff — post-mortem examination (see also Chapter 16)

Unless there is a compelling interest, which will often apply in post-transplant patients, post-mortem examination should not be carried out on patients who

302

are known to be infected with serum hepatitis virus. A limited autopsy will often suffice to provide the information required. When a full autopsy is required the pathologist should wear a complete enclosing boiler suit, waterproof boots, and a disposable plastic gown or long apron. A mask, gloves and plastic arm extension pieces should also be worn, and goggles or visor to prevent splashing of the eyes. Any assistant must be similarly clad. If the glove is punctured or the skin broken the glove must be removed immediately and the injury cleansed; anti-$HB_s Ag$ γ-globulin should be made available (see p. 305). After completion of the post-mortem the room must be decontaminated by washing down with hypochlorite solution. Instruments, bowls and trays should be disinfected by boiling before cleaning, or immersed in 2% glutaraldehyde in a sink for at least two hours, preferably overnight. If available, a pathologist known to be $HB_s Ag$ positive should carry out post-mortem examination on these patients.

Active immunization

There are now good prospects that an effective vaccine may, before long, become available for the protection of hospital staff likely to be at risk from hepatitis B.

References and Further Reading

Cosart, Yvonne E. (1977), *Virus Hepatitis and its Control*, Baillière Tindall, London.

Department of Health and Social Security (1972), *Safety in Pathology Laboratories*, HMSO, London.

Department of Health and Social Security (1978), *Code of Practice for Prevention of Infection in Clinical Laboratories and Post-mortem Rooms*, HMSO, London.

Department of Health and Social Security (1979), *Recommendations of an Expert Group on Hepatitis in Dentistry*, HMSO, London.

Department of Health and Social Security, Scottish Home and Health Department and Welsh Office: Rosenheim Advisory Group (1972), *Hepatitis and the Treatment of Chronic Renal Failure*, HMSO, London.

Provost, P. J. and Hilleman, M. R. (1979), Propagation of human hepatitis A virus in cell culture. *Proc. Soc. Exp. Biol.*, **160**, 213.

CHAPTER NINETEEN

Dialysis and Renal Transplantation Units

Prevention and control of hepatitis

Viral hepatitis is considered in some detail in Chapter 18, but the disease has been a particular problem in renal units and requires further comment in this context. Hepatitis in renal units has nearly always been due to hepatitis B virus, though a few mild outbreaks of non A-non B hepatitis have been reported.

Patients suffering from chronic renal failure and other conditions associated with immunological insufficiency (including those receiving immunosuppressive therapy) are often not made ill when infected with the hepatitis B virus, but become carriers of the virus. Healthy carriers in the general population usually carry virus in comparatively low titre in their blood, but patients with chronic renal failure, or those with grafted kidneys, often carry the virus in very high titre. Infection has, in the past, entered dialysis units by transfusion of blood from a carrier or through the introduction of an unsuspected patient carrier to the unit's treatment programme; the virus has then been spread from patient to patient by shared dialysis equipment.

Organ donors have also been a source of infection. Infection may be spread to staff by spilt blood getting into a scratch or eye, or by a prick from a contaminated needle. All blood donations in the United Kingdom are nowadays tested for hepatitis antigen HB_sAg, but no test can be guaranteed to exclude *all* infected donations.

In the absence of sensible precautions, hepatitis can become a major problem in renal units. In 1977, 23.5% of patients receiving hospital dialysis in Europe were infected (*Proc. Europ. Dialysis Transplant Ass.*, 1978); 671 members of staff were infected, with eight deaths. In the United Kingdom, where stringent precautions have been taken in the past ten years, the picture is entirely different, with very few hepatitis positive patients and no cases of hepatitis reported amongst staff in 1977 and 1978. Clearly preventive methods are worthwhile. The main procedures adopted in the UK have been based on the report of the Rosenheim Committee (DHSS, 1972).

Special measures for the prevention and control of hepatitis in renal units

(1) To prevent virus infection entering units

Screen patients before admission for the presence of HB_sAg and there-

304

after at monthly intervals while they are in-patients.

Give only blood transfusions screened by radioimmunoassay and use only screened organ donors. For some years it was normal practice to minimize or avoid blood transfusions to patients with chronic renal failure, to reduce the risk of introducing hepatitis. The demonstration that previous blood transfusion improves the success rate of cadaveric transplantation has changed this practice, hence the need for HB_sAg-screened blood.

Extend the use of home dialysis service.

Minimize transfer between dialysis units.

(2) To protect patients against transfer of virus within the unit

Use small volume dialysers primed with saline.

Use separate dialysers and dialysate proportionating and monitoring units for each patient whenever possible.

Screen patients for HB_sAg every month.

Segregate new 'acute' dialysis patients from those having 'chronic' dialysis.

Excreta (faeces and urine) may contain virus; for disposal see the section on *Standard isolation (excretion)*, in Chapter 9, p. 130.

Screen staff for HB_sAg and abnormal liver function tests before they start to work in the unit, and every three months.

Staff who get hepatitis or become antigen-positive must not return to work in a dialysis unit until three successive weekly blood samples have proved negative for HB_sAg.

(3) To enhance host-resistance of staff after accidental contamination

Vaccines are under trial, but not yet generally available. Ordinary pooled human γ-globulin has no prophylactic value, but γ-globulin prepared from plasma selected for its content of antibody to hepatitis B is available in limited supply, and gives good, but not infallible, protection against clinical hepatitis: 500 mg should be injected as soon as possible, but at least within ten days, into any person put at risk by accidental injection or splashing of infected blood into mouth, eyes or open skin lesions; stocks of this special γ-globulin are in the Region's Hepatitis Reference Laboratory. A second dose should be injected one month later.

General measures for prevention and control of hepatitis (see also Chapter 9, on patient isolation methods)

(1) Responsibility for safety

A member of the medical staff of the Renal Unit should be designated Safety Officer. Any accident or untoward happenings, illness etc., must be reported to him. He will also be responsible for seeing that agreed safety precautions are observed and ensuring that newly appointed staff are trained to work safely. Ultimate responsibility rests with the consultant in charge of the unit.

(2) Instruction of staff

New members must be instructed and trained in methods of work to minimize hazards of infection. The importance of neat and tidy working should be emphasized.

(3) Smoking, eating and drinking

These must be forbidden in the Unit.

(4) Overcrowding

Overcrowding in the unit must be avoided.

(5) Protective dressings

Staff must wear waterproof dressings over cuts or abrasions. Those with extensive untreated cuts or epithelial deficiency, e.g. eczema, should not work in renal units.

(6) Protective clothing

Surgical or disposable gloves must be worn on all occasions when taking blood, and when handling shunts or dialysis apparatus when the patient is on dialysis. The use of surgical gowns, masks, and disposable long plastic aprons is recommended when there is a risk that much blood may be shed, as for instance in setting up dialysis or declotting shunts. Contaminated aprons can be disinfected with hypochlorite solution (0.1% available chlorine, e.g. 1% 'Chloros') or 2% glutaraldehyde. *Change of clothing, gowns, etc.* — Gowns or uniforms must be changed if they become splashed with blood.

(7) Specimen collection

When taking blood with a syringe the specimen container should be filled from the syringe with the needle still attached. This is an exception to the general recommendation (DHSS, 1978 and p. 116) that the needle should be removed with forceps before discharging the contents of the syringe. Great care should be taken to avoid frothing. The syringe and attached needle should then be disposed of, placing them in a rigid box (e.g. the DRG box). Needles not attached to syringes (e.g. those of drip sets) should be discarded into an enclosed rigid box. Accidental cuts or pricks by sharp instruments are an important hazard and are the principal route of infection for staff. Sharp instruments must be disposed of with care.

(8) Spills

Any spilt blood from a patient must be mopped up and a wide area disinfected around the spill. A strong hypochlorite solution (see p. 99) is the best disinfectant to use except where its bleaching or destructive action, e.g. on metals, would be disadvantageous, when 2% glutaraldehyde is recommended. The 'mopping up' material should be autoclaved or burned.

(9) Decontamination of instruments

Surgical instruments used on the unit should be boiled or autoclaved before cleaning, or soaked in 2% glutaraldehyde for at least two hours.

(10) Hazard to others

Staff must ensure that contaminated material does not go to other departments (e.g. to Pharmacy or CSSD) before it has been disinfected.

(11) Accidents

There must be a routine to prevent accidents, and to deal with, report and record any accidents that do occur.

(a) **Cuts, pricks.** If a finger or hand is accidentally pricked the venous return should be occluded and the injury made to bleed if possible. The area should be treated with tincture of iodine (Tinct. iod. mitis BP). If the patient is antigen-positive and the member of staff is antigen negative when injured, human specific immunoglobulin should be offered; its administration should not be delayed if the person at risk cannot be tested for HB_sAg immediately. A very sensitive radio-immuno-assay test is available for testing patients whose antigen carriage may be in doubt.

(b) **Splashes in eyes.** If contamination of the conjunctiva occurs the eye should be immediately washed out with saline or tap water and anti-HB_sAg γ-globulin offered as above.

(12) Action when a patient is found to be antigen-positive

Isolate HB_sAg-positive patients.

Discharge HB_sAg-positive patients as soon as possible to home dialysis, or, if possible, to a special unit for HB_sAg positive patients.

Use disposable dialysers.

Burn or disinfect articles contaminated with blood or other secretions (e.g. menstrual discharge).

Linen should be transported to the laundry in sealed alginate bags contained in an outer bag labelled BIOHAZARD (see Chapter 11).

Clean and disinfect baths, toilet areas etc., possibly contaminated by HB_sAg-positive patients.

Limit laboratory investigations as far as possible.

(13) Staff in high risk areas

Specially trained staff should be selected for these duties.

(14) Consultation

There should be regular consultation and collaboration between staffs of the Renal Unit, the Microbiology Department and the Infection Control Team.

(15) Blood and blood products

These should be screened to exclude any that are found HB_sAg positive.

Prevention and control of bacterial infection

General preventive measures

The environment

The general measures designed to protect patients and staff from cross-infection are described elsewhere: these include meticulous attention to all aspects of bacterial suppression in the environment such as would normally be expected in an operating theatre suite. Unless this is done, gross contamination of the environment can occur, with attendant high risk of shunt infection.

In particular, extensive use of presterilized disposable dressing packs, syringes and instruments, strict control and safe disposal of soiled and fouled linen, and disinfection of bed, furniture and floors after use of a cubicle should be routine practice.

The patient

General. The patient's general cleanliness must be carefully assessed, and tactful guidance in these matters by the ward sister is invaluable. Bathing may present difficulties, in that keeping the shunt site dry is of paramount importance in the prevention of infection. Methods must be improvised to achieve this, depending upon the site of the shunt, and materials available.

Carrier sites. On acceptance of a patient for long-term dialysis, all carrier sites — nose, throat, axilla and groin — are swabbed. Where potential pathogens are found, in particular staphylococci resistant to antibiotics other than penicillin, appropriate measures are taken to eradicate them by topical application of ointments, e.g. 'Naseptin', to the nasal mucosa, and repeated use of an iodophor (e.g. povidone-iodine surgical scrub) or 4% chlorhexidine detergent solution ('Hibiscrub') or alcoholic chlorhexidine for disinfection of the skin. Swabs should be taken after such measures to ascertain their effectiveness.

This swabbing is repeated at monthly intervals in the first instance.

Nursing and medical staff

These are similarly screened for bacterial pathogen carriage on first appointment to the unit, and subsequently at three-monthly intervals.

Care of blood access sites

Access to the circulation is most commonly obtained by needle puncture of veins draining a subcutaneous arteriovenous fistula. This has largely replaced the external silastic-teflon arteriovenous shunt which poses special bacteriological hazards. Increasing use is being made of prosthetic devices to create subcutaneous

arteriovenous fistulae including grafts of bovine carotid artery and polytetra-
fluoroethylene (PTFE) ('Gortex' or 'Impra').

Subcutaneous arteriovenous fistulae

The subcutaneous fistula has a great advantage over the external shunt in that
there is no open wound once postoperative healing has occurred. The technique
for management is as follows:

(1) A wide area of the arm is cleaned with 0.5% chlorhexidine in 70% (or con-
    centrations up to 95%) ethyl alcohol. It is essential that this preliminary
    skin preparation should be very thorough, in order to avoid introduction of
    bacteria directly into the blood stream.
(2) Local anaesthesia is usually necessary in view of the wide bore of the needle
    to be inserted. Lignocaine 2% in 2 ml ampoules is recommended for this
    purpose.
(3) It is desirable to avoid inserting the needle through the identical point of
    insertion made during the preceding dialysis, where a small infected clot or
    scab may have formed.
(4) The fistula needle is strapped into position after reinsertion into the fistula
    site, but no dressing is necessary.
(5) Haemorrhage after withdrawal of the needle may be troublesome and severe
    blood loss can occur if adequate steps are not taken. To prevent this, a
    protamine-soaked swab is placed over the site and held in place with a firm
    bandage for 10 min. This is replaced by a sterile gauze square, and firmly
    bandaged for 2 h.

External arteriovenous shunts

The basic bacteriological problem presented by the external arteriovenous shunt
can be simply stated: it is how to avoid infection in a permanently open wound
containing a foreign body. This obviously presents considerable difficulties. Yet
prevention of infection at the arteriovenous shunt site is of major importance if
suppuration round the arterial limb of the shunt is to be avoided. This may lead
to destruction and abandonment of an important site when the number of sites
is strictly limited. Furthermore, the technical difficulties of the operation are
considerable and not to be undertaken lightly. Finally the risk of septic emboli
and fatal septicaemia has been reported in a number of papers. The organisms
concerned are most commonly coagulase-positive and coagulase-negative staphylococci, but Gram-negative bacilli, such as *Pseudomonas aeruginosa*, and haemolytic
streptococci may also be involved. The major pathogen in this context, however,
is the staphylococcus, and 80% of the strains isolated in one series were derived
from the patient's own carrier sites, the remainder being cross-infections acquired
from other patients.

In view of these considerations, the care of the arteriovenous shunt must be
seen to begin in the wider context of general hygiene and ward cleanliness, and
the measures used to control cross-infection in the general hospital ward situation should be applied perhaps even more rigorously in the Renal Unit.

Routine care of shunt site

The main object is to prevent introduction of pathogens. This is achieved by observance of strict aseptic principles in the dressing and handling of the shunt site, by an occlusive dressing, and by keeping the site dry at all times as far as possible.

Dressing technique

Standard aseptic practice must be used throughout. A dressing pack made up especially for shunt toilet by the CSSD is desirable. A pack containing two dressings and one waterproof towel, two gallipots, gauze squares and swab-mounted cotton wool 'buds' has been found suitable for this purpose.

The operator scrubs up, using an approved hand preparation, e.g. 4% chlorhexidine ('Hibiscrub') or povidone-iodine with detergent, or 10 ml of 0.5% chlorhexidine in 70 or 95% ethanol with 1% glycerol, rubbed into the skin till dry (the most effective method for single use); he wears a sterile gown, and gloves. The area around the shunt site is gently but thoroughly cleaned with a 4% chlorhexidine detergent solution, using cotton wool buds, and then dried. Finally it is painted with, preferably, a 10% solution of povidone-iodine in 70% ethyl alcohol.

The shunt ends are now separated, attached to the dialyser and dialysis commenced. The shunt site is covered with a loose sterile gauze square during dialysis.

At the end of dialysis the ends are disconnected from the machine and attached to each other once more. The area is again cleaned with a 4% chlorhexidine detergent solution ('Hibiscrub'), dried, and painted with povidone-iodine. A dry sterile gauze is placed over the shunt site and bandaged lightly.

It must be emphasized that techniques will vary with local practice and we are not at present able to present evidence that the method outlined gives appreciably better long-term results in sepsis control than any other. It is possible that excessive use of local skin disinfectants may, in some patients, devitalize tissue and later render it more liable to infection. Similarly, there may be a tendency to damage tissues by poking too vigorously with a cotton wool bud around the shunt site, so that unmounted cotton wool swabs may be preferred.

Training for home dialysis

Whilst it is important that home dialysis patients be trained to be self-sufficient, it is valuable in most circumstances for the spouse, relative or friend who may help the patient to be fully instructed in both the principles and practice of shunt care, bearing in mind that both they and the patient find the technique completely foreign and the aseptic precautions without apparent reason. Experience suggests that teaching is best done by example. At the same time, the dangers of autogenous infection must be stressed to encourage the highest standards of personal hygiene.

Infection in shunt site

When there is clinical evidence of infection at the site, a swab is taken for bacteriological examination, and swabs of nose, throat, axilla and groin are taken also.

If the clinical condition warrants antibiotic therapy pending the bacteriological report, antistaphylococcal drugs, and especially flucloxacillin, are started. Treatment is reviewed and altered if necessary on receipt of the bacteriological report. Avoid antibiotics that may accumulate to toxic levels in renal failure (see Chapter 12).

Treatment is continued until there is bacteriological evidence of clearance.

Carrier sites are treated as outlined above if found to carry pathogens.

Summary

The maintenance of an infection-free arteriovenous shunt depends upon rigorous attention to basic aseptic principles, to keeping the site dry, to prevention of colonization of carrier sites by pathogens and to a high level of personal and environmental hygiene.

Cleaning and sterilization of dialysis equipment

Although much attention has been focused upon the hepatitis risk, the greatest hazard to patients in dialysis units is bacterial infection. Techniques must take into account both factors.

The general measures required to avoid the introduction of hepatitis have been discussed in the first section of this chapter. This section will deal with (1) routine cleaning and sterilizing of dialysis equipment; (2) special measures in units treating patients carrying, or suspected of carrying, hepatitis.

In general, proportionating machines should be used for a designated small group of patients rather than at random, to confine the area of potential spread of infection. Non-disposable dialysers such as the Kiil should, whenever possible, be clearly numbered and each dialyser restricted to the treatment of one individual.

Adequate and safe boxes must be provided for the disposal of needles and cannulae.

Routine measures

The dialyser

(1) Disposable dialysers (coils, flat bed and hollow fibre) will normally be disposed of by incineration without dismantling.

It is the practice of many dialysis units to re-use these disposable items to reduce unit cost, and because they function well for several dialyses. When re-use is contemplated, the dialyser (with or without the blood lines) is thoroughly washed through to remove all traces of blood. The dialyser is then disinfected with 2% formalin. Before re-use the dialyser is thoroughly washed with sterile saline to remove all traces of formalin. There are machines available to perform the washing and disinfecting process. Tests should be made for formaldehyde in the effluent.

311

During dismantling and washing, staff should wear plastic aprons and gloves.

(2) The Kiil dialyser was designed as re-usable equipment. It is now less commonly used. It is washed through with saline and disinfected with 2% formalin for 24 h after one use and before the next.

Before rebuilding, the boards are scrubbed and the gaskets checked. They are then soaked in iodophor or hypochlorite solution.

The membranes are soaked in 0.2% benzalkonium chloride used as a wetting (but not disinfecting) agent.

Before use the blood compartment is washed through with sterile saline. The dialysate compartment may be washed with tap water. During dismantling staff will wear gowns and gloves. So far as possible, lines and membranes will be bagged for incineration without spilling contents. Kiil boards require thorough, but careful, scrubbing. Faulty gaskets must be replaced at once. Usually dialysers will be filled with 2% formalin or an iodophor solution for 24 h after building, before use. Membranes will be soaked in fresh 0.2% benzalkonium chloride solution before building, and not left soaking overnight. Benzalkonium chloride is used here as a wetting agent and should *not* be considered a suitable disinfectant. Alternatively a 'dry' technique may be applicable. A weekly soaking of Kiil boards in an idophor solution or a hypochlorite solution is recommended.

Proportionating machines

Dialysate for haemodialysis does not need to be sterile, but heavy bacterial growth leads to the dangers of contamination and changes the chemical composition of the solution.

There is now a wide choice of machines on the market. These employ one of three methods of sterilization or disinfection:

(a) Chemical sterilization usually with formalin;
(b) heat disinfection by hot water circulation at temperatures of 80–90° C (176°–194° F), or
(c) in a few models, 'autoclaving' of the dialysate circuit.

Whichever method is used, careful physical cleaning is required, particularly for units using chemical or hot water disinfection. For hot water systems a periodic thorough cleaning of the flow system is recommended followed by disinfection with a hypochlorite solution or by a period of recirculation with water for 4 h at 80° C (176° F).

Particular care is required to ensure the cleanliness of those parts of the circuit which, in some machines, are not included in the sterilizing or disinfecting pathway.

Pressure gauges

Particular danger attaches to 'blind' connections to pressure monitors which permit bacterial growth and subsequent contamination of the circuit, or, in the case of the venous pressure monitors, direct contamination by blood. The use of gauge isolators is essential, except with the newer machines fitted with pressure transducers which can be easily cleaned.

Contaminated gauges must be cleaned and if possible sterilized with ethylene oxide. Otherwise they should be replaced.

Measures required when hepatitis-positive patients are under treatment

Such patients should, if possible, be segregated on home dialysis or, if available, in special isolation units for HB_sAg-positive patients.

(1) Disposable dialysers should be used, and not re-used.
(2) Heat-sterilizing dialysis machines are preferred and should be treated weekly by the regime outlined in the section on Routine measures.

Peritoneal dialysis

Sterile pyrogen-free solutions and sterile cannulae and tubing are required for this procedure. Bottles of dialysate should be inspected for evidence of bacterial or fungal contamination. Abdominal drainage should be through a closed system.

Adequate skin preparation and stringent aseptic techniques are required for insertion of the peritoneal cannulae. A simple gauze dressing should be placed around the catheter and tied so that it cannot be pushed freely in and out by nursing staff.

Dialysate bottle tops should be adequately swabbed with alcoholic chlorhexidine or povidone-iodine solution before inserting needles.

Manual methods often include the use of a water bath or sink for warming the bottles of dialysate before use. This water is likely to become contaminated with Gram-negative bacilli, including *Pseudomonas* spp. The water should be changed frequently and a suitable disinfectant added.

Automatic systems for peritoneal dialysis usually include adequate instructions for sterilization.

Parts of the system likely to be in contact with dialysate must either be presterilized disposable items, or be autoclaved.

Routine addition of prophylactic antibiotics to peritoneal dialysis fluid is not recommended. It is desirable to send samples to the laboratory every 24 hours for culture (see Chapter 12).

Peritoneal dialysis for chronic renal failure requires the use of a permanent indwelling silicone rubber peritoneal catheter, usually of the Tenckhoff type. Such a catheter is plugged between uses except when continuous dialysis is practised. The insertion and care of these catheters closely resembles the care of external arteriovenous shunts. Whenever connections or disconnections are made, rigorous aseptic or no-touch techniques must be used. Peritonitis remains a common and serious complication of chronic peritoneal dialysis.

The technique of continuous ambulatory peritoneal dialysis (CAPD) requires the patient to change his bag of dialysate several times daily. Patients must be taught to avoid contaminating the connections during these changes. At the time of writing the type of connecting system used for CAPD is still undergoing development. The catheter connection is usually changed periodically by the staff of the 'parent unit' using full aseptic precautions. A type of connection is recommended which, while secure between bag changes, is easily undone by the patient with little risk of touching the parts coming in contact with dialysate.

Disinfection of equipment and materials (see also Chapter 7)

Equipment and materials should be autoclaved or heat-treated whenever possible. Chemical disinfection is less reliable. A strong hypochlorite solution yielding 1% available chlorine should be used for mopping up spilt blood and in containers for discarded specimens of blood. This solution may be obtained by diluting 'Chloros', 'Domestos', 'Sterite' or a similar strength hypochlorite solution, which contains 10–11% available chlorine (or 100 000 ppm, 1 part in 10). A weaker solution containing 0.1% available chlorine should be used for routine environmental cleaning in a dialysis unit, or in rooms occupied by patients with hepatitis. A compatible detergent should be added to the hypochlorite solution for all cleaning processes. Hypochlorite solutions may be corrosive to metals and fabrics, but some hypochlorite powders (e.g. 'Septonite', 'Diversol BX') are less so and may be preferred for use on equipment (see section above on cleaning and sterilization of dialysis equipment). 1% Solution w/v should give 1000 ppm available chlorine. Glutaraldehyde (2%) is less corrosive, but slower in action and less suitable for surface disinfection; it may cause skin sensitization on repeated use, and must not be used for skin disinfection. Glutaraldehyde is particularly useful for longer periods of disinfection (e.g. 1 to 2 hours), and should be freshly prepared (at least every week). Iodophors (e.g. 1% 'Wescodyne') are relatively non-corrosive and active against a wide range of bacteria. Their activity against enteroviruses is uncertain and at present hypochlorites are preferred if possible where a virucidal action is required in dialysis units.

Renal Transplant Units

The special problems associated with renal transplantation arise because of the effects of immunosuppressive agents used to prevent graft rejection. Most of the opportunistic infections in transplanted patients are due to organisms already carried by the patients, including the commoner bacteria, *M. tuberculosis*, fungi, *Pneumocystis carinii*, *Herpes simplex* virus and cytomegalovirus. The latter infection may sometimes be transmitted in the actual graft. It is unwise to use organs from grossly infected donors and a routine culture should be taken from the donor fat and perfusate at the time of grafting.

Isolation practice varies between different units, but strict protective isolation with barrier-nursing and positive pressure ventilation is not often used now because with less intensive immunosuppression, it is felt that the possible benefits of strict isolation are outweighed by the difficulties of ensuring adequate patient

314

care in this environment. Nevertheless, cross-infection can be a major problem and isolation in cubicles is desirable during the first two weeks, or when steroid dosage is increased for rejection episodes. Staff should take every sensible precaution to avoid transmitting infections from themselves or other patients as described elsewhere in the book.

References and Further Reading

Department of Health and Social Security, Scottish Home and Health Department and Welsh Office: Rosenheim Advisory Group (1972), *Hepatitis and the Treatment of Chronic Renal Failure*, HMSO, London.

Department of Health and Social Security (1978), *Code of Practice for the Prevention of Infection in Clinical Laboratories and Post-mortem Rooms*, HMSO, London.

Proceedings of the European Dialysis and Transplant Association (1978), 15, 66.

Selected Bibliography

Altemeier, W. A., Burke, J. F., Pruitt, B. A. and Sandusky, W. R. (eds) (1976), *Manual on Control of Infection in Surgical Patients*, Lippincott, Philadelphia.

Benenson, A. S. (ed.) (1975), *Control of Communicable Disease in Man*, 12th edn, American Public Health Association, New York.

Bennett, J. V. and Brachman, P. S. (eds) (1979), *Hospital Infections*, Little Brown and Company, Boston.

Brachman, P. S. and Eickhoff, T. C. (eds) (1971), *Nosocomial Infections*, American Hospital Association, Chicago.

Christie, A. B. (1980), *Infectious Diseases: Epidemiology and Clinical Practice*, Churchill Livingstone, London (3rd edn., in press).

Colbeck, J. C. (1962), *Control of Infections in Hospitals*, American Hospital Association, Chicago.

Cruickshank, R., Duguid, J. P., Marmion, B. P. and Swain, R. H. A. (eds) (1974), *Medical Microbiology* 12th edn, Churchill Livingstone, London.

Finegold, S. M. (1977), *Anaerobic Bacteria in Human Disease*, Academic Press, New York.

Gibson, G. L. (ed.) (1974), *Infection in Hospital: A Code of Practice*, Churchill Livingstone, London.

Hers, J. F. P. and Winkler, K. C. (eds) (1973), *Airborne Transmission and Airborne Infection*, Oosthoek, Utrecht.

Maibach, H. I. and Hildick-Smith, G. (eds) (1965), *Skin Bacteria and their Role in Infections*, McGraw Hill, New York.

Mandell, G. L., Douglas, R. Gordon and Bennett, J. E. (eds) (1979), *Principles and Practice of Infectious Disease*, J. Wiley, New York.

Maurer, I. M. (1978), *Hospital Hygiene*, 2nd edn, Edward Arnold, London.

Reeves, D. and Geddes, A. M. (eds) (1979), *Recent Advances in Infection*: Vol. 1, Churchill Livingstone, London.

Tyrrell, A. J., Phillips, I., Goodwin, C. S. and Blowers, R. (1979), *Microbial Disease: the Use of the Laboratory in Diagnosis, Therapy and Control*, Edward Arnold, London.

Williams, R. E. O., Blowers, R., Garrod, L. P. and Shooter, R. A. (1966), *Hospital Infection: Causes and Prevention*, 2nd edn, Lloyd Luke, London.

Williams, R. E. O. and Shooter, R. A. (eds) (1963), *Infection in Hospitals, Epidemiology and Control*, Blackwell, Oxford.

Willis, A. T. (1969), *Clostridia of Wound Infection*, Butterworth, London.

Willis, A. T. (1977), *Anaerobic Bacteriology: Clinical and Laboratory Practice*, 3rd edn, Butterworth, London.

Wilson, G. S. and Miles, A. A. (1975), *Topley and Wilson's Principles of Bacteriology and Immunity*, 6th edn, Edward Arnold, London.

316

Index

317